Hepatitis B
Vaccines in
Clinical Practice

INFECTIOUS DISEASE AND THERAPY

Series Editors

Brian E. Scully, M.B., B.Ch.   **Harold C. Neu, M.D.**

College of Physicians and Surgeons
Columbia University
New York, New York

Hepatitis B Vaccines in Clinical Practice

edited by

Ronald W. Ellis

Merck Research Laboratories
West Point, Pennsylvania

Marcel Dekker, Inc.   New York • Basel • Hong Kong

Library of Congress Cataloging-in-Publication Data

Hepatitis B vaccines in clinical practice / edited by Ronald W. Ellis.
     p.   cm. -- (Infectious disease and therapy; 7)
  Includes bibliographical references and index.
  ISBN 0-8247-8780-3
  1. Hepatitis B--Vaccination. 2. Hepatitis B vaccine. I. Ellis,
Ronald W. II. Series: Infectious disease and therapy ; v. 7.
  [DNLM: 1. Hepatitis B--prevention & control. 2. Viral Hepatitis
Vaccines. W1 IN406HMN v.7 / WC 536 H53355]
RC848.H44H485 1993
614.58'93623--dc20
DNLM/DLC
for Library of Congress   92-48753
                                                CIP

This book is printed on acid-free paper.

MARCEL DEKKER, INC.
270 Madison Avenue, New York, New York 10016

Current printing (last digit):
10 9 8 7 6 5 4 3 2 1

PRINTED IN THE UNITED STATES OF AMERICA

To my wife, Danielle, and children, Jacob and Miriam, for their love, patience, and support

Preface

The hepatitis B vaccine has several unique attributes among human vaccines. It is the world's first licensed recombinant-derived vaccine and also the first vaccine with potential for the prevention of a cancer in humans. It is the only vaccine used extensively outside the pediatric and geriatric populations. Its use was mandated recently by the Occupational Safety and Health Administration (OSHA) in the United States for the prevention of hepatitis B infection in adult populations at occupational risk of exposure and it is the vaccine most recently recommended for universal vaccination of infants.

Hepatitis B is one of the world's most prevalent infectious diseases. It is estimated that over 300 million people worldwide are chronically infected with the hepatitis B virus (HBV). The long-term sequelae of chronic hepatitis B include a high incidence of cirrhosis and hepatocellular carcinoma. Thus, the medical community has been highly interested for the past 20 years in the control, prevention, and eventual eradication of this serious disease.

The first-generation hepatitis B vaccines, derived from hepatitis B surface antigen (HBsAg) in plasma of chronic carriers, became available in the early 1980s (Chapter 2). The ongoing applications of recombinant DNA and biotechnology led to the development of recombinant-derived HBsAg into second-generation hepatitis B vaccines (Chapter 4), which were first licensed in 1986 and which constitute an ever-increasing percentage of hepatitis B vaccines used worldwide. These vaccines represent the first—and, at this time, only—recombinant-derived vaccines for humans. The use and availability of these vaccines in the field have been supported by studies of HBV structure and biology (Chapter 3), quality control tests on the vaccine (Chapter 5), and the development of antibody assays that enable a diagnosis of hepatitis B and interpretation of the success of vaccination (Chapter 6). In addition, as in all fields of biomedical product development, there is the realization that current vaccines have not fulfilled all needs and that there are groups who would benefit from a potential third-generation vaccine (Chapter 17). Research in this area is presented in Chapters 18–20.

The incidence and prevalence of HBV infection and the modes of viral transmission vary markedly in different parts of the world (Chapter 7). This has had an influence on clinical study designs for immunogenicity and efficacy in different locations (Chapters 8–12). The general conclusions from these studies are that the vaccines have been generally very well tolerated and highly efficacious in preventing hepatitis B disease. Since chronic hepatitis B infection is the most important determinant of liver cancer, the hepatitis B vaccine has the potential for prevention of a significant proportion of hepatocellular carcinoma worldwide (Chapter 13).

Several topics in this book are of particular interest to pediatricians and clinical practitioners. The current recommendations for vaccination, including use of HBIG, are presented for pre- and postexposure prophylaxis in all suitable target populations and groups (Chapter 1). In 1991, OSHA regulations were enacted that require employers in the United States to provide hepatitis B vaccine free of charge to those employees who have occupational exposure to blood or other infectious materials (Chapter 15). This group includes health care workers, paramedical personnel, police, and fire fighters. From 1991 through 1992, both the American Academy of Pediatrics and the Advisory Committee on Immunization Practices (Red Book) recommended universal vaccination of infants in the United States (Chapter 16), a recommendation previously enacted in other areas and countries, including Italy and New Zealand (Chapter 14). It is hoped that these recent recommendations will lead to a reduction in the incidence of HBV infections in the United States which was not manifest during the first decade in which the vaccine was available. Appropriate use of these and other long-term strategies for vaccination in other countries is expected to lead to a reduction in incidence and eventual eradication of hepatitis B disease.

I hope that this book will serve as a comprehensive reference on significant aspects of hepatitis B vaccines. Since vaccination remains a practical and cost-effective means of disease control, the widespread use of hepatitis B vaccines offers the long-term prospect of eradication of this serious disease. Given that the availability of these generally highly efficacious vaccines has had variable success in different countries or geographical areas in diminishing the incidence of new HBV infections, it has become increasingly clear that new vaccination strategies must continually be developed based on the epidemiology of disease incidence in a given area. In this respect, the new OSHA regulations and policies for universal infant immunization are positive steps which are expected to bear fruit long term in disease control.

I thank my many colleagues in the field of hepatitis B vaccines. I am especially grateful to Robert Gerety, Maurice Hilleman, and Edward Scolnick for their many stimulating discussions with me and their insights into this field. I thank Grayce Albanesius for her expert assistance with this book. The loving support and understanding of my wife, Danielle, and children, Jacob and Miriam, were very important to me throughout the course of preparation of this book. Most importantly, I thank all the authors for their insightful and professional contributions which have made this volume the key reference in the field of hepatitis B vaccines.

RONALD W. ELLIS

Contents

Contributors

Miriam J. Alter   Hepatitis Branch, National Center for Infectious Diseases, Centers for Disease Control, Atlanta, Georgia

Volker Bruss   Department of Medical Microbiology, University of Goettingen, Goettingen, Germany

Gary B. Calandra   Clinical Research, Merck Research Laboratories, West Point, Pennsylvania

Ding-Shinn Chen   Hepatitis Research Center, National Taiwan University, Taiwan, Republic of China

Pierre Coursaget   Faculté de Pharmacie, Laboratoire de Microbiologie, Tours, France

Michel De Wilde   Research and Development, SmithKline Beecham Biologicals, Rixensart, Belgium

Jules L. Dienstag   Department of Medicine, Harvard Medical School, and Gastrointestinal Unit, Massachusetts General Hospital, Boston, Massachusetts

Ronald W. Ellis   Virus and Cell Biology, Merck Research Laboratories, West Point, Pennsylvania

Wolfram H. Gerlich   Institute of Medical Virology, Justus Liebig University, Giessen, Germany

Victor P. Grachev   Biologicals Unit, World Health Organization, Geneva, Switzerland

Stephen C. Hadler   Division of Immunizations, Centers for Disease Control, Atlanta, Georgia

Tim J. Harrison   Department of Medicine, The Royal Free Hospital School of Medicine, University of London, London, United Kingdom

Pierre Hauser Department of Preclinical Development, SmithKline Beecham Biologicals, Rixensart, Belgium

Patricia L. Hibberd Department of Medicine, Harvard Medical School, and Infectious Disease Unit, Massachusetts General Hospital, Boston, Massachusetts

Maurice R. Hilleman Merck Institute for Therapeutic Research, Merck Research Laboratories, West Point, Pennsylvania

F. Blaine Hollinger Division of Molecular Virology, Baylor College of Medicine, Houston, Texas

Hsu-Mei Hsu Department of Health, Executive Yuan, Republic of China

Mark A. Kane Microbiology and Immunology Support Services, World Health Organization, Geneva, Switzerland

Chin-Yun Lee Department of Pediatrics, College of Medicine, National Taiwan University, Taiwan, Republic of China

Kwang-Juei Low Department of Internal Medicine, Veteran Administration, General Hospital, Taiwan, Republic of China

David I. Magrath Biologicals Unit, World Health Organization, Geneva, Switzerland

Harold S. Margolis Division of Viral and Rickettsial Diseases, National Center for Infectious Diseases, Centers for Disease Control, Atlanta, Georgia

Eric E. Mast Hepatitis Branch, National Center for Infectious Diseases, Centers for Disease Control, Atlanta, Georgia

Brian J. McMahon Department of Internal Medicine, Alaska Native Medical Center, Anchorage, Alaska

David R. Milich Department of Molecular Biology, Scripps Research Institute, La Jolla, California

William J. Miller Virus and Cell Biology, Merck Research Laboratories, West Point, Pennsylvania

Alexander Milne Hepatitis Research Unit, Hepatitis Control Centre, Whakatane, New Zealand

Christopher D. Moyes Hepatitis Research Unit, Hepatitis Control Centre, Whakatane, New Zealand

Robert H. Rubin Department of Medicine, Harvard Medical School, and Clinical Investigation Program, Massachusetts General Hospital, Boston, Massachusetts

Tineke Rutgers   Department of Research and Development, SmithKline Beecham Biologicals, Rixensart, Belgium

Robert D. Sitrin   Biochemical Process Research and Development, Merck Research Laboratories, West Point, Pennsylvania

Juei-Low Sung   Department of Internal Medicine, College of Medicine, National Taiwan University, Taiwan, Republic of China

Catherine L. Troisi   Division of Molecular Virology, Baylor College of Medicine, Houston, Texas

Robert B. Wainwright   Arctic Investigations Program, Centers for Disease Control, Anchorage, Alaska

D. Eugene Wampler   Biochemical Process Research and Development, Merck Research Laboratories, West Point, Pennsylvania

David J. West   Clinical Research, Merck Research Laboratories, West Point, Pennsylvania

E. K. Yeoh   Hospital Authority, Hong Kong

Betty Young   Queen Elizabeth Hospital, Kowloon, Hong Kong

Arie J. Zuckerman   WHO Collaborating Centre for Reference and Research on Viral Diseases, The Royal Free Hospital School of Medicine, University of London, London, United Kingdom

Hepatitis B
Vaccines in
Clinical Practice

1

Recommendations for Prevention of Hepatitis B with Vaccine

Gary B. Calandra and David J. West

*Merck Research Laboratories,
West Point, Pennsylvania*

I. INTRODUCTION

Guidelines for the prevention of hepatitis B with vaccine are issued by a number of organizations. In the United States, the use of hepatitis B vaccine is addressed in publications of the Immunization Practices Advisory Committee (ACIP), the American Academy of Pediatrics (AAP), and the American College of Physicians (ACP) (1–3). Similar government or professional society–based advisory groups formulate recommendations for vaccine usage in other countries. Worldwide, the Technical Advisory Group (TAG) of the World Health Organization (WHO) has recommended the addition of hepatitis B vaccine as a component of the Expanded Programme on Immunization (EPI) in all countries with moderate to high endemicity of infection (4).

This chapter reviews the settings in which transmission of hepatitis B virus (HBV) is likely to occur and the populations for whom immunoprophylaxis may be indicated. These topics are illustrated with particular reference to current recommendations of the ACIP, an organization that advises the U.S. Public Health Service on immunization policies and practices. The chapter concludes with an overview of the strategies and prospects for controlling hepatitis B infection and disease through immunization in both high- and low-incidence areas of the world.

II. PREEXPOSURE PROPHYLAXIS

Hepatitis B virus (HBV) is commonly present in the blood, semen, or other body fluids of infected persons and may be transmitted through percutaneous or mucosal exposure to these substances. Consequently, vaccination should be considered for persons at risk of these kinds of exposure.

A. Populations for Whom Vaccine is Indicated

Preexposure immunization with hepatitis B vaccine is recommended for a number of groups at risk for hepatitis B because of occupation, environment, medical condition, or lifestyle (Table 1). Vaccination of high-risk adults, especially health-care workers, has been a primary objective since vaccine became available in 1982 (reviewed in Chapter 15). Considerable effort has also been made to vaccinate paramedical personnel such as firemen and police officers, who may come into contact with blood and blood contaminated body fluids. Through 1990, sufficient hepatitis B vaccine had been distributed in the United States to immunize more than 4 million adults, most of them health-care or paramedical personnel (M. Sanyour, Merck Vaccine Division, and E. Beruff, SmithKline Beecham Pharmaceuticals, personal communication). Vaccination has probably contributed to a reduction in the proportion of health-care workers among reported cases of hepatitis B over the past few years (5). Continued efforts are needed to improve the immunization status of this population, with emphasis given to the vaccination of health-care workers in training.

Sexual transmission (related to both homosexual and heterosexual activity) and intravenous drug abuse have emerged as major factors in the occurrence of hepatitis B within the United States (5). Few people with these risk factors have been vaccinated, and greater effort is needed to deliver vaccine to susceptible high-risk individuals in a variety of settings such as prisons, STD clinics, and drug rehabilitation centers.

Children may also be exposed to HBV in a variety of ways. Infants born to mothers with acute or chronic HBV infection are at very high risk (see Sec. III). Horizontal transmission of HBV to children from infected siblings, playmates, or other members of the household or community often occurs in populations where infection is endemic. Routine vaccination of infants and children is imperative where HBV infection is highly endemic. In some areas of the world this includes entire countries. In the United States, routine vaccination has previously been recommended for infants in populations of Alaskan natives, Pacific Islanders, refugees from HBV-endemic areas, and for infants of women born in areas where HBV infection is prevalent (6). Catch-up vaccination of children through 6 years of age is also recommended in these high-risk settings.

New guidelines from the AAP and ACIP now recommend universal immunization of infants in the United States against hepatitis B (1,7). The intent

Table 1   ACIP Recommendations for Preexposure Immunization with Hepatitis B Vaccine

1. *Persons with occupational risk.*
   Vaccination is indicated for health-care or public-safety workers whose tasks involve contact with blood or blood-contaminated body fluids. For public-safety workers whose exposure to blood is infrequent, timely postexposure prophylaxis should be considered rather than routine preexposure vaccination. Vaccination should be completed for students of the health-care professions before they have blood contact.

2. *Clients and staff of institutions for the developmentally disabled.*
   Susceptible clients and staff who work closely with clients should be vaccinated. So should susceptible clients and staff who live or work in smaller residential settings with known HBV carriers. Vaccination is recommended for staff of nonresidential daycare programs enrolling HBV carriers. Vaccination of susceptible clients in daycare programs may be considered and is recommended when there is an HBV carrier classmate with aggressive behavior or special medical problems that increases the risk of exposure to his/her blood or serous secretions.

3. *Hemodialysis patients.*
   Vaccination of patients with chronic renal insufficiency prior to dialysis treatment is recommended where possible.

4. *Recipients of certain blood products.*
   Patients who receive clotting factor concentrates should be vaccinated as soon as their specific clotting disorder is identified.

5. *Household contacts and sex partners of HBV carriers.*
   All susceptible household and sexual contacts of persons identified as HBsAg+ should be vaccinated.

6. *Adoptees from countries of high HBV endemicity.*
   Adoptees should be screened for HBsAg. If the children are HBsAg+, then family members should be vaccinated.

7. *International travelers.*
   Vaccination should be considered for travelers to areas with high endemicity of HBV infection if they will reside there for >6 months and have close contact with the local population. Vaccination should also be considered for short-term travelers to these areas if they are likely to have either blood or sexual contact with residents.

8. *Injecting drug users.*
   All susceptible members of this group should be vaccinated.

9. *Sexually active homosexual and bisexual men.*
   All susceptible members of this group should be vaccinated.

Table 1   *(continued)*

10. *Sexually active heterosexual men and women.*
     Vaccination is recommended for persons who are diagnosed as having recently
     acquired sexually transmitted diseases, for prostitutes, and for persons who have a
     history of sexual activity with multiple partners in the previous 6 months.

11. *Inmates of long-term correctional facilities.*
     Vaccination is recommended for susceptible persons with histories of high-risk
     behavior.

Source: Adapted from Ref. 1.

here is to integrate hepatitis B vaccine with other pediatric vaccines given in the
context of established health-care contacts. This will create broad-based immunity before individuals enter occupations, develop medical conditions, or engage in
behaviors that place them at high risk of infection, and so will compensate for
poor immunization of adult risk groups (Chapter 16). Similar initiatives to
vaccinate all infants against hepatitis B in areas of low to moderate endemicity
have previously been implemented in New Zealand and Italy (8; G. Da Villa,
University of Naples, personal communication).

B.   Vaccines: Dosages and Schedules

Two licensed hepatitis B vaccines are currently available in the United States.
Both are comprised of alum-adsorbed particles of hepatitis B surface antigen
(HBsAg) synthesized by a genetically engineered strain of *Saccharomyces cerevisiae*. A series of at least three doses given by intramuscular injection in the
anterolateral thigh of infants or the deltoid muscle of children and adults is
recommended to achieve optimal protection. The dosage of each vaccine to be
used for preexposure prophylaxis for various populations is shown in Table 2.
Manufacturers of both vaccines currently endorse administration of successive
doses at intervals of 0, 1, and 6 months. ENGERIX B® also has an alternate
four-dose schedule for healthy subjects with vaccine given at intervals of 0, 1, 2,
and 12 months. This schedule may be considered when there is a desire for more
rapid induction of immunity. The fourth dose typically induces a sizable boost to
ensure prolonged persistence of antibody. There is, however, no clear evidence
that the four-dose regimen provides any greater protection than the standard
three-dose regimen. For dialysis patients, a four-dose regimen of ENGERIX B®
is standard (vaccine administered at 0, 1, 2, and 6 months), while for RECOM-
BIVAX HB®, a three-dose regimen is recommended (vaccine administered at 0,
1, and 6 months).

   In recommending universal immunization of infants against hepatitis B, both

Table 2   Recommended Dosages and Schedules for Preexposure Prophylaxis with Hepatitis B Vaccines Licensed in the United States[a]

Group	RECOMBIVAX HB® dose in μg (ml)	ENGERIX B® dose in μg (ml)
Infants and children ($\leq$10 years)[b]	2.5 (0.25)	10 (0.5)
Adolescents (11–19 years)	5 (0.5)	20 (1.0)
Adults ($\geq$20 years)	10 (1.0)	20 (1.0)
Dialysis patients/other immunocompromised persons	40 (1.0)[c]	40 (2.0)[d]

[a]Vaccine should be given i.m. in the anterior thigh muscle of infants or the deltoid muscle of children and adults. Both vaccines are recommended to be given to healthy subjects at intervals of 0, 1, and 6 months; ENGERIX B® also has an alternate four-dose schedule with vaccine administered at intervals of 0, 1, 2, and 12 months.
[b]For infants of HBsAg– mothers.
[c]Special dialysis formulation of RECOMBIVAX HB® to be administered as a three-dose regimen at 0, 1, and 6 months.
[d]Two 1.0-ml injections are given at different sites; a four-dose schedule is recommended with vaccine given at intervals of 0, 1, 2, and 6 months.
Source: Refs. 1, 9, 10.

the AAP and the ACIP suggest a range of schedules for administration of vaccine (Table 3). This was done to facilitate integration with other pediatric immunizations, so that additional clinic or physician visits will not be required to administer hepatitis B vaccine. That should improve acceptance and minimize the cost of immunization against hepatitis B.

Under the AAP and ACIP recommendations, hepatitis B vaccine may be administered to infants starting at birth. If that option is selected, then the second dose should be given 1–2 months later, with the third dose given at 6–18 months of age. Alternately, vaccination may commence at approximately 2 months of age when an infant would normally receive the first dose of OPV, DTP, and Hib vaccines. A second dose of hepatitis B vaccine is then given in conjunction with the second doses of DTP, OPV, and Hib vaccines at 4 months of age, and the third dose may be given at any time between 6 and 18 months of age.

Currently, a number of the vaccination schedules encompassed by the AAP and ACIP recommendations are outside the schedules endorsed by the vaccine manufacturers, but changes in the product circulars to accommodate flexible scheduling are anticipated.

Table 3 Schedules Recommended by AAP and ACIP for Administration of Hepatitis B Vaccine to Infants Born of HBsAg– Women

Schedule	Age
Schedule 1[a]	
Dose 1	Birth (before discharge from hospital)
Dose 2	1–2 months
Dose 3	6–18 months
Schedule 2	
Dose 1	1–2 months
Dose 2	4 months
Dose 3	6–18 months

[a]The AAP recommends Schedule 1 where possible; the ACIP considers both schedules to be equally acceptable.
Source: Refs. 1, 7.

III. POSTEXPOSURE PROPHYLAXIS

Where possible, immunization before exposure to HBV is preferred. However, there are a number of settings in which postexposure prophylaxis with hepatitis B vaccine is either necessary or acceptable. Postexposure prophylaxis should be given in the following situations:

1. Perinatal exposure of an infant born to an HBsAg+ mother.
2. Sexual exposure to an HBsAg+ person.
3. Household exposure of an infant <12 months of age to a primary caregiver who has acute hepatitis B.
4. Accidental percutaneous or permucosal exposure to HBsAg+ blood.

Recommended prophylactic regimens vary by type of exposure. Many of these regimens combine immediate passive immunization with hepatitis B immune globulin (HBIG) and active immunization induced by hepatitis B vaccine.

Before the advent of vaccine, passive immunization with anti-HBs in immune globulin was the sole option for postexposure prevention of HBV infection. A single dose of HBIG at birth was 50% effective in preventing chronic HBV infection among infants born to HBsAg+/HBeAg+ women, while multiple doses of HBIG were up to 75% effective (11). Two doses of HBIG doses, one given after exposure and one a month later, were about 75% effective in preventing HBV infection following percutaneous exposure, while a single dose of HBIG had similar efficacy when used following sexual exposure (12–14).

When hepatitis B vaccine first became available, a combination of passive and active prophylaxis involving a dose of HBIG at birth followed by active immunization with three doses of vaccine proved to be highly effective, reducing the rate of chronic HBV infection in infants of HBsAg+/HBeAg+ mothers by 90–98% (15). Recent studies with currently available yeast recombinant hepatitis B vaccines also suggest that similar levels of protective efficacy may be obtainable using regimens of vaccine only without concomitant HBIG (16, 17). This approach is especially important for many areas of the world with high endemicity of HBV infection where it is not feasible to screen women for HBsAg or to employ the combination of passive and active prophylaxis.

Formal assessment of the efficacy of passive-active prophylaxis following percutaneous or sexual exposure to HBV has not been done. However, it is recommended in these postexposure settings based on the excellent efficacy of combined HBIG plus vaccine for the prevention of perinatal HBV infection.

A. Perinatal Hepatitis B Infection

An infant born to an infected mother is at high risk of becoming infected with HBV, and most infants infected at this time will become chronic carriers of the virus. In 1988, the ACIP recommended that all pregnant women in the United States be screened for HBsAg during the prenatal period and that infants born to HBsAg+ women be given immediate immunoprophylaxis (18). Current recommendations of the AAP and the ACIP for prevention of perinatal infection in these high-risk infants are summarized in Table 4. A 0.5-ml injection of HBIG should be given on the day of birth (preferably within 12 hours) and a series of at least three doses of vaccine should also be administered. The first dose of vaccine is preferably given within 12 hours of birth but at a different site than that used for administration of HBIG.

In the event that a woman gives birth before the result of her HBsAg test becomes available, the ACIP recommends that the infant be given the first dose of vaccine using the dosage appropriate for an infant of an HBsAg+ mother (Table 4). If the mother subsequently proves to be HBsAg+, then her infant should receive the additional protection of HBIG as soon as possible and within 7 days of birth (although the efficacy of HBIG given after 48 hours of age is not known), and immunization should be completed as shown in Table 4. If the mother's test for HBsAg proves to be negative, then immunization of the infant should be completed using the dosage of vaccine recommended for infants of HBsAg− mothers (see Table 2) (1).

B. Sexual Exposure

Sexual partners of HBsAg+ persons are at increased risk of HBV infection. ACIP recommendations for immunoprophylaxis of susceptible persons whose

Table 4 ACIP Recommendations for Postexposure Immunoprophylaxis of Infants Born to HBsAg+ Mothers or Persons Having Sexual Contact with an HBsAg+ Person

	HBIG		Vaccine	
Exposure	Dose	Recommended timing	Dose	Recommended timing
Perinatal	0.5 ml i.m.	Within 12 hours of birth	0.5 ml i.m.[a]	Within 12 hours of birth[b]
Sexual	0.06 ml/kg i.m.[c]	Single dose within 14 days of last sexual contact	1.0 ml i.m.[d]	First dose at time of HBIG treatment

[a]5 μg of RECOMBIVAX HB® or 10 μg of ENGERIX B®.

[b]The first dose can be given at the same time as HBIG but at a different site. Subsequent doses should be given at 1 and 6 months (RECOMBIVAX HB® or ENGERIX B®) or at 1, 2, and 12 months (ENGERIX B® alternate four-dose schedule).

[c]An alternate treatment for the sexual partner of a person with an acute HBV infection is to administer a single dose of HBIG. If the infection resolves, then no further treatment is required. However, if the index case is still HBsAg+ 3 months later, then the contact should receive a second dose of HBIG plus a standard vaccine series.

[d]10 μg of RECOMBIVAX HB® or 20 μg of ENGERIX B® for healthy adults. See Table 2 for dosage recommendations for other groups.

Source: Ref. 1.

sexual partners have either acute or chronic HBV infection are summarized in Table 4. If the last sexual contact with an HBV-infected person occurred within 14 days, then a single dose of HBIG (0.06 ml/kg i.m.) should be administered. A course of hepatitis B vaccine should also be initiated at this time (see Table 2 for appropriate dosages and schedules).

ACIP has also recommended an alternate treatment regimen for persons whose regular sexual partners have acute rather than chronic HBV infection. In this case, the contact may be given just a dose of HBIG. No further treatment is needed if the sexual partner becomes HBsAg- within the following 3 months. However, if the partner remains HBsAg+, then the contact should receive passive/active prophylaxis with a second dose of HBIG and vaccine as indicated in Table 4 (1).

C. Household Contacts

Household contacts of an individual with acute HBV infection are not considered to be at increased risk of infection *unless*:

1. The contact has had identifiable blood exposure to the index patient (e.g., sharing toothbrushes or razors). In that case, the contact should be given prophylaxis similar to that following sexual exposure (see above).

2. The contact is an infant <12 months of age and the index case with acute
    HBV infection is the infant's mother or other primary caregiver. In that
    case, the infant should be given combined passive/active prophylaxis as
    indicated for the prevention of perinatal HBV infection (see Table 4).

As noted previously (see Sec. II), vaccination is routinely recommended for
household contacts of persons with chronic HBV infection.

D.   Acute Exposure to Blood

Immunoprophylaxis against hepatitis B infection may be indicated following
accidental percutaneous (needlestick, laceration, or bite) or permucosal (ocular
or mucous membrane) exposure to blood. The appropriate action to take depends
on several factors:

1. Whether the source of blood is available for testing.
2. The HBsAg status of the blood.
3. The hepatitis B vaccination and vaccine response status of the exposed
    person.

Since such exposures generally involve persons for whom preexposure vaccination is recommended (see Table 1), any exposed unvaccinated person should be
given vaccine. Depending on the factors noted above, consideration must be
given to the administration of HBIG in addition to or, rarely (if the person is a
known nonresponder after a complete vaccination series plus booster doses),
instead of vaccine. Recommendations of the ACIP for immunoprophylaxis
against hepatitis B following blood exposure are summarized in Table 5.

IV.   OTHER ISSUES REGARDING HEPATITIS B
          VACCINE

A.   Pre/Postvaccination Testing for Antibody

Whether or not to test vaccine candidates for susceptibility is essentially an issue
of cost-effectiveness. In populations with a high prevalence of HBV serological
markers (e.g., >20% as in many groups of male homosexuals, intravenous drug
abusers, or sexual/household contacts of carriers), prevaccination screening is
appropriate, while it is typically not cost-effective in low-prevalence populations
such as health professionals in training or the routine immunization of children
and most adolescents.

Hepatitis B vaccine can be expected to induce a protective level of anti-HBs
(10 mIU/ml, approximately equal to 10 SRU or 10 S/N as determined by
radioimmunoassay or a positive test by enzyme immunoassay) in >90% of
healthy subjects (19). Consequently, routine testing for antibody after vaccina-

Table 5 ACIP Recommendations for Hepatitis B Immunoprophylaxis After Percutaneous or Permucosal Exposure to Blood

		Status of Exposed Person		
	Unvaccinated	Vaccinated		
Blood		Responder	Nonresponder	Unknown
HBsAg+	HBIG × 1[a] plus vaccine[b]	Test for anti-HBs; if adequate[c] then no treatment, if not adequate then booster dose of vaccine	HBIG × 2[d] *or* HBIG × 1 plus 1 dose vaccine	Test for anti-HBs; if adequate then no treatment, if not adequate then HBIG × 1 plus dose 1 vaccine
HBsAg–	Vaccine[b]	No treatment	No treatment	No treatment
Unknown	Vaccine[b]	No treatment	If blood from high-risk source, *treat as if HBsAg+*	Test for anti-HBs; if adequate then no treatment, if not adequate then booster dose of vaccine

[a]HBIG dose 0.06 ml/kg i.m.
[b]See Table 2 for dosages and schedules.
[c]Adequate anti-HBs is ≥10 mIU/ml or 10 SRU by RIA or positive by EIA.
[d]Two doses of HBIG one month apart.
Source: Ref. 1.

tion is not needed. The ACIP does recommend postvaccination antibody testing of persons whose management depends on knowing their immune status (e.g., dialysis patients and staff, infants born to HBsAg+ mothers, and persons with HIV infection). Postvaccination testing should also be considered for persons at occupational risk who may have needlestick exposures necessitating postexposure prophylaxis (1). When necessary, the test for anti-HBs should generally be done 1–6 months after completion of the vaccine series. Infants born to carrier mothers should be tested 3–9 months after completion of the vaccine series.

B. Revaccination of Nonresponders

The ACIP recommends revaccination with one or more additional doses of vaccine for persons who fail to respond to the primary series (1). The responses of nonresponders to further vaccination have been varied (see also Chapter 17). The proportion of nonresponders developing ≥10 mIU/ml of anti-HBs after an additional dose of vaccine has ranged from as little as 18% to as great as 54%, while 33–83% of hyporesponders (positive for anti-HBs at a level less than 10 mIU/ml after the initial vaccine series) achieved this level of antibody after a single booster dose of vaccine (20, 21). In several other groups of nonresponders or mixed nonresponders and hyporesponders, 44–75% developed a protective level of anti-HBs after a complete three-dose course of revaccination (22–25).

C. Booster Doses

Antibody level does wane after vaccination (see also Chapter 17). However, healthy responders to vaccine in early efficacy studies have been almost completely protected against clinical hepatitis B or antigenemia over periods of 5–8 years, even though in some cases up to half of the vaccinees failed to maintain at least 10 mIU/ml of anti-HBs during this time (26–29). The basis for continuing protection in the face of declining antibody is the presence of long-lived memory cells, partially differentiated B and T lymphocytes that on later restimulation with antigen differentiate further to rapidly produce antibody. Persistence of immunological memory can be demonstrated by a rapid anamnestic antibody response to a booster dose of vaccine in persons given a primary vaccine series several years before. For example, 48 healthy adults given a booster dose of recombinant hepatitis B vaccine 5–7 years after responding to a primary series of plasma-derived hepatitis B vaccine all displayed an anamnestic antibody response, even though 44% had less than 10 S/N and 19% had no detectable antibody at all when the booster dose was given (30). Similar long-lived immunological memory has been demonstrated in children, including those who received the primary vaccine series using either a standard schedule (intervals of 0, 1, and 6 months) or an accelerated schedule (intervals of 0, 1, and 2 months) (31, 32).

Because of immunological memory, the ACIP does not recommend routine booster doses for healthy recipients of hepatitis B vaccine. A booster dose may be appropriate in certain cases after exposure to percutaneous or permucosal exposure to blood (see Table 5).

In dialysis patients, protection may last only as long as the anti-HBs titer remains above 10 mIU/ml. The ACIP recommends that dialysis patients be tested annually following receipt of vaccine and a booster dose be given whenever the anti-HBs titer is <10 mIU/ml (1).

V. PREVENTION OF HEPATITIS B WITH VACCINE: AN OVERVIEW

Hepatitis B virus infection and disease is a major public health problem. Worldwide, it is estimated that 300 million people are carriers of HBV, and more than

1 million deaths annually are attributed to serious sequelae of chronic HBV infection (33). Since there is no established therapy for hepatitis B, control efforts are focused on immunization with hepatitis B vaccine.

The epidemiology of hepatitis B infection varies markedly in different parts of the world (reviewed in Chapter 7), and this has implications for the immunization strategies that may be considered (Table 6). At one end of the spectrum lie areas with a very high endemicity of HBV infection, such as many countries of Southeast Asia, the western Pacific, and Africa. Here the prevalence of chronic HBV infection is typically greater than 5% and may exceed 20%. Of particular concern is the prominence of virus transmission from an infected mother to her child in the perinatal period and horizontal transmission from infected siblings, playmates, or other members of the family or community to susceptible infants and children. In this setting, universal immunization of infants is the obvious strategy of choice. Since 1987, WHO has recommended that hepatitis B vaccine be administered to all infants in areas with moderate to high endemicity of HBV infection (4). In many countries, it is not feasible to screen pregnant women for HBsAg or to utilize HBIG. Consequently, efforts to control HBV infection in much of the world depend on timely immunization with vaccine alone. WHO recommends that hepatitis B vaccine be given in conjunction with other pediatric vaccines in the EPI (Table 7). In areas where there is substantial risk of perinatal transmission, the first dose of vaccine should be given as soon as possible after birth. Subsequent doses of vaccine should be given to infants at times when they would normally receive OPV and DPT or measles vaccine.

What immunization strategies make sense for lower-incidence countries such as the United States and most of the countries of Western Europe? There is considerable heterogeneity here. In the United Kingdom and in Scandinavia, for

Table 6   Strategies for Prevention of Hepatitis B with Vaccine

Incidence of Infection:	High (HBsAg+ >5%)	Low (HBsAg+ <2%)
Transmission of HBV:	Mother —-> child Horizontal in infancy/ childhood	Sexual contact Intravenous drug abuse Work exposure Mother —-> child Horizontal in infancy/ childhood
Immunization strategies:	Universal immunization of infants	Immunization of high- risk adult populations Universal immunization of infants/adolescents

Table 7 Recommendations of the World Health Organization for the Immunization of Infants with Hepatitis B Vaccine

Three doses of hepatitis B vaccine should be given to all infants within the Expanded Programme on Immunization in countries with moderate to high incidence of infection (carrier rate > 2%)

Schedule:____

Dose 1	Birth (or as soon as possible)
Dose 2	4–12 weeks after first dose
Dose 3	2–12 months after second dose

Source: Ref. 4.

example, the carrier rate is <0.1% (34). In the United States and many countries of Western Europe, the prevalence of HBV carriers is intermediate, ranging from 0.1% to about 0.5%, while some of the Mediterranean countries have rates that exceed 1%.

The epidemiology of hepatitis B is actually more complex in many lower-incidence countries with multiple modes of HBV transmission (Table 6). In the United States, for example, most HBV infections occur in adults, and a large portion of these are attributable either to sexual transmission or to intravenous drug abuse (5). As discussed earlier, vaccination is indicated for persons at risk of exposure to virus by these routes. However, vaccination only of specific high-risk adult populations is not sufficient. Members of these populations often are difficult to identify or access. When identified, a substantial portion may already be infected with HBV, and those who are susceptible are often reluctant to accept vaccine or fail to complete the full recommended vaccination regimen. Consequently, the use of established health-care contacts to effect broad-based immunity in infants and children, before they enter occupations or engage in other behaviors that place them at high risk of exposure to HBV, appears to be a good way to compensate for poor delivery to or acceptance of vaccine by older populations. Universal vaccination of infants along with screening of pregnant women for HBsAg and passive/active immunization of infants born to infected women will also eliminate the HBV infections that occur at an early age. While relatively few infants and children become infected in low-incidence countries, the propensity for these infections to become chronic means that they make a disproportionate contribution to the reservoir of virus carriers and the burden of serious liver disease. Vaccination of infants will first have an impact by reducing the size of the HBV carrier pool. As the number of carriers is reduced, there will be less transmission of virus and a lower incidence of infection. Since serious liver diseases such as cirrhosis and hepatocellular carcinoma are sequelae of chronic HBV infection, a long-term reduction in the prevalence of HBV carriers will eventually be manifested in lower rates of these diseases.

The hepatitis B immunization policies that are actually adopted and implemented will differ from country to country and can be expected to reflect the local epidemiology of HBV infection and disease, the structure of the health-care delivery system, and available resources. Cost-benefit assessments should precede the implementation of large-scale immunization programs. In very high-incidence areas of the world, such as Asia and Africa, the long-range benefits of universal infant immunization against hepatitis B are undisputed. However, inadequate delivery systems and high vaccine costs are impediments to broad implementation of universal immunization in these areas.

In lower-incidence countries like the United States, universal screening of pregnant women for HBsAg and passive-active prophylaxis of the infants whose mothers are HBsAg+ as well as universal immunization of infants born to HBsAg− women appear to have strong positive benefit-to-cost ratios (35; Dr. H. Margolis, U.S. CDC, personal communication). The benefit-to-cost ratio of universal infant immunization has not yet been determined for the lowest-incidence countries such as the United Kingdom and Scandinavia, and such programs may not be warranted there. In these countries, efforts are now focused on voluntary vaccination of health-care workers and other well-defined high-risk groups plus the screening of foreign-born pregnant women and the vaccination of infants born to carrier mothers (34).

REFERENCES

1. Centers for Disease Control, Hepatitis B virus: A comprehensive strategy for eliminating transmission in the United States through universal childhood vaccination. Recommendations of the Immunization Practices Advisory Committee (ACIP), *MMWR*, *40*(RR-13): 1 (1991).

2. Committee on Infectious Diseases—American Academy of Pediatrics, *Report of the Committee on Infectious Diseases*, 22nd edition, American Academy of Pediatrics, Elk Grove Village, IL (1991).

3. American College of Physicians, *Guide for Adult Immunization*, 2nd ed., American College of Physicians, Philadelphia (1989).

4. World Health Organization, Progress in the control of viral hepatitis: Memorandum from a WHO meeting, *Bull. WHO*, *66*: 443 (1988).

5. M. J. Alter, S. C. Hadler, H. S., Margolis, et al., The changing epidemiology of hepatitis B in the United States. Need for alternative vaccination strategies, *JAMA*, *263*: 1218 (1990).

6. Centers for Disease Control, Protection against viral hepatitis. Recommendations of the Immunization Practices Advisory Committee (ACIP), *MMWR*, *39*(RR-2): 1 (1990).

7. D. Fleischman, Committee outlines universal strategy to counter hepatitis B, *AAP News*, *7*(7): 1 (1991).

8. C. Salmond and D. Bandaranayake, Progress of the neonatal hepatitis B immunisation programme in Northland, *NZ Med. J.*, *104*: 233 (1991).
9. RECOMBIVAX HB® (Hepatitis B Vaccine (Recombinant), MSD), Prescribing information, Merck & Co., Inc., issue date March 1990.
10. Engerix-B® (Hepatitis B Vaccine (Recombinant)), Prescribing information, SmithKline Beckman Corp., issue date September 1989.
11. R. P. Beasley, L. Y. Hwang, C. E. Stevens, et al., Efficacy of hepatitis B immune globulin for prevention of perinatal transmission of the hepatitis B virus carrier state: Final report of a randomized double-blind, placebo-controlled trial, *Hepatology*, *3*: 135 (1983).
12. L. B. Seeff, E. C. Wright, J. J. Zimmerman, et al., Type B hepatitis after needle-stick exposure: Final report of the Veterans Administration Cooperative Study, *Ann. Intern. Med.*, *88*: 285 (1978).
13. G. F. Grady, V. A. Lee, A. M. Prince, et al., Hepatitis B immune globulin for accidental exposures among medical personnel: Final report of a multicenter controlled trial, *J. Infect. Dis.*, *138*: 625 (1978).
14. A. G. Redeker, J. W. Mosley, D. J. Gocke, et al., Hepatitis B immune globulin as a prophylactic measure for spouses exposed to acute type B hepatitis, *N. Engl. J. Med.*, *293*: 1055 (1975).
15. R. P. Beasley, L-Y. Hwang, G. C-Y. Lee, et al., Prevention of perinatally transmitted hepatitis B virus infection with hepatitis B immune globulin and hepatitis B vaccine, *Lancet*, *2*: 1099 (1983).
16. Y. Poovorawan, S. Sanpavat, W. Pongpunlert, et al., Comparison of a recombinant DNA hepatitis B vaccine alone or in combination with immune globulin for the prevention of perinatal acquisition of hepatitis B carriage, *Vaccine*, *8* (Suppl.): S56 (1990).
17. R. J. Gerety and D. J. West, Current and future hepatitis B vaccines, *Progress in Hepatitis B Immunization* (P. Coursaget and M. J. Tong, eds.), Colloque INSERM/John Libbey Eurotext Ltd., London, Vol. 194, pp. 215–225 (1990).
18. Centers for Disease Control, Recommendations of the Immunization Practices Advisory Committee. Prevention of perinatal transmission of hepatitis B virus: Prenatal screening of all pregnant women for hepatitis B antigen, *MMWR*, *37*: 341 (1988).
19. Centers for Disease Control, Recommendations of the Immunization Practices Advisory Committee. Update on hepatitis B prevention, *MMWR*, *36*: 353 (1987).
20. W. Jilg, M. Schmidt, and F. Deinhardt, Immune response to hepatitis B vaccine, *J. Med. Virol.*, *24*: 377 (1988).
21. D. J. West, L. Kersh, V. Ioli, et al., Anti-HBs responses to a booster dose of hepatitis B vaccine in healthy adult nonresponders and hyporesponders to primary vaccination, *1990 International Symposium on Viral Hepatitis and Liver Disease*, Houston, TX, Abstract No. 304.
22. P. Wismans, J. van Hattum, T. Stelling, et al., Effect of supplementary vaccination in healthy non-responders to hepatitis B vaccination, *Hepato-gastroenterol.*, *35*: 78 (1988).
23. J. Y. Weissman, M. M. Tsuchiyose, M. J. Tong, et al., Lack of response to recombinant hepatitis-B vaccine in nonresponders to the plasma vaccine, *JAMA*, *260*: 1734 (1988).

24. L. Butterly, E. Watkins, C. A. Hinkle, et al., Response to recombinant yeast hepatitis B vaccine, *Hepatology*, *5*: 1007 (1985).

25. D. G. Ostrow, J. Goldsmith, S. B. Kalish, et al., Nonresponse to hepatitis B vaccine in homosexual men, *Sex. Transm. Dis.*, *14*: 92 (1987).

26. R. B. Wainwright, B. J. McMahon, L. R. Bulkow, et al., Duration of immunogenicity and efficacy of hepatitis B vaccine in a Yupik Eskimo population, *JAMA*, *261*: 2362 (1989).

27. S. C. Hadler, F. N. Judson, P. M. O'Malley, et al., Studies of hepatitis B vaccine in homosexual men, *Progress in Hepatitis B Immunization* (P. Coursaget and M. J. Tong, eds.), Colloque INSERM/John Libbey Eurotext Ltd., London, Vol. 194, pp. 165–175 (1990).

28. M. J. Tong, C. E. Stevens, P. E. Taylor, et al., Prevention of hepatitis B infection in infants born to HBeAg positive HBsAg positive carrier mothers in the United States. An update, 1989, *Progress in Hepatitis B Immunization* (P. Coursaget and M. J. Tong, eds.), Colloque INSERM/John Libbey Eurotext Ltd., London, Vol. 194, pp. 339–345 (1990).

29. L-Y. Hwang, C-Y. Lee, and R. P. Beasley, Five year follow-up of HBV vaccination with plasma derived in neonates—evaluation of immunogenicity and efficacy against perinatal transmission, *1990 International Symposium on Viral Hepatitis and Liver Disease*, Houston, TX, Abstract No. 247.

30. S. Krugman and M. Davidson, Hepatitis B vaccine: Prospects for duration of immunity, *Yale J. Biol. Med.*, *60*: 333 (1987).

31. C. D. Moyes, A. Milne, and J. Waldon, Very low dose hepatitis B vaccination in the newborn: anamnestic response to a booster at four years, *J. Med. Virol.*, *30*: 216 (1990).

32. A. Milne, Hepatitis B vaccination in high risk children: Five year efficacy and booster studies, presented at the 2nd National Immunisation Conference, Public Health Association of Australia, Canberra, 27–29 May, 1991.

33. Y. Ghendon, WHO strategy for the global elimination of new cases of hepatitis B, *Vaccine*, *8* (Suppl.): S129 (1990).

34. A. Goudeau and the European Regional Study Group, Epidemiology and eradication strategy of hepatitis B in Europe, *Vaccine*, *8* (Suppl.): S113 (1990).

35. J. S. Arevalo and A. E. Washington, Cost-effectiveness of prenatal screening and immunization for hepatitis B virus, *JAMA*, *259*: 365 (1988).

2

Plasma-Derived Hepatitis B Vaccine: A Breakthrough in Preventive Medicine

Maurice R. Hilleman

Merck Research Laboratories,
West Point, Pennsylvania

I. HUMAN HEPATITIS B

Human hepatitis B virus (HBV) infection causes liver diseases of immense importance to people in most parts of the world. Though the acute viral infection may cause severe illnesses and sometimes death in a small percentage of infected persons, the more serious consequences are related to a viral carrier state that often progresses to chronic liver disease with cirrhosis and hepatocarcinoma 15–30 years after initial infection. There are presently about 300 million carriers of hepatitis B virus in the world population, and it is estimated that 75–100 million of them will die of liver cirrhosis and/or liver cancer. The probability of developing the carrier state following HBV infection is greatest in early life and diminishes with increasing age. Up to 90% of babies born to carrier mothers may become carriers themselves.

It is something of a miracle in modern medicine, perhaps, that HBV infection is now preventable by vaccination, even in the great majority of babies born to mothers who are carriers of the virus. The first HBV vaccine (1–12), licensed in the United States in 1981, was prepared in these laboratories using viral surface antigen purified from the plasma of human carriers of the infection. Having demonstrated remarkable safety and efficacy, this vaccine became the world standard for all hepatitis B vaccines that followed, including more recent preparations made using recombinant technology (see also Chapter 4). In the short span of less than a decade after its development, hepatitis B vaccine is being used worldwide, and the effort is being initiated, first, to eliminate hepatitis B as a disease of major importance and, second, to eradicate hepatitis B from the planet. These objectives are achievable. Because the vaccine prevents hepatitis B infection, it will also prevent the liver cirrhosis and hepatocarcinoma caused by the virus, and it represents the first vaccine against cancer in human beings.

The scope of this chapter is limited to the plasma-derived hepatitis B vaccine that was pioneered and developed in our laboratories (1–12). The substance of the chapter is a description of the evolution of concepts, problem definition, and stepwise resolution of each defined objective in an area in which a product was targeted, starting from a woefully inadequate database and the lack of any meaningful precedents to follow. New ground needed to be broken each step of the way, and the creation of the vaccine was a venture in combined basic exploratory and applied research endeavors. Other hepatitis B vaccines prepared using plasma-derived or recombinant-produced hepatitis B antigen have since been described. They are well recorded in reviews, textbooks, and individual publications (13–15) and will not be made part of this chapter.

II. QUEST FOR A HUMAN HEPATITIS B VACCINE

A. Etiological Discovery

Historically, vaccines began in 1798 with Jenner's cowpox vaccine against human smallpox. That vaccine, and all the viral vaccines that followed to the midpoint of the twentieth century, consisted of live or killed whole virus, and the virus used to prepare vaccine was derived from the infected organs or tissues of animals or embryonated hens' eggs. The breakthrough renaissance of tissue culture by Enders et al. (16) opened the door to use of viruses grown in vitro in cell culture. All of these viral vaccines acted by stimulating production, in the vaccinee, of specific antibodies that were known or presumed to be neutralizing and that prevented viral infection. Some of the vaccines, principally those consisting of live virus, may also have induced cytotoxic T-lymphocyte immunity, which is of importance in immune clearance of already infected cells.

Control of the complex of viral agents causing hepatitis has piqued the interest of vaccinologists since the beginning of the present century, but, until recently, the responsible agents were undefined and nonpropagable in the laboratory. Hence, there was no source of antigen for vaccine, and the prehistory of hepatitis B vaccine was centered on the discovery of the agent and its means of propagation, an elusive objective that has not been achieved to this date.

Hepatitis, a disease of many etiologies that manifests jaundice, had its roots in antiquity. The earliest medical writings probably included hepatitides of viral etiology. Parenterally transmitted jaundice was documented in 1885 (17). It became evident during World War II that there were two kinds of hepatitis: epidemic infectious hepatitis and human serum–transmitted jaundice, termed hepatitis A and hepatitis B, respectively, by MacCallum in 1947 (18). These two entities were clearly delineated and defined in 1967 in the clinical research investigations carried out by Krugman et al. (19) at the Willowbrook State School for the Mentally Handicapped.

These fundamental discoveries still did not permit the development of a vaccine against hepatitis B. The vaccine became possible with the discovery of an antigen and its association with hepatitis B infection by Blumberg et al. (20) and by Prince et al. (21) in the mid-1950s. Blumberg called this antigen Australia antigen, because it was found in the serum of an Australian aboriginee, and Prince called the antigen SH antigen based on its presence in cases of serum hepatitis. This antigen was soon found to be a subunit of HBV present in the blood of acute cases and carriers of HBV infection. The virus itself, the Dane particle, was described by Dane et al. in 1970 (22).

B. Development of a Hepatitis B Vaccine

1. Concept

The existence of hepatitis B surface antigen in the blood of carriers of hepatitis B infection suggested a far-out and unprecedented possibility that it just might be feasible to develop a vaccine based on isolation and utilization of the 22-nm surface antigen particles from human plasma. Work was started in our laboratories in 1968 to explore and pursue this possibility.

It was recognized at the outset that the evolution of a satisfactory product must rest on the provision of technical solutions to a number of critical needs:

1. The antigen must be essentially pure, to avoid adverse reactions and to assure lack of interference with the inactivation by chemical agents of any residual life form.
2. The antigen must contain no living or viable unconventional infectious entity, such as agents of the scrapie family.
3. The antigen incorporated in proper amount into a vaccine must be capable of eliciting an antibody response that is sufficient in kind and amount to afford protection against infection on exposure to the virus.
4. The vaccine must induce protective immunity in the great majority of human recipients against all HBV strains following a practical and clinically acceptable immunization regimen.
5. Protective immunity following vaccine must be of at least several years duration, and it would be expected that an acceptable immunological adjuvant would be needed.
6. The vaccine must cause no more than minimal and clinically acceptable reactions.

7. The vaccine and its preparation must be totally controllable with respect to purity, safety, potency, and efficacy using in vivo and in vitro tests that would include use of animals. It must have a reasonable stability on storage at 4°C.
8. The cost for vaccine, per dose, must be economically acceptable, assuming selection of plasma of highest possible antigen content, and use in the vaccine of the least amount of antigen needed to immunize.

These objectives were achieved.

An indication of the economics of a vaccine was provided in the important studies on HBV inactivation by Krugman and colleagues (23). In 1971, Krugman reported that a crude HBV-containing serum that had been diluted 1:10 and heated at 98°C for one minute induced measurable antibody in a majority of human recipients following one or more injections of the preparation. The virus in the serum was incompletely inactivated since it induced anti-hepatitis B core conversion in some children, indicating that infection had occurred in some of the recipients. The infection, however, was clinically inapparent. Subsequent challenge with infectious unheated serum showed complete protection against hepatitis B in 59% of the 29 children who had received the heated plasma and subclinical transient infection in 10%. Krugman kindly furnished a small sample of heat-treated material to us, and it was found that there was about 1 μg of hepatitis B surface antigen (HBsAg) per ml. This provided a basis for belief that the plasma-derived vaccine we were developing would likely be in an economically acceptable range, in answer to critical need 8 listed above. These important early studies by Krugman gave, in addition, a first indication that antibody, stimulated artificially by surface antigen, was relevant to induction of immunity against HBV.

2. Antigen Purification, Virus Inactivation, and Adjuvantation (1–12).

Plasma from carriers of HBV contain varying amounts of HBsAg spheres (22-nm particles) or tubules, Dane (virus) particles, and normal human plasma components that may or may not be contaminated with additional living agents (Fig. 1). It was evident from the first exploratory experiments that preliminary precipitation with ammonium sulfate, followed by rate zonal centrifugation and isopycnic banding, would provide starting material in which about 10% of the total protein content was HBsAg and from which the bulk of large virus particles, particularly those of hepatitis B, were removed. Development, at that time, of the Electronucleonics KII ultracentrifuge greatly facilitated large-scale processing.

Further purification was needed and special attention was required to evolve procedures that would inactivate all possible life forms, including nondetectable agents. Sequential continuous flow ultraviolet light and heat inactivation in a closed system were tried, but it was soon found possible to effect both high-level purity (ultimately more than 99% purity) as well as viral inactivation in a se-

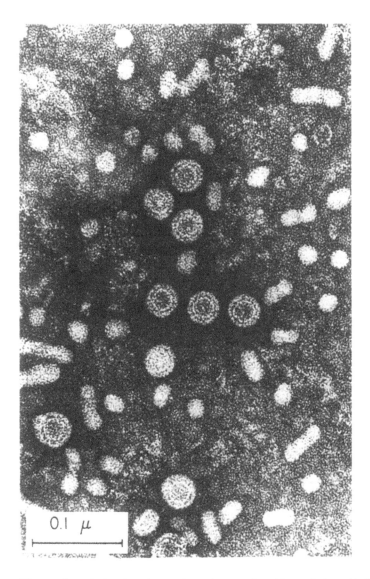

Figure 1 Viral and surface antigen elements found in crude hepatitis B preparations from infected plasma from a human hepatitis B carrier.

quence of steps (Fig. 2) that depended mainly on digestion with pepsin, denaturation with urea and renaturation, and, finally, treatment with formaldehyde. Each step in the whole process was carried out in a closed system in separate and isolated facilities in order to guarantee freedom from possible contamination with material from an earlier step in the process. The steps in the process were

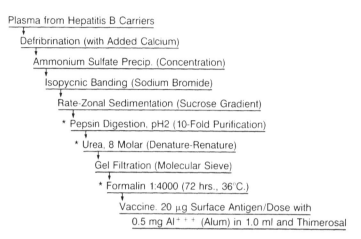

Plasma from Hepatitis B Carriers
Defribrination (with Added Calcium)
Ammonium Sulfate Precip. (Concentration)
Isopycnic Banding (Sodium Bromide)
Rate-Zonal Sedimentation (Sucrose Gradient)
* Pepsin Digestion, pH2 (10-Fold Purification)
* Urea, 8 Molar (Denature-Renature)
Gel Filtration (Molecular Sieve)
* Formalin 1:4000 (72 hrs., 36°C.)
Vaccine. 20 μg Surface Antigen/Dose with
0.5 mg Al^{+++} (Alum) in 1.0 ml and Thimerosal

Figure 2   Key steps in preparing human hepatitis B vaccine (*see Table 1).

each shown, in laboratory studies and in the published literature, to destroy all possible microbial life forms that could be present in human blood (Table 1). Importantly, the infectious agent(s) causing transmissible spongiform encephalopathy, as exemplified by scrapie virus of sheep, were shown to be susceptible to destruction by treatment with concentrated urea (24). Total inactivation of scrapie agent may be difficult to demonstrate owing to use of crude brain suspensions as source of agent; with purified hepatitis B antigen, the material is essentially pure. The late appearance of the retrovirus HTLV-III (HIV-I), causing AIDS in human beings, threatened the concept of safety of the hepatitis B vaccine, even though the virus was readily inactivated by the procedures used to prepare the vaccine (25).

The purified surface antigen consists of a homogeneous suspension of 22-nm particles (Fig. 3) consisting of S antigen alone and free of the pre-S components that may be present in small and variable amount in the native surface antigen.

Studies of the immunogenicity of the purified surface antigen in animals revealed that immunizing potency was improved by formulation in aluminum hydroxide adjuvant. To achieve the best possible adjuvantation, the alum and antigen were coprecipitated from a mixed aqueous solution to give floccules of aluminum hydroxide in which the antigen was occluded by as well as absorbed to the alum.

3.   Preclinical Testing

Quality Control   Control procedures developed to measure the purity, uniformity, potency, and safety of the hepatitis B vaccine are summarized in Table 2. Development of an extinction dilution potency assay in mice, in which the

Table 1 Inactivation of Animal Viruses by Reagents

Treatment	Family	Example
Pepsin digestion at pH 2	Hepadnavirus	Hepatitis B
	Rhabdovirus	Vesicular stomatitis
	Poxvirus	Vaccinia
	Togavirus	Sindbis
	Reovirus	Reovirus
	Herpesvirus	Herpes simplex
	Coronavirus	Infectious bronchitis
	Picornavirus	Mengovirus
Urea	Hepadnavirus	Hepatitis B
	Rhabdovirus	Vesicular stomatitis
	Poxvirus	Vaccinia
	Togavirus	Sindbis
	Reovirus	Reovirus
	Herpesvirus	Herpes simplex
	Coronavirus	Infectious bronchitis
	Picornavirus	Mengovirus
	Myxovirus	Newcastle disease virus
	Slow viruses	Scrapie
Formalin	Most viruses, including parvovirus, retrovirus, delta agent, and hepatitis A	

minimal amount of antigen needed to seroconvert 50% of ICR/Ha or BALB/c mice following a single intraperitoneal dose of vaccine was measured, made it possible to control the immunizing potency of the vaccine. Development of the chimpanzee model for HBV infection (26) permitted routine testing of all lots of vaccine for safety from live HBV contamination (27) and also opened the door to a test to study protective efficacy of the vaccine (Table 3).

Immune Response and Protective Efficacy in Animals Studies in mice, guinea pigs, monkeys (Table 4), and chimpanzees (Fig. 4), in which the animals were given varying amounts of antigen in aqueous or alum formulation and in different regimens, all showed the immunizing capability of the purified antigen, especially when given with alum.

Protective efficacy was established in tests in which susceptible chimpanzees were given three doses of vaccine a month apart and were then challenged with 1000 chimpanzee infectious doses of the virus (Table 5). The chimpanzees were solidly protected against induction of liver histopathology, liver enzyme eleva-

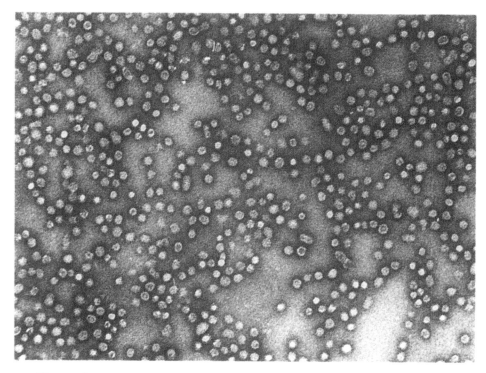

Figure 3   Hepatitis B vaccine, lot 560 (×56,000).

tion, the appearance of a hepatitis B antigenemia, and the carrier state. A single chimpanzee that failed to develop detectable antibody following vaccination was, nevertheless, protected, even though there was transient infection indicated by the appearance of antibody to hepatitis B core antigen that is not present in the vaccine. Studies by others (28) of serotype crossing showed that cross-protection was afforded when chimpanzees were vaccinated with serotype *adw* vaccine and challenged with *ayw* virus and vice versa. Similar cross-protection was afforded by infection (29).

4.   Early Clinical Tests in Human Beings

The vaccine was considered to be sufficiently well developed by 1975 to justify first trials in humans. In an arranged collaborative study to test for safety, Dr. Saul Krugman gave a first injection of the vaccine to nine salaried employees of Merck & Co. and to two nonemployees. On November 3, 1975, these persons were given one dose of vaccine, and they were followed for a period of 6 months for the development of markers of hepatitis B infection. All remained free of infection, and this opened the door to larger-scale studies in humans, with

Table 2 Principal Quality Control Tests for Hepatitis B Vaccine

Plasma pool	Purified bulk antigen	Final container tests
Animal tests	Microbial sterility	Microbial sterility
Adult mouse (i.p.,	Blood group substance	Mouse and guinea pig
i.c.)	Human IgM (im-	(general safety)
Suckling mouse (i.p.,	munodiffusion)	Free formaldehyde
i.c.)	DNA polymerase	Thimerosal
	Gel electrophoresis	Aluminum
Chick embryo	Lowry protein with RIA	Identity
Yolk sac	antigen assay	
Allantoic sac	Specific absorption (UV)	
	Formaldehyde	
Cell culture	Limulus pyrogen (LAL)	
Grivet monkey kidney	Chimpanzee safety	
(vero)	Mouse potency (on	
WI-38 (human diploid)	alum)	
cells		

i.p. = intraperitoneal; i.c. = intracerebral; UV = ultraviolet light.

Table 3 Assay for Infectivity (Safety) of Lot 559 Formalin-Treated Hepatitis B Vaccine Given i.v. to Susceptible Chimpanzees Observed for 40 Weeks

		Findings during 40-week observation period[a]				
			Enzyme	Antibody		Hepatitis
		Antigenemia	elevation	Surface	Core	histo-
Material injected	Chimpanzee	(HBsAg)	(SGPT)	anti-HBs	anti-HBc	pathology
Control: Human	804	+[b]	+	+	+	+
hepatitis B live	805	+	+	0	+	+
virus given in-	806	+	0	+	0	0
travenously	702	+	0	+	0	0
(1000 chimpan-	748	0	0	+	0	0
zee infectious						
doses)						
Test: Lot 559 vac-	815	0[b]	0	0	0	0
cine given in-	816	0	0	0	0	0
travenously, 20	817	0	0	0	0	0
μg/dose	763	0	0	0	0	0

[a]HBsAg by Ausria II test; anti-HBs by Ausab test; anti-HBc test by Drs. Hoofnagle and Schulman; histopathology by Dr. M. J. Iatropoulos (ICES).
[b]Positive (+) at some time(s) during the 40-week period or negative (0) during the entire period.

Table 4 Potency Assays in Grivet Monkeys Given Three Doses of Hepatitis B Vaccine in Aqueous or Alum Formulation

| | | | Hepatitis B antibody response (AUSAB®) following dose[a] | | | | | |
| | | | 1 | | 2 | | 3 | |
Lot no.	Formulation	Antigen Dose (μg)	No. Positive/ Total	Geo-metric Mean Titer	No. Positive/ Total	Geo-metric Mean Titer	No. Positive/ Total	Geo-metric Mean Titer
727	Aqueous	40	2/4	4	3/4	21	3/4	26
	Alum	40	4/4	163	4/4	113	4/4	192
		20	4/4	326	4/4	234	4/4	291
723	Alum (lot	40	4/4	102	4/4	272	4/4	289
	560	20	3/4	48	4/4	198	4/4	265
	aqueous)							

[a]Vaccine given subcutaneously in 1-ml amount at 0, 4, and 8 weeks.

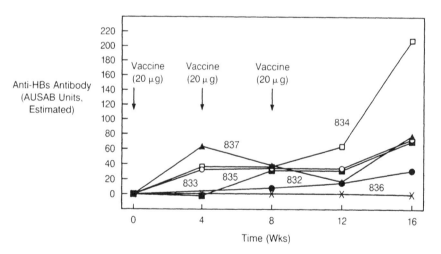

Figure 4 Hepatitis B antibody response, according to time, in six chimpanzees given three does, subcutaneously, of 20 μg each (1 ml) of aqueous lot 559 vaccine at monthly intervals. (*Note*: None of the animals developed anti-HBc antibody.)

Table 5 Protective Efficacy of Hepatitis B Vaccine in Chimpanzees

Animal no.	Hepatitis B antibody before challenge	Findings after challenge with HBV			
		Hepatitis B antigenemia	Transaminase elevation	Antibody development vs.	
				Surface antigen	Core antigen
Vaccinated[a] animals					
1	+	0	0	0	0
2	+	0	0	0	0
3	+	0	0	0	0
4	+	0	0	0	0
5	+	0	0	0	0
6	0	0	0	+	0
Unvaccinated controls					
7	0	+	0	+	+
8	0	+	0	+	+
9	0	+	0	+	+
10	0	+	+	0	+
11	0	+	0	0	0

+Indicates positive; 0, negative.

[a]Three doses, 20 μg per dose.

emphasis, initially, on development of an optimal dose and time regimen for giving the vaccine.

It was shown that 75–85% of normal human adults (Fig. 5) developed antibody against hepatitis B after only two doses of the vaccine given a month apart, and more than 90% of persons had antibody after a third or booster dose given 5 months after the primary vaccinations. This regimen has been used routinely in administering the plasma-derived vaccine. The booster dose is of importance (Fig. 6) not only in increasing the percentage of persons who respond, but also in increasing the antibody titer and immunological memory.

Antibody characteristically declines following recovery from viral infections and especially following vaccines. However, recovery from infection (Fig. 7) or vaccination (Fig. 8) induces a very strong capability for immediate anamnestic recall. Anamnestic sensitization has lasted for 7 or 8 years following vaccine, even though antibody has declined to low and undetectable levels. Persons exposed to the virus at such late times are solidly protected against disease and

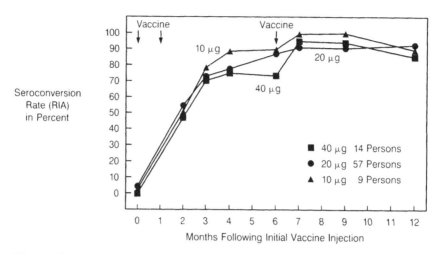

Figure 5 Seroconversion rates in adult human subjects given lot 751 human hepatitis B vaccine in graded doses in alum formulation (Study 542).

the carrier state, though a few may develop a core antibody response indicating transient infection (30,31).

Very young children and adults greater than 40 or 50 years of age (Fig. 9) show a lessened ability to mount an antibody response against hepatitis B antigen. Individuals who are immunologically compromised may show a severely depressed ability to respond to vaccine.

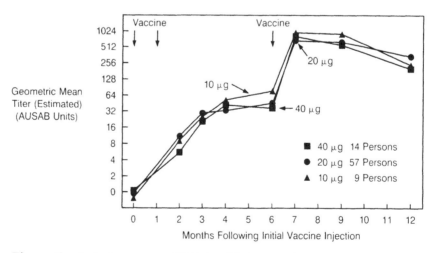

Figure 6 Antibody responses (RIA) in adult human subjects given lot 751 human hepatitis B vaccine in graded doses in alum formulation (Study 542).

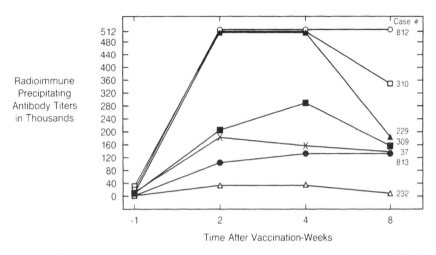

Figure 7 Representative examples of radioimmune precipitating antibody (AUSAB) responses to a single dose of lot 727 hepatitis B vaccine in alum given to seven initially seropositive donors with low titers of antibody.

5. Alternative Hepatitis B Vaccine Produced from Human Hepatocarcinoma Cells in Culture, Producing HBsAg

Recognizing the limitation in supply of suitable carrier plasma to prepare hepatitis B vaccine, our group carried out studies to explore the use of Alexander cells (32) in culture as a source of antigen. The Alexander cell (33) is a continuous line

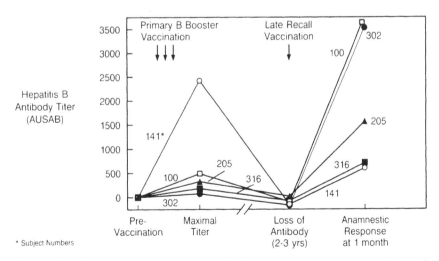

Figure 8 Anamnestic response to hepatitis B vaccine among persons who lost their antibody and were given a 20-μg recall dose of vaccine.

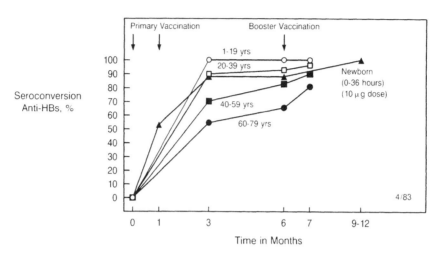

Figure 9 Antibody response, according to age and time, to three 20-µg doses of hepatitis B vaccine.

of hepatocarcinoma cells derived from a patient with liver cancer who was also a carrier of hepatitis B.

The Alexander cell grows readily in cell culture and normally secretes HBsAg in a relatively small amount. Our group was able to increase the yield of antigen to an economically competitive level with that of the plasma source by propagating the cells in Vitafiber pseudocapillary units in which the cellular metabolism was slowed by addition of 10^{-4} M caffeine to the circulating medium and by lowering of temperature of incubation to 32°C. The antigen, purified by immune affinity chromatography, digestion with DNase and pepsin, and Sephadex G-150 separation, was found to be indistinguishable in all measurable aspects from that derived from human plasma.

The formalin-treated antigen was formulated in 20-µg dose on alum adjuvant with thimerosal added as a preservative. This cell culture vaccine was as potent as human plasma-derived vaccine as measured in a mouse potency assay. The vaccine proved safe in tests in chimpanzees and in human subjects who were in late stages of cancer of the central nervous system and who were receiving therapy for their condition. None of five subjects who received the vaccine developed untoward clinical reactions. Two of the subjects who received all three doses of vaccine developed antibody against HBsAg. Three persons—two given only the primary doses and one given all three doses but lost to follow-up—demonstrated no response. The slow and relatively low antibody responses to the vaccine were similar to those in other immunosuppressed persons given vaccine of human plasma origin.

Though this vaccine was highly promising because of its simplified technology, it was not acceptable at the time to use any biological preparation made from continuous mammalian cells, even when highly purified and treated to remove any possible oncogenic DNA (see Refs. 34, 35). The more recent developments in cell culture safety (35–37) have revolutionized this restrictive concept and would now allow use of continuous mammalian cells, even those containing substantial amounts of contaminating DNA.

The Alexander cell vaccine was not pursued further. The issue had become academic through the breakthroughs in recombinant technology that led to the development by our laboratories of the world's first recombinant-produced vaccine (38–39)—that against hepatitis B, using antigen produced in transfected yeast cells in culture. The yeast-produced vaccine, first licensed in 1986, has rendered all previous hepatitis B vaccines obsolete because of the superior and simplified technology used to produce it.

III. VACCINE PROTECTION

The final test for the vaccine was measuring its ability to protect against disease, infection, and the carrier state. The first clinical efficacy trial was initiated in 1978 by Szmuness et al. (40) in a study conducted among male homosexuals in New York City. The 0-, 1-, 6-month dose regimen was employed, and all individuals who received the vaccine and responded serologically were protected against the disease and the carrier state. A second study was performed by Francis et al. (41) of the Centers for Disease Control. Similar findings were obtained, though the levels of the antibody responses in some locations were lower than in others. This was possibly due to inadvertent freezing of vaccine in shipping. Many additional studies of the vaccine were carried out, which are the subject of other chapters of this text and were reviewed recently by Hollinger (13).

IV. VACCINE APPLICATION

While possibilities for fine-tuning present hepatitis B vaccines to effect minor improvement do exist, the far greater issue is in the area of vaccine utilization. Clearly, hepatitis B is an eradicable disease. There is no animal reservoir, the protective antigen is stable (see below for possible second serotype), and the vaccine is highly effective. It is of special importance that vaccine, given to the newborn of carrier mothers, is highly effective (greater than 90%) in breaking the chain of transmission by this route (13–15).

In the United States (see Refs. 42, 43), there are about 300,000 new hepatitis B infections each year. The vaccine, although licensed in 1981, has seen such limited use in high-risk persons that the rate for new virus infections is increasing annually. To state it simply, the vaccine for the most part sits on the shelf, where it is quite ineffective in preventing hepatitis B. Further, most infections occur outside the total of the defined high-risk groups. For this reason, nothing short of a universal immunization program will bring the epidemic to a halt. This kind of approach has been very successful in native Americans (Indians and Eskimos in Alaska), and plans are being laid for the time when this kind of approach can be brought to the entire country.

Worldwide (44–46), hepatitis B vaccine has been applied to an even lesser extent than in the United States, except for small pilot programs that have been started in some countries to vaccinate all newborns, especially those born to *e* antigen–positive (highly infectious) mothers. Wherever possible, hepatitis B vaccine is being added to the World Health Organization's Expanded Programme on Immunization (EPI). There are two principal deterrents to achieving the desired end: the cost of vaccine and finding funding for and establishing the vaccine delivery system in many developing nations. The World Health Organization will not likely be capable of implementing any worldwide program for immunization until such time that the vaccine becomes more affordable and funds are available for supply of vaccine on a routine basis. Delivery of the vaccine can be facilitated, substantially, by adjusting schedules to fit into the existing regimens for immunization against the other EPI vaccines. Additionally, immunization will be greatly facilitated by developing polyvalent formulations in which the hepatitis B vaccine is combined with DTP, inactivated poliovirus vaccine, and possible other immunogens. This is all difficult but doable in the long term.

V.   POSTSCRIPT

As stated above, the plasma-derived vaccine, though still manufactured in some countries, became obsolete with the introduction of the yeast recombinant vaccine in 1986 (38,39). During the latter time period, however, additional studies have been made that are pertinent to hepatitis B vaccine, irrespective of how it is manufactured. Some of these developments will be reviewed briefly here.

A.   Duration of Immunity

Concern is now being expressed as to how long immunity will last following vaccination and whether there is a need for a late booster dose of vaccine at present or in the future (see also Chapter 17). One view calls for surveillance of antibody levels in vaccinated persons and reimmunization at a calculated time period or when the measured level of antibody decreases to a prescribed low level. A second view is that immunity does not depend upon detectable circulating antibody, but, rather, upon a retained capability for lymphocytes to give an immediate anamnestic response upon encounter with the virus. The latter judgment accords with the majority view and with current WHO and U.S. Public Health Service policy not to pursue routine reimmunization. However, there can be no harm from reimmunization for those persons whose resources permit reimmunization.

The lack of need, at this time, for reimmunization is supported by the best available knowledge of the function of the immune system (Fig. 10) in retaining capability for specific immunological memory. Two primary doses of vaccine given a month apart elicit an initial IgM response that quickly switches to IgG. After a few months, the antibody reaches a low level, at which time a third or booster dose of vaccine is given, which results in very rapid antibody response to a very high level. The antibody then falls again to a low level or entirely disappears after 5–7 years. At this time, a late booster dose of vaccine or experience with the virus itself quickly sends the antibody soaring to very high levels in a highly effective anamnestic response. Persons exposed to virus at this time show no disease and do not develop a carrier state, though a few may experience very transient infection with antigenemia of short duration plus development of antibody against the core antigen of the virus that is not present in the vaccine. They are protected from clinical disease and from becoming carriers.

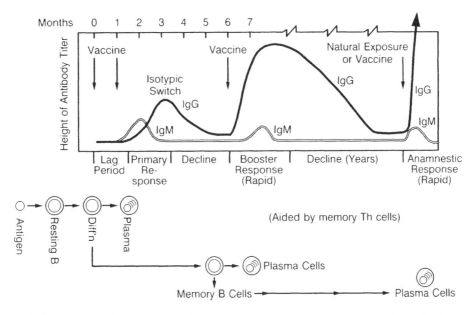

Figure 10 Primary, anamnestic, and memory responses of B cells producing antibodies.

Understanding the durability of protection may be facilitated by review of the memory cell system (see Fig. 10). Resting B lymphocytes that respond to HBsAg rapidly differentiate to antibody-producing plasma cells upon contact with antigen. The plasma cells are terminally differentiated, have a finite life span, and die. As presently conceived, the immune system retains a number of partially differentiated lymphocytes, called memory cells, that are long-lived and are available for rapid recall and for producing antibody when needed. These consist both of specific B-memory cells and specific T-helper cells. On each experience with antigen or virus, the memory cell pools are called upon to respond immunologically, and with each cessation, new banks of memory cells are retained. Thus, immunity is memory! When a late booster dose of vaccine will be needed, if ever, remains to be determined by future experience.

Alternative concepts for retention of immunological memory are based on retention of antigen in the immune system, persistence of vaccine virus in subclinical infection, and repeat immune stimulation on experience in nature. These latter theories, in this author's judgment, are lacking in substance. Killed antigens cannot induce persistent infection, and long-term immunity exists even in persons geographically isolated from natural exposure. Just how and where unprocessed or processed antigen would be stored and passed on to succeeding generations of B and T lymphocytes has not been established.

B. Improving the Immune Response

Considerable attention has been and is being paid to increasing the immune response to hepatitis B vaccine, especially in genetic nonresponders, in the immunocompromised such as renal dialysis patients, and in the elderly.

One concept being explored is that of inclusion of polypeptides of the Pre-S1 and Pre-S2 regions in the vaccine with the idea that these might increase the epitope repertoire, especially for T-helper epitopes (discussed in Chapter 20). It is known that the Pre-S2 polypeptide binds to albumin and includes an epitope that induces neutralizing antibody, though of short-term retention. Pre-S1 sequences include the ligand that binds the virus to receptors on liver cells. Various approaches to utilization of Pre-S antigens include the preparation of vaccines that contain whole sequences or selected epitopes from the Pre-S1 and Pre-S2 regions. Though unsuccessful in the past, recent studies reported at the 1990 International Symposium on Viral Hepatitis and Liver Disease (47) suggest that there may be promise in this approach.

The findings of Meuer et al. (48) are of considerable importance in attempts to understand the failure of immune responses in uremic hemodialysis patients. Meuer and colleagues postulated a defect in the antigen-presenting cells of the macrophage/monocyte series (possibly resulting in failure of release of interleukin-1 or other lymphokines). Meuer et al. were able to circumvent the defect and to obtain normal antibody responses in such immunodeficient patients by immediate second dosing at the injection site with T-helper lymphokine, IL-2.

The route of vaccine administration may also be of considerable importance in influencing the immune response. In the early period, persons with kidney failure who are being dialyzed commonly show far less antibody than do normal individuals. This may be expected, since such persons are often immunodeficient. Findings showed, however, that the poor antibody response was exaggerated by the fact that such individuals were commonly vaccinated into the buttocks rather than into the deltoid muscle. Injection into the buttocks commonly results in deposition of the vaccine into fat rather than into muscle, resulting in poor antigen distribution to the immune system. Response in such individuals was greatly improved by injection of vaccine into the muscles of the arm.

C.   Hepatitis B Escape Mutant, a New Serotype

Hepatitis B virus is a double-stranded DNA virus with the ability to proofread its genetic replication to maintain its genetic integrity. However, it passes through a RNA stage in its replication in which error-prone replication may occur. Even though there has been but a single immunological serotype of HBV, it was very surprising and potentially alarming when Carman and coworkers (49) uncovered a second serotype of HBV that is not protected against by the hepatitis B vaccine. This variant was first detected in southern Italy and may be moving outside its focal area. Investigation of the basis for immunological change revealed (Fig. 11) a single-point mutation from guanosine to adenosine at nucleotide position 587, resulting in an amino acid substitution from glycine to arginine in the second *a* antigen loop. The mutation is stable. It is far too early to assess the practical importance of this observation, but it must be borne in mind that a second serotype S antigen might need, eventually, to be included in hepatitis B vaccine (discussed in Chapter 18).

VI.   SUMMARY

It is worthy of note that the 21 years since work on hepatitis B vaccine was first initiated has seen the development of two effective vaccines against HBV infection with excellent safety profiles. The first-generation plasma-derived hepatitis B vaccine represented the first subunit viral vaccine of any kind and has provided the world standard for all future HBV vaccines. The second-generation recombinant DNA hepatitis B vaccine represents the first vaccine produced by recombinant technology and has provided the technological approach and basis for all future recombinant-produced vaccines. Though fine-tuning to effect improvement in the recombinant vaccine is being pursued, this

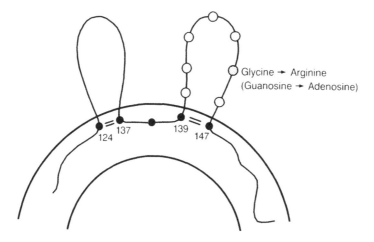

Figure 11 Hepatitis B escape mutant, a new serotype. (From Ref. 49.)

vaccine already provides feasibility and practicality in vaccine manufacture whereby the worldwide eradication program for hepatitis B can be achieved. The immediate important objective must be to implement the worldwide immunization program whereby hepatitis B elimination and eventual eradication will be brought about. The Expanded Program for Immunization of the World Health Organization has added hepatitis B to its battery of vaccines and is giving initial focus to vaccination of newborn infants, especially those born to hepatitis B carrier mothers.

Since the technology for preventing hepatitis B now exists, a major technical focus for future research ought to be given to the development of means for treatment and cure of the very large world population of carriers who are at high risk to death from cirrhosis and liver cancer.

REFERENCES

1. E. B. Buynak, R. R. Roehm, A. A. Tytell, A. U. Bertland, G. P. Lampson, and M. R. Hilleman, Development and chimpanzee testing of a vaccine against human hepatitis B, *Proc. Soc. Exper. Biol. Med.*, *151*: 694 (1976).
2. E. B. Buynak, R. R. Roehm, A. A. Tytell, A. U. Bertland, G. P. Lampson, and M. R. Hilleman. Vaccine against human hepatitis B, *J. Am. Med. Assoc.*, *235*: 2832 (1976).
3. M. R. Hilleman, A. U. Bertland, E. B. Buynak, G. P. Lampson, W. J. McAleer, A. A. McLean, R. R. Roehm, and A. A. Tytell, Clinical and laboratory studies of HBsAg vaccine, *Viral Hepatitis* (G. N. Vyas, S. N. Cohen, and R. Schmid, eds.), Franklin Institute Press, Philadelphia, p. 525 (1978).

4. M. R. Hilleman, New developments with new vaccines, *New Developments with Human and Veterinary Vaccines*, Progress in Clinical and Biological Research Series (A. Mizrahi, I. Hertman, M. A. Klingberg, and A. Kohn, eds.), Alan R. Liss, New York, Vol. 47, p. 21 (1980).

5. M. R. Hilleman, E. B. Buynak, W. J. McAleer, A. A. McLean, P. J. Provost, and A. A. Tytell, Hepatitis A and hepatitis B vaccines, *Viral Hepatitis. 1981 International Symposium* (W. Szmuness, H. Alter, and J. Maynard, eds.), Franklin Institute Press, Philadelphia, p. 385 (1981).

6. M. R. Hilleman, E. B. Buynak, W. J. McAleer, A. A. McLean, P. J. Provost, and A. A. Tytell, Newer developments with human hepatitis vaccines, *Perspect. Virol.*, *XI*:219 (1981).

7. M. R. Hilleman, W. J. McAleer, E. B. Buynak, and A. A. McLean, The preparation and safety of hepatitis B vaccine, *J. Infect.*, *7*(S1): 3 (1983).

8. M. R. Hilleman, W. J. McAleer, E. B. Buynak, and A. A. McLean, Quality and safety of human hepatitis B vaccine, *Develop. Biol. Standard*, *54*: 3 (1983).

9. M. R. Hilleman, Immunologic prevention of human hepatitis, *Perspect. Biol. Med.*, *27*: 543 (1984).

10. M. R. Hilleman, W. J. McAleer, E. B. Buynak, A. A. McLean, P. J. Provost, and D. E. Wampler. Future vaccines against hepatitis, *Viral Hepatitis B Infection* (S. K. Lam, C. L. Lai, and E. K. Yeoh, eds.), World Scientific Publ. Co., Singapore, p. 237 (1984).

11. M. R. Hilleman, E. B. Buynak, W. J. McAleer, and A. A. McLean, Preparation and testing of human hepatitis B virus vaccine, *Viral Hepatitis B Infection* (S. K. Lam, C. L. Lai, and E. K. Yeoh, eds.), World Scientific Publ. Co., Singapore, p. 131 (1984).

12. M. R. Hilleman, Vaccines against viral hepatitis, *Intl. Rev. Army, Navy Air Force Med. Serv.*, *57*: 11 (1984).

13. F. B. Hollinger, Hepatitis B virus, *Virology*, 2nd ed. (B. N. Fields, D. M. Knipe, et al., eds.), Raven Press, New York, Ch. 77, p. 2171 (1990).

14. S. Krugman, Hepatitis B vaccine, *Vaccines* (S. A. Plotkin and E. A. Mortimer, Jr., eds.), W. B. Saunders, Philadelphia, Ch. 21, p. 458 (1988).

15. A. J. Zuckerman, ed., *Viral Hepatitis and Liver Disease*, Alan R. Liss, New York (1988).

16. J. F. Enders, T. H. Weller, and F. C. Robbins, Cultivation of the Lansing strain of poliomyelitis in virus cultures of various human embryonic tissues, *Science*, *109*: 85 (1949).

17. A Lurman, Eine Icterusepidemie, *Berl. Klin. Wochenschr.*, *22*: 20 (1885).

18. F. O. MacCallum, Homologous serum jaundice, *Lancet*, *2*: 691 (1947).

19. S. Krugman, J. P. Giles, and J. Hammond, Infectious hepatitis: Evidence for two distinctive clinical, epidemiological and immunological types of infection, *J. Am. Med. Assoc.*, *200*: 365 (1967).

20. B. S. Blumberg, Australia antigen and the biology of hepatitis B, *Science*, *197*: 17 (1977).

21. A. M. Prince, An antigen detected in the blood during the incubation period of serum hepatitis, *Proc. Natl. Acad. Sci. USA*, *60*: 814 (1968).

22. D. S. Dane, C. H. Cameron, and M. Briggs, Virus-like particles in serum of patients with Australia-antigen-associated hepatitis, *Lancet*, *1*: 695 (1970).

23. S. Krugman, L. R. Overby, I. K. Mushahwar, C-M. Ling, G. G. Frosner, and F. Deinhardt, Viral hepatitis, type b. Studies on natural history and prevention reexamined, *N. Engl. J. Med.*, *300*: 101 (1979).

24. G. D. Hunter, R. A. Gibbons, R. H. Kimberlin, and G. C. Millson, Further studies of the infectivity and stability of extracts and homogenates derived from scrapie affected mouse brains, *J. Comp. Path.*, *79*: 101 (1969).

25. Centers for Disease Control, Hepatitis B vaccine: Evidence confirming lack of AIDS transmission, *M.M.W.R.*, *33*: 685 (1984).

26. L. F. Barker et al., Transmission of serum hepatitis, *J. Am. Med. Assoc.*, *211*: 1509 (1970).

27. E. Tabor, E. Buynak, L. A. Smallwood, P. Snoy, M. Hilleman, and R. J. Gerety, Inactivation of hepatitis B virus by three methods: Treatment with pepsin, urea, or formalin, *J. Med. Virol.*, *11*: 1 (1983).

28. V. J. McAuliffe et al., Type B hepatitis: A review of current prospects for a safe and effective vaccine, *Rev. Infect. Dis.*, *2*: 470 (1980).

29. B. L. Murphy et al., Viral subtypes and cross-protection in hepatitis B virus infections of chimpanzees, *Intervirology*, *3*: 378 (1974).

30. Centers for Disease Control, Leads from the M.M.W.R. Recommendations of the Immunization Practices Advisory Committee update on hepatitis B prevention, *J. Am. Med. Assoc.*, *258*: 437 (1987).

31. S. Krugman and M. Davidson, Hepatitis B vaccine: Prospects for duration of immunity, *Yale J. Biol. Med.*, *60*: 333 (1987).

32. W. J. McAleer, H. Z. Markus, D. E. Wampler, E. B. Buynak, W. J. Miller, R. E. Weibel, A. A. McLean, and M. R. Hilleman, Vaccine against human hepatitis B virus prepared from antigen derived from human hepatoma cells in culture, *Proc. Soc. Exp. Biol. Med.*, *175*: 314 (1984).

33. J. Alexander, G. Macnab, and R. Saunders, Studies on *in vitro* production of hepatitis B surface antigen by a human hepatoma cell line, *Perspectives in Virology* (M. Pollard, ed.), Raven Press, New York, p. 103 (1978).

34. M. R. Hilleman, Line cell saga—An argument in favor of production of biologics in cancer cells, *Cell Substrates* (J. C. Petricciani, H. E. Hopps, and P. J. Chapple, eds.), Plenum Publishing, New York, p. 47 (1979).

35. M. R. Hilleman, History, precedent, and progress in the development of mammalian cell culture systems for preparing vaccines: Safety considerations revisited, *J. Med. Virol.*, *31*: 5 (1990).

36. WHO Study Group Report: Acceptability of Cell Substrates for Production of Biologicals. Technical Report Series 747. World Health Organization, Geneva (1987).

37. A. J. Zuckerman and F. Deinhardt, Vaccines, cells and nucleic acids, *Bull. W.H.O.*, *68*: 139 (1990).

38. W. J. McAleer, E. B. Buynak, R. Z. Maigetter, D. E. Wampler, W. J. Miller, and M. R. Hilleman, Human hepatitis B vaccine from recombinant yeast, *Nature*, *307*: 178 (1984).

39. M. R. Hilleman, Yeast recombinant hepatitis B vaccine, *Infection*, *15*: 3 (1987).

40. W. Szmuness, C. E. Stevens, E. A. Zang, E. J. Harley, and A. Kellner, A controlled clinical trial of the efficacy of the hepatitis B vaccine (Heptavax B): A final report, *Hepatology*, *1*: 377 (1981).

41.   D. P. Francis, S. C. Hadler, S. E. Thompson, et al., The prevention of hepatitis B with vaccine: Report of the Centers for Disease Control multi-center efficacy trial among homosexual men, *Ann. Int. Med.*, *97*: 362 (1982).

42.   F. B. Hollinger and the North American Regional Study Group, Controlling hepatitis B virus transmission in North America, *Vaccine*, *8* (S): S122 (1990).

43.   Centers for Disease Control, Protection against viral hepatitis. Recommendations of the Immunization Practices Advisory Committee (ACIP), *M.M.W.R.*, *39* (RR-2): 1 (1990).

44.   Y. Ghendon, WHO strategy for the global elimination of new cases of hepatitis B, *Vaccine*, *8* S: S129 (1990).

45.   J. E. Maynard, Hepatitis B: Global importance and need for control, *Vaccine*, *8* (S): S18 (1990).

46.   J. E. Maynard, M. A. Kane, and S. C. Hadler, Global control of hepatitis B through vaccination: Role of hepatitis B vaccine in the Expanded Programme on Immunization, *Rev. Infect. Dis. 11* (S3): S574 (1989).

47.   Miscellaneous abstracts. Scientific Program and Abstract Volume, The 1990 International Symposium on Viral Hepatitis and Liver Disease, April 4–8, 1990, Houston, Texas, pp. 116–119.

48.   S. C. Meuer, H. Dumann, K. H. Meyer zum Buschenfelde, and H. Kohler, Low dose interleukin-2 induces systemic immune responses against HBsAg in immunodeficient non-responders to hepatitis B vaccine, *Lancet*, *1*: 15 (1989).

49.   W. F. Carman, A. R. Zanetti, P. Karayiannis, J. Waters, G. Manzillo, E. Tanzi, A. J. Suchkerman, and H. C. Thomas, Vaccine-induced escape mutant of hepatitis B virus, *Lancet*, *2*: 325 (1990).

3

Functions of Hepatitis B Virus Proteins and Molecular Targets for Protective Immunity

Wolfram H. Gerlich

Justus Liebig University, Giessen, Germany

Volker Bruss

Goettingen University, Goettingen, Germany

I. INTRODUCTION

The medical term "immunity" is classically used to define a state in which a host organism will not develop disease after repeated encounters with a defined pathogenic agent. This acquired property is brought about by the cells of the immune system and their products. Today, all induced activities of the immune system are considered to be immune reactions, whether these reactions mediate protection or not. In fact, many immune reactions are more detrimental to the host than they are beneficial, and often protection cannot be separated from pathogenic events. Hepatitis B virus is one of those agents that is pathogenic mostly, though not exclusively, due to the immune response of the host. One of the major goals in modern vaccine development is to separate those immune reactions that are more pathogenic from those that are more protective.

The immune system detects proteins of a virus in two principal ways: (a) the B lymphocytes recognize directly structures that are accessible on the surface of virus proteins or virus particles (B-cell epitopes) by their membrane-bound immunoglobulin receptor; (b) T cells recognize proteolytic fragments of the virus proteins which have been generated by host cells during virus infection (T-cell epitopes). These virus-derived peptides are trapped within grooves of the proteins of the major histocompatibility complex (MHC; or human leukocyte antigen, HLA) and are then transported to the cell surface where they are presented to T lymphocytes. Cytotoxic or suppressor CD8-positive T-cells recognize such peptide antigens preferentially when they are presented by class I MHC proteins, which are found on most cell types. Helper CD4-positive T cells recognize peptides that are presented by class II MHC molecules, most commonly found on the cells of the immune system itself. Class II molecules predominantly entrap peptides that have been generated by the antigen-presenting cell after endocytosis of the foreign protein (for a brief review, see Ref. 1). Given this complex mechanism of immune recognition, it would be inappropriate to restrict this chapter to the B-cell epitopes of hepatitis B surface antigen. Due to endocytosis of antigens and presentation of internal peptides, virtually all protein sequences encoded by an infectious agent can theoretically be targets of immune reactions.

Antibody-dependent immunity requires the exposure of the corresponding B-cell epitopes on the surface of viral particles or virus-infected cells. However, development of this immunity usually also depends on internal amino acid sequences of the same particle, since the induction of B-cell immunity requires (with certain exceptions) T-helper cells, which, in an MHC-dependent manner, preferentially recognize internal structures. If a cell surface molecule is the target of a cytotoxic immune reaction (either a virus protein in the case of antibody-dependent cytotoxicity or an MHC-presented viral peptide in case of cytotoxic T cells), protection against further viral activity and cell death cannot be separated.

In natural infections by noncytopathogenic agents like hepatitis B virus (HBV), both B- and T-cell immunity are equally required to eliminate the agents. Infectivity-neutralizing antibodies would prevent the agent from spreading to not yet infected target cells, but they could not stop the already infected cells from persistently producing new infectious progeny virus. Finally, detrimental immune complexes would accumulate in the host organism as in the case of HBV-associated immune complex diseases such as periarteriitis nodosa or glomerulonephritis. Cellular immunity alone might kill the infected cells but could not neutralize the infectious agent, which would in fact even be liberated by cell lysis in addition to normal export. Continuous new infection and damage of cells would result, as is the case in chronic hepatitis B.

Current vaccination strategies against hepatitis B are based upon the observation that the presence of actively produced antibodies against one of the three surface proteins of HBV ("anti-HBs") indicates immunity against a challenge with infectious HBV. Passive administration of anti-HBs also confers a certain degree of transient immunity—in the classical sense—to the recipient. However, evidence is accumulating that protection by active immunization with the small surface protein of HBV is mediated not only by humoral but possibly also by cellular immunity. Moreover, certain failures of passive and active immunization have been reported in spite of significant anti-HBs levels in the vaccinated person. To facilitate the discussion of perspectives for further development of hepatitis B vaccines, a brief description of all the known viral proteins and their functions shall be given in this chapter. From the occurrence and function of these proteins, their potential suitability as candidates for a vaccine component shall be deduced at the end of the chapter. For a detailed discussion of B- and T-cell epitopes and peptide vaccines, see Chapter 19. A thorough description of the molecular biology of HBV is given in two recent monographs (2,3).

II. STRUCTURAL COMPONENTS OF HBV

A. HBV and HBs particles

During the late 1960s it was recognized that sera with high titers of infectious HBV contained an antigen (4), originally named Australia antigen (5). This antigen is found on three types of particles: on pleomorphic spheres of approximately 20 nm diameter, on filaments of variable length and approximately 20 nm diameter, and on spherical double-shelled particles of approximately 42 nm diameter (Fig. 1A). The latter particles are often referred to as Dane particles after their discoverer (6). The inner protein shell of the Dane particle is called the core particle (7). Only this particle contains nucleic acid (8). The core particle is the capsid of HBV, which is highly immunogenic. The corresponding antigen is named hepatitis B core antigen (HBcAg); its antibody is anti-HBc. The antigen present on the outer protein shell of the Dane particle is referred to as hepatitis B surface antigen (HBsAg); its antibody is called anti-HBs. (Some authors prefer the terminology envelope protein or "env" instead of HBs as it is used for most enveloped viruses.) We suggest use of the designation HBc or HBs *protein* instead of *antigen* unless the antigenic properties of these proteins are specifically addressed.

B. HBs Proteins

Early studies on the structure of the HBs proteins were mainly done with the 20-nm HBs spheres, assuming that the surface structure of the Dane particle would be identical. The first results of denaturing polyacrylamide gel electrophoresis from different laboratories were quite divergent. Some authors described as many as 11 bands in purified HBs spheres, others only two. As a constant feature two major protein bands were found which had an apparent molecular weight of 22–26 and 25–30 kilodaltons (kD). Peterson (9) showed that the larger protein was the N-glycosylated version of the unglycosylated smaller protein. As shown in Figure 1B, we refer to these proteins as P24 and GP27 (P for protein, GP for glycoprotein, the number gives the apparent molecular weight in kilodaltons).

The amino- and carboxy-terminal sequences of P24 and GP27 were elucidated by classical protein analysis (10). Soon after the HBV genome was cloned, its complete DNA sequence was determined. Four open reading frames (ORF)

Hepatitis B Virus (Dane Particles)   Filaments   20nm Particles

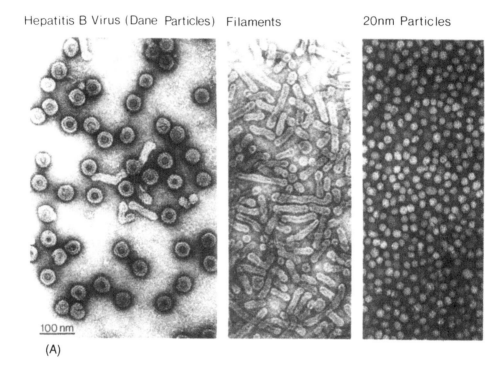

(A)

Figure 1 Particles and proteins associated with hepatitis B virus. (A) HBs particles were isolated from the plasma of a typical chronic HBV carrier with high viremia. Twenty-nm particles were separated from the larger HBs particles by size chromatography and purified further by isopycnic cesium chloride centrifugation. Dane particles and filaments were separated by sucrose density gradient centrifugation. The particles were stained with uranylacetate for electron microscopy. The approximate ratios of Dane particles:filaments:20-nm particles was 1:10:10 000.

encoding proteins larger than 50 amino acids were identified (Fig. 2A). One of these ORFs was found to code for the sequences of P24/GP27 at its 3' end. From these data the complete amino acid sequence of P24 could be deduced (11). P24 is a protein made up of 226 amino acids and unusually rich in cysteins, tryptophans, and hydrophobic amino acids. Many authors consider P24 and its derivative GP27 as *the* HBsAg or HBs proteins. However, this view does not agree with the original definition of HBsAg as the entity of all antigenic components on the viral surface.

A more refined analysis of HB virion proteins showed, in addition to P24 and GP27, at least four more bands that come from the virion surface: GP33, GP36, P39, and GP42 (12) (Fig. 1B). A combination of biochemical and genetic methods allowed elucidation of their amino acid sequence. The analysis of the ORFs in the HBV DNA sequence showed that P24 occupies only the last 226 of

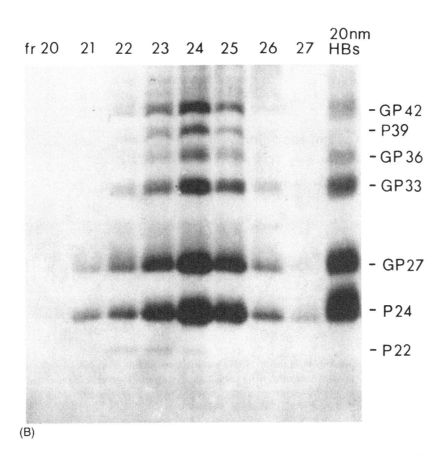

(B)

Figure 1   (B) Proteins of purified HBs particles were denatured by SDS/dithiothreitol, separated by polyacrylamide gel electrophoresis, and stained with silver as described by Heermann et al. (12). The different lanes show the fractions of the density gradient that were used for partial separation of Dane particles from filaments. Fraction 22 was used for the staining of Dane particles in part A, fraction 24 for staining of filaments. The HBs proteins are more intensely stained by silver than the core protein (P22).

389 or 400 codons in its ORF (13, 14). Initially, the function of the upstream sequence was unknown. It was named preS because it was upstream of the gene for P24/GP27 (gene S) (15). There were two or three additional start codons for protein synthesis upstream. It turned out that the sequence of the middle-sized proteins GP33 and GP36 started 55 amino acids upstream of the start of P24/GP27 in the preS sequence (16). The sequence of the largest HBs proteins P39/GP42 covers the entire ORF S (12). We suggest the use of the widely accepted terms small (SHBs), middle (MHBs), and large (LHBs) hepatitis B surface proteins, and not the term preS *proteins* because this suggests a nonexis-

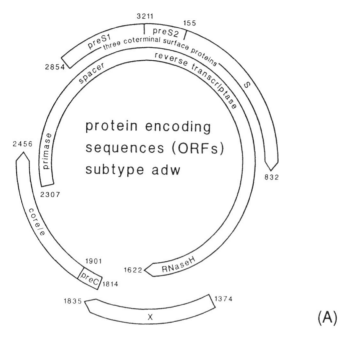

(A)

Figure 2 Genome organization of HBV, transcription pattern of covalently closed HBV DNA, and physical structure of virion DNA. (A) The four open reading frames (ORFs) of the circular HBV genome encode four protein sequences, which start with a AUG codon for initiation of protein synthesis and end with a stop codon. The core/e ORF encodes HBe protein if translation starts at the first AUG upstream of the preC sequence, or the core protein if translation starts at the second AUG at the end of the preC sequence (for details see text). Similarly, the ORF S encodes three coterminal proteins as outlined in Figure 3. The numbers indicate the base position of the starts and stops of the ORFs for a typical HBV genome of subtype adw (H. G. Köchel, EMBL Data Library number X 51970). (B) In the nucleus of infected hepatocytes, the virion DNA is converted to a covalently closed circle. The start sites for transcription of the mRNAs encoding the various HBV proteins are shown as triangles. Black triangles show mRNAs that are transcribed efficiently only in liver cells, while open triangles show mRNAs that are transcribed ubiquitously in animal cells. All mRNAs are 3' coterminal because transcription stops only at the TATAAA signal. The mRNAs for HBe and HBc protein run through this transcription stop signal at the first pass, thus presenting more than genome-length molecules with a terminal redundancy R. Transcription activity is not only governed by signals upstream of the start sites (i.e., promoters) but also by the enhancer sequences and the glucocorticoid-responsive elements (GRE). The mRNA for the HBc protein also allows for translation of the polymerase protein by internal initiation. This mRNA also carries a signal for reverse transcription (SRT), which is recognized by the polymerase. (C) In the virion, the HBV genome is present as an unusual composite molecule of DNA, RNA, and protein. The (–) strand has a constant length of 3221 bases in the case of HBV

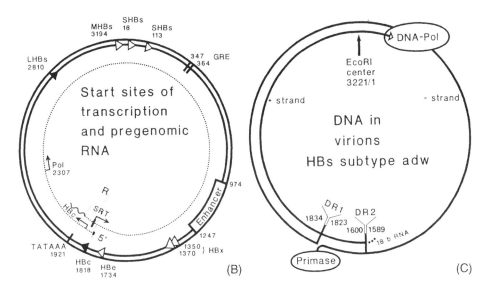

Figure 2 *(continued)* adw, a covalently bound protein at the 5' end named terminal protein (TP) or primase. The (+) strand has an 18-base RNA primer at its 5' end. Its 3' end is variable and noncovalently linked with the HBV polymerase. The circular structure comes from the cohesive overlaps of the two strands between bases 1589 and 1834. Two direct repeats DR1 and DR2 of 11 bases are at the ends of the cohesive region. The cleavage site of restriction endonuclease Eco RI was taken arbitrarily as number 1 (or 3221), as suggested by Galibert et al. (13). The complicated structure of HBV DNA is generated by its mode of replication, as outlined in Figure 9.

tent precursor function of the L and M protein for the S protein. The term preS1 should be reserved for the domain only present in the LHBs protein, and preS2 only for the next domain present in LHBs and forming the amino-terminal end of the MHBs protein. Only the S domain is present in all three HBs proteins. The domain structure and the glycosylation pattern of the three HBs proteins are shown in Figure 3. It is noteworthy that asparagine 146 of the S domain is in part glycosylated in all three HBs proteins, and that the asparagine 4 of the preS2 domain is completely glycosylated in the M protein but not at all in the L protein. The other three potential N-glycosylation sites in the ORF S are not used (12).

C.   Proteins of the Virion

The relative proportion of the HBs proteins is not the same in virions, filaments, and spheres. All three particle types contain the SHBs proteins as the major component and M proteins as minor components. However, the L protein is most abundant in virions, still present in moderate amounts in filaments, but a very

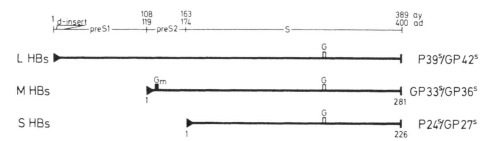

Figure 3   Organization of the ORF-S that encodes the three HBs proteins. The adw subtypes of HBV genomes carry a 11-codon insertion with a 5'-terminal AUG codon, which is missing (or deleted) in ayw subtypes. Thus, the ORF has a different length for the two subtypes. Gm: Triantennary N-linked glycan of the hybrid type with one mannose antenna. G: Biantennary N-linked glycan of the complex-type present in half of the HBs molecules.

minor component in spheres. The relative composition varies between different isolates, but the order is always S > L > M in virions and filaments and S > M > L in spheres (12). Some authors refer to SHBs protein as major HBs protein. However, L protein is not a minor component in virions and filaments. On the other hand, virions and filaments are indeed minor species compared to HBs spheres in the blood.

A model of the virion structure is shown in Figure 4. The virion contains, in addition to the three above-mentioned HBs proteins, one kind of core protein P22 (12), its DNA genome (8), a DNA polymerase, which is also a reverse transcriptase/RNase H (RT) (17), and a terminal protein (TP) linked to the 5' end of the protein-coding DNA-strand (18). The latter two proteins are derived from the polymerase ORF (19, 20). The proteolytic processing of the polymerase polyprotein into its functional products has not yet been elucidated, but in Fig. 4 it is assumed that the RT and TP are separated. Furthermore, a protein kinase is present within the capsid, which phosphorylates the core protein (21). The nature of this serine kinase (22) is not yet definitely known, but it is probably host encoded. It has been proposed that the viral HBx protein has a serine/threonine kinase activity and that it is also a structural component of virions (23). However, these data have not yet been confirmed by other groups.

Natural liver-derived virions that circulate in the blood of infected individuals contain at least one host protein bound to their surface: human serum albumin (HSA) (24). Furthermore, epitopes of the viral surface, mainly the preS1 antigen, are often covered by immunoglobulins (25) once the immune system has started antibody production. Due to the difficulty in isolating natural HBV particles in sufficient amounts and purity, it cannot be excluded that they contain further protein components.

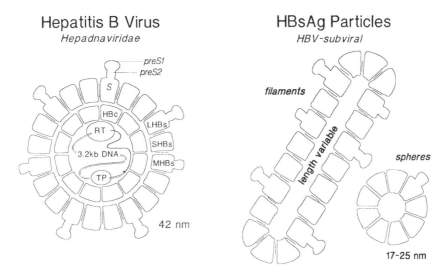

Figure 4 Model of the hepatitis B virus particle, HBs filaments, and HBs 20-nm spheres. RT: Reverse transcriptase; TP: terminal protein.

III. BIOSYNTHESIS AND TOPOLOGY OF HBsAg

As mentioned above, a prerequisite for a B-cell epitope is its exposure on the outside of the antigen. To rationalize which parts of the HBs proteins are external, we shall have a closer look at the biosynthesis and morphogenesis of HBs particles and the viral envelope.

A. ER Translocation Signals and Topogenesis

HBs proteins are initially synthesized as transmembrane proteins at the endoplasmic reticulum (ER) membrane. To study this process, the gene encoding the protein of interest was inserted downstream of a phage promoter (e.g., from the SP6 phage) on a plasmid. An RNA copy of the gene was then synthesized in vitro by addition of phage SP6 RNA polymerase to this plasmid. This RNA was used as mRNA to program protein synthesis in a cell extract, which is often prepared from reticulocytes because these cells contain relatively little endogenous mRNA. Newly synthesized proteins were labeled, e.g., by ^{35}S-methionine, and visualized after polyacrylamide gel electrophoresis by autoradiography. The translocation process at ER membranes can be studied in such a system by adding vesicle preparations of such membranes (usually isolated from dog pancreatic tissue). Parameters indicating the translocation of a protein are (a) the cleavage of signal peptides by the ER luminal signal peptidase resulting in a mobility shift on the gel, (b) the glycosylation of proteins, which is also catalyzed by ER luminal enzymes, or (c) the resistance of protein domains to exogenously added proteases due to protection by the ER membrane.

Experiments of this kind showed that the transmembrane topology of MHBs and SHBs proteins is generated by the effect of at least two translocation signals in the S chain. Signal I comprises the hydrophobic sequence 8–22 of SHBs. It directs the N-terminus of the protein into the lumen of the ER, which is topologically equivalent to the outside of HBs particles or virions (26). The 55-amino-acid preS2 domain of the MHBs protein, which does not contain topogenic signals, is translocated into the ER lumen by the action of the downstream signal I in its S domain. This was an exceptional finding, because usually sequences upstream of translocation signals like signal I are much shorter (27). The second signal around the hydrophobic sequence 80–98 in the S domain anchors the protein into the ER membrane and causes downstream sequences to enter the ER lumen and upstream sequences to remain in the cytoplasm (28). The combination of these two signals generates a complex topology of the S and MHBs proteins traversing the ER membrane at least twice with a cytoplasmic loop between residues 24 and 79 of the S domain and a luminal domain containing the hydrophilic sequence 120–160, which forms the major B-cell epitope of SHBs. It is unclear whether the hydrophobic C-terminus of SHBs downstream of amino acid 170 contains further signal sequences for the interaction of the protein chain with the ER membrane, but it is probably inserted in the lipid bilayer. A mutant SHBs protein without the hydrophobic C-terminal domain is no longer able to form 20-nm HBsAg particles. However, when this mutant is coexpressed with wild-type SHBs, it becomes a component of mixed 20-nm HBsAg particles (29). Circular dichroism spectra of purified HBs particles suggested that a large proportion of the SHBs protein has an alpha-helical conformation (30). It appears likely that the membrane-associated carboxy-terminal sequence has the conformation shown in Figures 5 and 6. The models of SHBs and MHBs proteins shown in these figures predict that the preS2 domain and the hydrophilic region between amino acids 120 and 160 are exposed at the surface of HBs particles. Reactivity of these sites with specific antibodies, enzymes, or surface-specific chemical reagents confirm this prediction (31).

B. The Topology of the LHBs Protein

The topology of the LHBs protein in the ER membrane is less clear. Its glycosylation site at asn 146 in the S domain is used in more than half the molecules (12). Since glycosylation is catalyzed by enzymes at the inner side of the ER membrane, it is apparent that this region of the protein resides in the ER lumen and is probably translocated by the action of signal II. While signal I is capable of translocating the 55-amino-acid sequence upstream of the S domain in the case of the MHBs protein, it is doubtful whether this signal can act in a

S-Epitopes

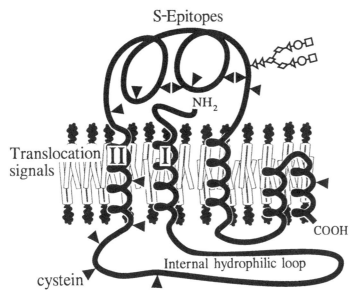

Figure 5 Topological model of SHBs at the membrane of the endoplasmic reticulum (ER). The cytoplasmic side is at the bottom, the luminal side on top. The structure at top right shows the biantennary complex glycan at Asn 146. The roman numerals designate the two topological signals for membrane insertion.

similar way on the 174-amino-acid preS region of LHBs (P. Ostapchuk and D. Ganem, personal communication). So far no translocation signals have been identified in the preS1 domain. The fact that Asn 4 in the preS2 domain of LHBs is not glycosylated, whereas this site is always glycosylated in MHBs protein, may be explained by a model where this sequence of LHBs is not translocated into the ER lumen. However, amino acids 31–34 of preS1 forming the epitope of monoclonal antibody MA 18/7 (Pumpen et al., in preparation) are accessible on the viral surface, and Arg 100 (in subtype *ay*) is sensitive to trypsin cleavage (32). Therefore, these sequences are assumed to be surface-oriented, as shown in Figure 7. Only the amino-terminal myristic acid (33) is assumed to be part of the lipid layer. Possibly the translocation of the preS domain does not occur cotranslationally but at a later step during virus maturation.

The current model of HBsAg morphogenesis assumes that during and after synthesis the transmembrane HBs proteins mature by formation of intramolecular disulfide bridges, oligomerization, and appearance of intermolecular S-S bridges. This process is characterized by a progressively developing protease

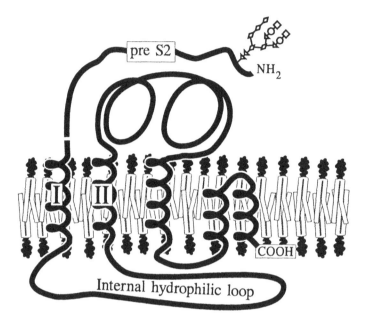

Figure 6 Topological model of MHBs. The S domain of MHBs is assumed to be slightly rearranged in comparison to SHBs, with its NH₂ terminus being more exposed. The sequence of preS2 is assumed to cover most of the SHBs epitopes. The triantennary glycan of preS2 is shown at top right.

resistance of the in vitro synthesized transmembrane proteins (34). Following these steps, the HBs proteins are released from the ER membrane with the inclusion of membrane lipid, forming either 20-nm spheres or virions by enveloping a core particle during a budding process. By this process cytoplasmic domains become internal parts of the HBs particles and luminal domains become exposed to the surface.

C.   HBs Particle Secretion

The SHBs (35) and MHBs (36) proteins are able to form 20-nm spheres without participation of other viral proteins. The LHBs protein is not secreted from cells by itself. Rather, the secretion of SHBs and MHBs is inhibited when the proportion of LHBs protein is too high (37–40). Both the myristylation and retention signal(s) in the preS1 sequence contribute to the secretion inhibition. The HBV subtypes with an 11-amino-acid deletion at the start of preS1 (corre-

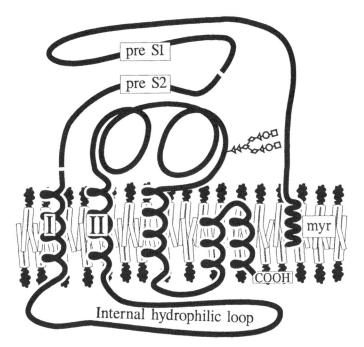

Figure 7 Topological model of LHBs. The S and preS2 domains are assumed to be similar as in MHBs, but the preS2 domain is not glycosylated and covered partially by the preS1 domain. The NH$_2$-terminus of LHBs is coupled with myristic acid, which probably inserts to the ER membrane.

sponding to HBsAg subtype *ay*) are obviously retained preferably by the myristic acid (41), while the longer preS1 types (corresponding to HBsAg subtype *ad*) are retained by the peptide sequence as well (42, 43). The cell type in which the HBs proteins are expressed is probably also important for the efficiency of the secretion.

The proportion of LHBs to SHBs regulates the morphology of the secreted HBs particles. At less than 5% LHBs, only 20-nm particles are formed, at higher concentrations filaments are secreted, and at still higher concentrations the secretion of filaments is prevented (44).

D. Ground Glass Hepatocytes

Continuous low-level production of nonsecreted LHBs seems to occur in many low-symptomatic HBsAg carriers and to generate the so-called ground glass cells

(45). The ground glass appearance of these hepatocytes is caused by the large number of HBs filaments in the dilated ER. The pathological consequences in humans of this storage phenomenon are not clear. In mice that express LHBs profusely as a transgene product, the storage leads to hepatocyte malfunction, inflammation, hepatic adenomas, and finally carcinomas (46).

E.   Virion Morphogenesis

In order for core particles to become enveloped, the participation of the SHBs as well as LHBs protein is necessary (47), although the whole protein sequence of SHBs is present in LHBs. It is unclear why both proteins are necessary for virion morphogenesis. The inhibitory effect of LHBs on SHBs secretion is not required because LHBs deletion mutants that no longer prevent the secretion of SHBs still allow formation of virions (47). The dual dependence of virion maturation on SHBs as well as LHBs protein can be explained by different models. One model assumes that both proteins have to form a mixed oligomer in the ER membrane to which the core particle can bind for budding. Another model predicts that the LHBs and SHBs proteins have different but complementary functions, e.g., binding of the core particle by LHBs and driving of the budding process by SHBs. It has been reported that the presence of MHBs protein is dispensable for this morphogenesis process (47), although another report contradicts this finding (48).

Virions and 20-nm spheres are transported from the ER lumen by the ordinary secretory pathway of the cell. They pass the Golgi apparatus (49), where the glycoside at asn 146 is modified to a mixed complex type, and finally reach the outside of the cell.

IV.   FUNCTIONS OF HEPATITIS B SURFACE PROTEINS

A.   Lack of In Vitro Infectivity Systems

Surface proteins are the viral tools that facilitate attachment to and penetration into the cell. The current vaccination strategy is to achieve induction of antibodies against the attachment and/or penetration-activating sites of the viral surface. These antibodies would impede the initial steps of the infection process and promise the safest and most reliable protection. Modern techniques of gene analysis generally permit rapid mapping of essential attachment and penetration sites, provided that an efficient and medically relevant in vitro system for the measurement of viral infectivity is available. Unfortunately, infectivity of HBV can be measured only by inoculation into chimpanzees. Comparison of the number of HBV genomes per ml with the number of infectious doses in chimpanzees suggests that at least one in ten virions is indeed infectious (50). However, if one adds a serum with 10^8 or more virions/ml to a culture of the human hepatoma cells HepG2, the yield of newly synthesized virus is relatively low (51) if detectable at all. Also, primary cultures of human hepatocytes can only be infected with low efficiency (52, 53). In spite of the inability to become efficiently infected, the same HepG2 cells quite efficiently produce infectious HBV after artificial introduction of cloned HBV DNA (54). Thus, it appears that early steps of the authentic infection process do not take place in this cell line.

B. PreS1 Attachment Site

Several authors have used the HepG2 cell to study liver-specific attachment of HBV. Neurath et al. (55) reported specific adherence of suspended HepG2 cells, but not of cell types from other organs or species, to immobilized HBsAg preparations containing LHBs. Adherence could be specifically competed for by preS1 peptide 21–47 and was blocked by antibodies to virions or antibodies to preS1 peptide 21–47 (56). Pontisso et al. (57) showed that recombinant LHBs from yeast bound to plasma-cell membranes of human liver biopsies while MHBs and SHBs did not. Purified virions or HBs filaments also bound while purified spheres did so much weaker (58). The binding of virions could be inhibited by the monoclonal antibody MA 18/7 against an epitope formed by the amino acids 31 to 34 Asp-Pro-Ala-Phe, thus confirming the preS1 specificity of the binding. While attachment via the site around position 30 of preS1 to natural liver membranes suggests some in vivo relevance, this attachment site is not exclusively liver specific. Several other cultured human cell lines and monocytes from peripheral blood were found to bind preS1 (59).

The receptor for the preS1 attachment site has not been identified. It has been proposed to be a novel IgA receptor (60). The sequence 21–47 has indeed a detectable, although low, sequence homology with the alpha 1C sequence 28–55 of human IgA, but the receptor itself has not yet been characterized (61).

The best evidence that this preS1 site is essential for the viral life cycle in vivo comes from protection experiments with antibodies against preS1 [12–47] (62) and from direct immunization with such a peptide (63).

Another surface-accessible site is the sequence around amino acid 100 of preS1. This site is recognized by antibodies from chronic HBV carriers (64). It appears that this antigenic site does not induce protective antibodies. Immunization of chimpanzees with this peptide induced only weak protection (63).

C. PreS2 Attachment Site and Albumin Binding

The preS2 domain of MHBs is exposed on the surface of virions or 20-nm particles (65). This can be demonstrated (a) by an efficient surface iodination of Tyr 21 of the preS2 sequence, (b) by binding of preS2 specific antibodies to native HBsAg, and (c) by the sensitivity of the preS2 domain of MHBs to cleavage by trypsin at arg 15, 17, and 47. Much attention has been drawn to the preS2 domain since it was discovered that this sequence binds to artificially polymerized human serum albumin (pHSA) (66). This binding was reported to be specific for albumin of human or chimpanzee origin, the only organisms that can be infected by HBV. Since binding of pHSA was also observed on liver cell membranes (67), it was hypothesized that the attachment of HBV to its host cell might be mediated by a bridge of modified serum albumin. Furthermore, denatured human serum albumin is internalized by hepatocytes, antiserum against the preS2 domain is able to neutralize HBV infectivity (68), and preS2 peptides elicit protective immunity (69, 70).

The albumin-bridge hypothesis was hampered by the fact that only artificially modified albumin showed the above-mentioned effects (71). However, recent observations showed that natural HSA contains a very small amount of a monomeric subspecies, which binds to preS2 (24). HBsAg levels higher than 10 μg/ml totally absorb this form of HSA and exhibit free HSA-binding sites. Polymeric HSA has, however, a higher affinity (24) and may possibly replace monomeric HSA. Such a polymeric HSA is not found in serum, but it may be bound to liver membranes where it can absorb HBs particles or virions (58). HepG2 cells contain no pHSA receptors in contrast to natural liver cells. This may be one of the deficiencies of HepG2 cells that make them uninfectable by HBV.

D.   pHSA Binding and Immunity

Another potential function of HSA binding may be the induction of T-suppressor cells. B lymphocytes that expose anti-HBs-specific IgM receptor molecules would internalize not only HBV proteins but also the self-molecule HSA. Such B cells present HSA self-peptides to hypothetic suppressor T cells, which may overrun HBV specific T-helper cells. Such an immune suppressive effect of adsorbed HSA may explain the disappointing results in primates and humans with experimental HBV vaccines (72) containing preS2 in addition to the S domain. In mice, where the interaction with serum albumin does not occur, preS2 increased the T- and B-cell response considerably (see Chapter 19).

E.   PreS2 Glycan-Dependent Binding

The preS2 domain contains, in addition to bound HSA, a further host-derived structure. Asn 4 carries a hybrid-type glycan. At least two mouse monoclonal antibodies are known that preferably bind glycan-linked peptide sequences around asn 4 of preS2: Q19/10 (73) and F124 (74). Both antibodies react much more weakly with the unglycosylated preS2 sequence. Q19/10 reacts also with a cell surface structure of HepG2 cells. This suggests a molecular mimicry of HBV by the epitope of Q19/10 (X. Y. Lu and W. H. Gerlich, unpublished). The amino-terminal glycopeptide part of MHBs binds in a species- and organ-specific manner to HepG2 cells. MHBs from HBV carrier plasma does not bind to cultured mouse hepatocytes or HeLa cells. These cells obviously lack the receptor for MHBs. MHBs expressed by transfected mouse fibroblasts has a high-mannose glycan structure in preS2 and does not bind to HepG2 cells. These observations suggest that a novel lectin of HepG2 cells recognizes a liver-derived glycan also occurring in HBV (X. Y. Lu, unpublished). This lectin is not identical with the known hepatic lectins, such as the asialoglycoprotein receptor, the galactose receptor, or the mannose receptor.

F. Proteolysis-Induced Membrane Insertion

The preS2 domain of MHBs, and to a lesser degree of LHBs, is very sensitive to protease. Digestion of natural HBs particles with trypsin cleaves MHBs more rapidly than LHBs, while SHBs is virtually resistent (32). The size of the digestion product suggests cleavage at Arg 47 of preS2. V8 protease cleaves MHBs at Glu 2 of the S domain (16). If one incubates V8- or trypsin-treated HBs particles from HBV carriers with various mammalian cells, a nonspecific irreversible binding to the cell membrane occurs. This binding is optimal at pH 5.5. Our current hypothesis is that the proteolytic cleavage exposes the hydrophobic sequence GFLGPLLVLQAG, which resembles fusion peptides of surface proteins from other viruses like influenza or measles viruses. Such sequences induce fusion of virion membranes with cell membranes. The fusion peptides are often activated by proteases and/or pH changes. The fusion hypothesis is supported by the fact that chymotrypsin cleaves MHBs within the putative fusion sequence and abolishes nonspecific membrane binding (X. Y. Lu, unpublished). The same fusion sequence is present without any protease cleavage in SHBs, but as mentioned above it is obviously not surface exposed. The amino-terminal methionine of SHBs next to Glu 2 cannot be removed from native HBs particles by V8 protease (X. Y. Lu, unpublished). Accordingly, the amino end of SHBs is drawn in Figure 5 as a hidden structure surrounded by the transmembranous alpha-helices and the HBs-antigen loops. The topology of the amino-terminal preS domain of MHBs of LHBs would necessitate a different structure whereby the amino end of the S domain in MHBs or LHBs can be exposed after proteolysis.

G. Penetration of HBV

The above-mentioned (still hypothetical) model suggests that proteolysis would play a central role in the penetration of HBV into hepatocytes. One reason for the fact that HepG2 cells cannot easily be infected may be the absence of a suitable protease. The low pH optimum of the membrane binding suggests that it occurs in endosomes. Thus an endosomal protease may be necessary. This is turn would require receptor-mediated endocytosis. Denatured HSA would be a first candidate for a ligand that could induce such a liver-specific endocytosis, whereas preS1 may be a first attachment site at a receptor without endocytotic capacity.

The proteolysis site itself may be a target for neutralizing antibodies. Prevention of proteolysis at the transition site between preS2 and S would prevent viral penetration. This site is quite variable among various HBV isolates, and in addition, it seems to form T-cell epitopes (see Chapter 19). Antibodies against this site should directly block proteolysis.

H.   Protective Epitopes of SHBs

One of the positive surprises in HBV vaccine development is the great success of HBV vaccines that consist predominantly or exclusively of SHBs. Currently, the great efficiency of SHBs vaccines is not at all understood at the molecular level. SHBs was found to bind to Vero cells (75), but it appears doubtful whether this interaction is relevant during natural infection. Other studies (76) that suggest binding of SHBs to primary liver cells may be misleading because they were done with yeast-derived SHBs. These particles were not produced by natural assembly processes and may have exposed the putative fusion sequence of SHBs. A direct interaction of natural SHBs with hepatocytes or a role of SHBs in penetration has not yet been convincingly shown.

Nonetheless, SHBs carries at least one neutralizing epitope. One of the most stringent ways to map neutralizing epitopes is the isolation and sequencing of escape mutants. Such mutants of HBV were first observed in HBV-vaccinated children who developed HBs antigenemia in spite of relatively high anti-HBs levels (77). Due to the nature of the vaccine, the mutation could only be in the S domain. It was found in position 145, which was mutated from gly to arg. This position is located within the disulfide-stabilized peptide loop 139–147, which is considered to form the HBV-group–specific determinant "a" (78). It is interesting to note that this antigen loop is also the site of glycosylation in the S domain. Obviously, the nonglycosylated part of this determinant is essential for the infectivity process. Theoretically, nonglycosylated vaccines like those from yeast would provide more of the neutralizing epitope.

The constant occurrence of exactly this mutation in many escape mutants (A. J. Zuckerman, personal communication) suggests that there are no other reliably protective group-specific epitopes in the SHBs. It remains unknown whether subtype-specific epitopes can confer protection against the homologous subtype. The occurrence of the escape mutant in many regions of the world with different SHBs subtypes (Italy, United States, Taiwan) suggests that subtype-specific immunity may not play an important role if SHBs is the only vaccine component. The repeated appearance of one and the same escape mutant suggests furthermore that HBV has not much freedom of mutation in this gene region. Thus, one may cope with this escape mutation by addition of an Arg 145 variant to the vaccine.

I. HBsAg Subtypes

Two further determinants have been described for HBsAg. One determinant has either "d" or "y" specificity, and the other has either "w" or "r" specificity. All combinations of determinants are found resulting in four subtypes: adw, adr, ayw, and ayr. Sequence comparison of SHBs proteins from different subtypes revealed that amino acid 122 is important in specifying the d/y phenotype: A lysine is found in all d subtypes, whereas an arginine is present in all y subtypes (79). Correspondingly, for the w/r subtype amino acid 160 is crucial: all w subtypes carry a lysine, while all r subtypes have an arginine at this position (80). When an amino acid other than lysine or arginine is present at position 122 or 160, no d/y or w/r subtype, respectively, is expressed. The subtypes do not strictly reflect a phylogenetic relationship of the isolates. Some SHBs sequences are more closely related to SHBs sequences from a different subtype than to some SHBs sequences of the same subtype.

Subtype-specific epitopes also occur in the preS2 domain. They can be distinguished by monoclonal antibodies (81), but no clear nomenclature has been developed.

In rare cases mixed HBsAg subtypes like adwr or aydwr are found. These mixed subtypes probably are the result of double infections or spontaneous mutations of one subtype to another during the course of infection. When mixed subtypes are found on the same particles (phenotypic mixing), a double infection of the same host cell has to be assumed.

V. FUNCTIONS OF CORE AND POL PROTEINS

The expression and function of the two proteins core and *pol* are closely linked together. They are both expressed from the same mRNA (Figs. 2B and 8). The synthesis of the 185-amino-acid long core protein starts with a high efficiency at the 5' terminal AUG codon of the mRNA. The first AUG of the *pol* ORF is a second, less efficient initiation site for protein synthesis (19, 82a). A core-*pol* frameshift and fusion that occurs in retroviruses is not an essential mechanism for the synthesis of the HBV polymerase.

The *pol* protein is multifunctional (see Fig. 2A). Its amino-terminal part forms the terminal protein for initiating DNA minus strand synthesis; the central part forms the reverse transcriptase for the synthesis of the DNA minus strand and most likely also the DNA-dependent polymerase for synthesis of the DNA plus strand; the carboxy-terminal part forms the RNase H, which is necessary for the degradation of the RNA pregenome during the synthesis of the DNA minus strand. It is not known whether these three domains need to be separated from each other by proteolysis, and whether an HBV-encoded protease activity catalyzes such processing. A 68-kD *pol* protein has been described in HB virions (84), which reacted with antibodies against the carboxy-terminal sequence of *pol*

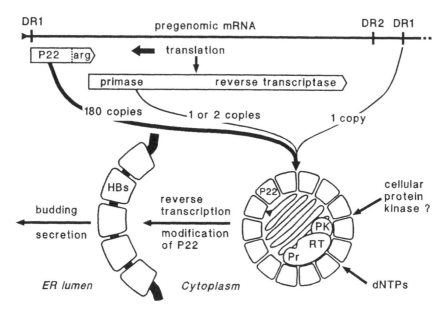

Figure 8 Assembly of hepatitis B core particles. The mRNA for HBc protein has a threefold function: (a) it serves as highly efficient template for the translation of HBc protein (P22) with an arginine-rich carboxy-terminal domain; (b) it serves with low efficiency as template for translation of the HBV polymerase with its two principle domains primase and reverse transcriptase; (c) the two proteins coassemble with their own template and a cellular (?) protein kinase as shown. The reverse transcription (see Fig. 9) and modification of P22 require nucleotide triphosphates (dNTPs), which can diffuse into the core particle. Thereafter the core particle associates with the cytoplasmic side of the HBs proteins, which have been produced at and inserted into the ER membrane. The core particle becomes enveloped, buds to the ER lumen, and can be secreted as complete virion.

(85). This would suggest the existence of a protease that would cleave the pol protein into an approximately 30-kD terminal protein and a 68-kD reverse transcriptase/RNase H. Recently, a 40-kD RNase H has also been described (S. Oberhaus, personal communication).

A. Assembly of Core Particles

It has been suggested that a newly synthesized *pol* protein molecule would directly after completion interact with its own RNA template, whereby this RNA would become destined for encapsidation (86). After encapsidation, this mRNA has a second function as RNA pregenome. The encapsidation signal on the RNA pregenome was localized at the 5'-terminal 137 nucleotides (87). It appears likely that this region is recognized by the polymerase (88). After these steps, the core protein subunits assemble around the RNA–*pol* protein complex and form the core particle. In absence of the *pol* protein, the core protein is also able to encapsidate up to 3300 bases of RNA (89), however, without sequence specificity (V. Bruss unpublished). Thus, an interaction between core and *pol* protein has to be assumed for efficient generation of pregenome-containing core particles.

Core particles are often found in high numbers in the nuclei of hepatocytes of persistently infected HBV carriers. Theoretically, it would be possible that these core particles originate from infecting HBV particles that were phagocytized from the bloodstream. However, these particles have a low density (1.31 g/ml) and a low content of nucleic acid as suggested by their UV spectrum (W. Gerlich, unpublished). Nucleic acid hybridization suggested furthermore that they contain very little HBV-specific nucleic acid (V. Bruss, unpublished). Core particles formed by recombinant DNA techniques in *E. coli* efficiently encapsidate RNA and have a density of 1.37 g/ml in CsCl solution. Blotted core protein from *E. coli* binds RNA efficiently (89, 91), but natural core protein does not (90). Core protein can assemble into core particles without any packaging of RNA. Removal of the arginine-rich carboxy-terminal domain abolishes packaging of RNA but still allows particle formation (89–91). However, core protein from human liver nuclei has the same size as full-length core protein expressed in *E. coli* (92). Thus, core protein expressed in hepatocytes seems to be modified in a way that it loses its ability to encapsidate RNA.

B. Phosphorylation of Core Protein

Natural core particles, both from liver nuclei and from serum-derived virions, contain an endogenous protein kinase activity (21, 22). This protein kinase phosphorylates core protein in its arginine-rich domain (93). The modification seems to abolish the affinity of core protein for RNA. Core particles can be disassembled by low ionic strength buffer. In this state recombinant core protein can be phosphorylated in vitro by protein kinase A. After in vitro phosphorylation, RNA is no longer bound (M. Kann, personal communication). The arginine-rich domain contains target sequences both for protein kinase A and C. Which of the two kinases or whether yet another kinase is encapsidated during assembly of the core particle is not yet clear. The occurrence of complete virions that contain the RNA-derived genome, *pol* protein, and protein kinase suggests that encapsidation of RNA occurs in the presence of *pol* protein more rapidly than phosphorylation of the core protein. In the absence of the *pol* protein, assembly may be slower than phosphorylation and transport to the nucleus. Assembly of phosphorylated core protein in the nucleus would no longer lead to encapsidation of HBV RNA.

C.   Reverse Transcription (Fig. 9)

The *pol* protein recognizes specifically, probably before encapsidation, the 5'-terminal region of the pregenome. Probably after encapsidation, a site at the 3' end of the pregenome interacts with the amino terminal domain of the *pol* protein in such a way that a tyrosine of this region becomes part of the priming structure for DNA-minus strand synthesis. Reverse transcription starts at the center of the 3'-terminal 10-base direct repeat sequence (DR), which occurs three times in the pregenome. The reverse transcription stops 18 bases before the 5' end of the pregenome, thus generating a redundancy of nine bases in the DNA minus strand. The RNase H activity degrades the RNA pregenome into oligo-ribonucleotides in connection with the proceeding DNA synthesis. Finally, only the 18-base RNA fragment of the 5' terminus remains. This fragment is translo-cated to the DR2 sequence in the minus DNA strand and is then used as primer for the synthesis of the DNA-plus strand. The *pol* protein, which acts now as DNA-dependent DNA polymerase, passes DR1 generating a short triple DNA strand region of nine bases at this point. The plus strand synthesis proceeds further to variable points leaving a large gap of several hundred to 2000 bases. The resulting DNA structure (shown in detail in Fig. 2C) is identical with the one found in virions. The polymerase stops at numerous "pause" sites, which are formed by short hairpin loops. It is not known whether the space within the core particle is too limited to accommodate a fully double-stranded DNA structure or whether the process of envelopment, budding, and secretion is coupled to the progress of DNA-plus strand synthesis, thus removing the virion from the dNTP-rich cytoplasm. A detailed discussion of HBV genome replication is given by Seeger et al. (94).

The secretion of naked core particles by transfected cells (95) and by naturally infected liver in the absence of anti-HBc (96) has been reported, but the findings could not be confirmed by our groups (29, 97).

D.   Effects on the Interferon System

Besides their crucial role in viral replication, core and pol proteins may have important effects on the host's defense system. A not yet exactly defined product of the core ORF was reported to suppress induction of the beta-interferon promoter (98). There is, however, no evidence that HBV would otherwise be able to induce beta-interferon. More important for the host defense may be the inhibitory effect of the terminal protein on the induction of interferon-responsive genes (99).

VI.   THE HBe PROTEIN

HBeAg was discovered when sera from high- and low-viremic HBsAg carriers were allowed to react with each other in agar gel immunodiffusions (100). The

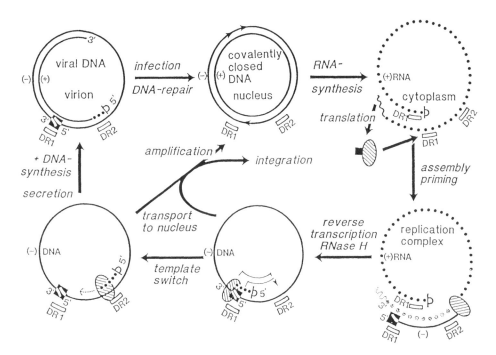

Figure 9 Replication cycle of the HBV genome. The virion DNA (top left, described in detail in Fig. 2C) enters the nucleus of the infected cells and is converted to a covalently closed circle, probably by cellular enzymes of DNA repair. This DNA is template for a pregenomic mRNA, which in turn is translated to core protein and polymerase protein. These three components assemble as shown in Fig. 8. The polymerase (shown as black square and hatched oval) recognizes a sequence around the 3'-terminal DR1 in the pregenomic RNA (top right). Within the core particle, reverse transcription of the RNA pregenome generates a growing DNA(−) strand, which is linked to the primase protein (black square). The RNase H function of the reverse transcriptase degrades the already transcribed RNA, finally leading to a single DNA(−) strand. The remaining 5'-terminal piece of the pregenomic RNA is shifted from DR1 to DR2, where it serves as primer for the DNA(+) strand (bottom left). As soon as the discontinuity in the (−) strand is passed, the DNA structure present in the virion is generated and the core particle is ready for envelopment and secretion.

high-viremic sera contained much HBeAg, while the low-viremic sera had antibodies to HBeAg (anti-HBe). The role of HBeAg has remained enigmatic. Today, the structure and biosynthesis of HBeAg are known, but as to the function, not much has been learned since 1972.

A. Biosynthesis (Fig. 10)

The amino acid sequence of the unprocessed HBe protein is almost identical to that of the HBc protein (101). The only difference is that 29 additional amino acids of the so-called preC sequence precede the HBc protein sequence. In this case (and in contrast to the preS sequences) the prefix means in fact that the presequence is partially removed from the larger precursor protein to yield a smaller product. The preC sequence functions as a signal for the translocation of the subsequently synthesized polypeptide to the lumen of the ER (102). In a manner similar to that of many other signal peptides of secreted proteins, it can be partially cleaved off by the luminal ER-protease signalase at amino acid 19 of the preC sequence, leaving 10 amino acids of the preC sequence at the HBe

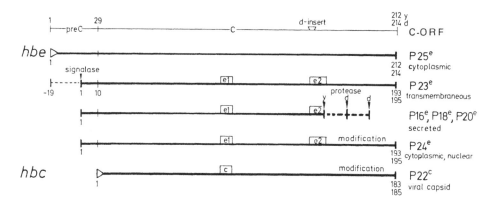

Figure 10 Biosynthesis and intracellular distribution of HBe protein. Translation of the complete C-ORF generates a P25^e, which may be either cytoplasmic or inserted into the ER membrane. At the ER, P25^e can be cleaved by the signalase to a transmembraneous P23^e. This protein may become a part of the plasma membrane. If the arginine-rich carboxy-terminal part of P23^e is cleaved at variable loci, a secretable form of HBe is generated (P16^e, P18^e, P20^e). The P23^e may also flip back to the cytoplasm. There it becomes phosphorylated, whereby it migrates like a P24^e in electrophoresis. Finally P24^e can migrate to the nucleus. Translation of C-ORF beginning at the second AUG leads to the core (or HBc) protein. The DNA sequences encoding HBe and HBc protein may be termed *hbe* and *hbc*. HBe protein has two major epitope regions, e1 and e2. The major epitope region of assembled HBc particles overlaps with e1 but has a different antigenicity (c).

protein (103). The arginine-rich domain of the core protein, which is also present in the newly made HBe protein, seems to prevent complete translocation (102) or secretion. In the secreted HBe protein, this domain is either completely (104) or partially removed (103, 105). Besides this pathway, nascent HBe protein may slip back to the cytoplasm (106) and may migrate to the nucleus (107), or it remains in the ER and reaches the plasma membrane later (108). When expressed in animal cells, HBe protein cannot form core particles (109), and it exposes an antigenicity, "HBe," different from the core protein ("HBc"). From these data it is clear that the combined preC and core sequence encodes a pre-HBe protein and not a precursor for the core protein; preE instead of preC would be a more appropriate nomenclature, but is not used.

B. HBe—A Nonessential Protein

The start codon for the preC sequence upstream of the core sequence and the HBe protein is conserved in the family of hepadnaviridae. Thus, the preC sequence appears to provide, by leading to an HBe protein, an evolutionary advantage for this virus family. However, transfection experiments with HBV genomes in which the preC sequence has been mutated away yielded viable virus in absence of HBe protein (82, 83). Furthermore, patients without HBe protein but with high viremia contain an HBV variant with a destroyed preC sequence. Typical is the introduction of a stop codon at base 1819 (77, 110).

C. HBe—An Immunomodulator?

The frequent association of HBe-negative HBV variants with severe chronic or fulminant acute hepatitis B suggests that HBe has some not yet understood effect on the host's immune response. Currently, it is believed that cytotoxic immune reactions against the HBc protein predominantly contribute to the pathogenesis of chronic hepatitis B (111). In many HBV carriers with high viremia, this cytotoxic immune reaction seems to be very weak, and they are almost asymptomatic. These carriers are virtually always HBeAg positive. Seroconversion from HBe antigenemia to anti-HBe in such persons is usually connected with a rise of transaminases and a decrease in viremia. If liver disease and viremia persist, thereafter, an HBe-negative HBV variant can usually be isolated. Thus, HBe protein seems to favor long-term survival of carriers highly productive for HBV. One way that HBe could possibly generate tolerance against HBc and HBe antigen is by transplacental transmission of HBe protein from mother to child, and subsequent elimination of HBe/c-specific T cells in the fetus, because HBe is mistaken as a self-protein (112). The transplacental transmission, however, has not yet been convincingly demonstrated in humans. Furthermore, HBe seems to have also a tolerogenic function in subjects who have been infected postnatally.

Since T lymphocytes recognize proteolytically degraded protein, they may not distinguish clearly between HBe and HBc protein because the major T-cell epitopes seem to be in sequences common to both proteins (111). On the other hand, the different intracellular distribution of the two proteins may lead to different presentation patterns. HBc as a cytoplasmic protein may be degraded by a cytoplasmic protease complex and be captured by MHC class I molecules. HBe as ER-associated molecule may be degraded by an endosomal protease of different specificity and would be captured by MHC class II molecules. After HBV infection, hepatocytes may possibly express class II molecules because HBx protein seems to transactivate their expression (113). For some unknown reason, however, HBe protein seems to have an adverse effect on T-cell immunity.

VII.   THE HBx PROTEIN

A.   HBx—A Nonessential Protein?

If the "e" in HBeAg stands for "enigma," the "x" for the designation of this protein is even more justified. The first indication for the existence of HBx protein came from the sequence analysis of cloned HBV genomes. The function of three ORFs could immediately be identified, but the existence of a fourth ORF was surprising (Fig. 2). The ORF is conserved in the mammalian hepadnaviruses from woodchucks and ground squirrels, but it is not present in the two well-characterized avian hepadnaviruses from ducks or grey herons. These observations suggest that the HBx protein is not directly involved in the biochemistry of genome replication, which is very similiar in all members of the hepadnaviridae.

HBx protein has been produced (with some difficulties) in various vector/host systems. Using recombinant HBx antigen, anti-HBx was found in a varying proportion of acutely or chronically HBV-infected persons. Antibodies against recombinant HBx protein or partial peptides of HBx have been used for search of HBx protein in liver tissue, serum, or HBV particles. Due to the high degree of nonspecificity of these antibodies, results have to be considered with some reservation. The mRNA for HBx protein has been found in naturally infected liver only at very low levels.

There are no clear reports that HBx is essential for viral infectivity or replication in the natural host. Transfection of the human hepatoma cell Huh7 with an HBx-deficient mutant yielded the same level of HBV particles as transfection with the wild-type genome. Transfection of the more differentiated HepG2 cell still yielded HBV particles but at a lower level (114). It appears possible that HBx is a nonessential protein like HBeAg or MHBs (H. Will, personal communication), but it may increase viability of the virus in its natural host to the extent that it can spread through the population.

B. Transcription Activation by HBx

Numerous studies have demonstrated the transcription-activating properties of HBx protein on a wide variety of target DNA sequences like the HBV enhancer itself, the HIV LTR (115), beta-interferon (116), HLA-D (113), c-myc (117), or c-fos promoter/enhancer (S. Schaefer and W. H. Gerlich, unpublished). It appears unlikely that HBx binds directly to these target sequences. It has been suggested that HBx would be a serine/threonine kinase, which would activate cellular transcription factors by phosphorylation (23). Another study suggested that HBx would directly or indirectly activate protein kinase C, which in turn would activate transcription factors (A. Kekule et al., personal communication). Still another theory suggests that HBx would, as a coactivator, link specific enhancer-binding transcription factors with promoter-binding transcription factors (118). Furthermore, a sequence similarity of HBx with nucleotide diphosphate kinase was noted (Y. Shaul, personal communication). These various observations do not exclude each other, but they clearly demonstrate that the effect of HBx on transcription is not yet understood. Since HBx activates the transcription of mRNAs and the pregenome, an enhancement of viral protein production is most likely one major function of HBx.

C. HBx—A Viral Oncoprotein

In contrast to the retroviridae, hepadnaviridae need not be integrated into the host chromosome. However, as a side effect of viral replication variable fragments of HBV DNA are often integrated into the host chromosome. Mono- or oligoclonal integration patterns of HBV DNA are frequently found in HBV-associated liver carcinomas. A typical integrated HBV DNA fragment contains a truncated version of the HBx gene, the product of which can still activate transcription. Since HBx has been shown to transactivate cellular oncogenes such as c-myc (117, 119) or c-fos, this might provide an explanation for the manner in which HBx contributes to development and progression of liver tumors.

An oncogenic effect of HBx in the absence of other HBV proteins has been made likely in a transgenic mouse strain that expressed HBx under control of its own enhancer/promoter. These mice frequently develop liver carcinoma after one year of life (120). Premalignant hepatocyte cultures that have been transformed by SV40 Tumor antigen can be converted to fully malignant growth by transfection with HBV DNA. These cells express large amounts of HBx protein (121). The HBx gene under control of its enhancer/promoter can also induce malignant growth if the HBx protein is expressed at high levels (122). A mutant HBx gene with a stop codon instead of codon 23 could not induce malignant growth (123), although it expressed large amounts of HBx mRNA. In the HBx-transformed hepatocytes, but not in the control cells with the mutant HBx gene, the growth suppressor protein p53 is retained in the cytoplasm where it cannot fulfill its function (M. Höhne and W. H. Gerlich, in preparation).

The HBx protein corresponds in many respects to other tumor proteins of DNA viruses, such as E1A and E1B of adenoviruses, E6/7 of papillomaviruses, or SV40 tumor antigen. They have some rather nonspecific transcription-activating properties, and they inactivate a growth suppressor protein. HBx protein is certainly not sufficient for transformation of normally growth-controlled cells. Adenoviruses and papillomaviruses have at least two viral oncoproteins, if not more. In our experiments, transfection with complete HBV DNA was more oncogenic than transfection with the hbx gene alone, although the latter expressed more HBx protein. This suggests that the HBV genome contains further transforming proteins.

Most DNA tumor viruses are not acutely transforming. Thus, the long latency period of HBV-associated liver carcinoma does not exclude the presence of expressed oncogene(s) during HBV infection. After integration of these oncogenes and subsequent dysregulation, they may develop their fatal activity in conjunction with cellular factors.

VIII. TARGET PROTEINS FOR PROTECTIVE IMMUNITY

Since the first immunization attempts in the 1970s, hepatitis B vaccines have generally consisted of SHBs. Experience with plasma-derived vaccines and with the first generation of recombinant vaccines suggests that 20-nm particles composed of SHBs are able to induce protection with high efficiency. Early studies confirmed the obvious expectation that protection was coupled to detection of anti-HBs in the vaccine recipients, but the protective mechanisms may be more complex. The possible inclusion of additional HBV antigens or proteins in future vaccines is also discussed in Chapter 20.

A. Neutralizing SHBs Epitopes

As mentioned above, the manner in which anti-HBs protects against HBV is not well understood, since a function of SHBs during attachment or penetration of HBV has not yet been identified. One monoclonal antibody (RF1) against SHBs was able to neutralize 3000 infectious doses of HBV in vitro, as was shown by inoculation of the antibody-HBV mixture into chimpanzees (124). The epitope of RF1 is present only on dimers or oligomers of SHBs (125). Fortunately, accurate assembly as it occurs in the infected hepatocyte is not absolutely required for the generation of protective epitopes. The absence of glycan in the yeast-derived SHBs vaccine may be even advantageous because the major group-specific epitope around glycine 145 would be masked by glycan.

B. T-Cell Immunity Against SHBs

It is not completely clear whether anti-HBs is the sole or even the predominant protective factor induced by the SHBs vaccine. Studies in newborn children from highly viremic mothers suggest that active vaccination with a potent SHBs vaccine from yeast is as efficient as combined passive-active immunization with an SHBs vaccine and anti-HBs immune globulin (126). Passive immunization with anti-HBs was only effective when it was given at high doses within 48 hours after birth. However, active production of anti-HBs after vaccination takes much longer.

Studies in chimpanzees that had received infectious HBV showed that shortly after this exposure, active vaccination protected better (127) than passive immunization (128). These observations suggest indirectly that cellular immunity induced by the SHBs vaccine may be as important or even more important than the actual presence of anti-HBs. Since the activation of anti-SHBs producing B lymphocytes would require T-helper lymphocytes, the presence of anti-SHBs would be an indicator not only for neutralizing antibody but also for SHBs inducible T-helper lymphocytes. The surprisingly high efficiency of the yeast-derived vaccine may be in part the result of the less condensed structure of the particles, which may be more accessible to proteolytic degradation in antigen presenting cells. Denatured SHBs was reported to be presented more efficiently than native HBs particles to T-helper cells (129).

It appears that SHBs will remain one essential component of future hepatitis B vaccines because of its tremendous success. It may, however, be worthwhile to optimize the tertiary and quarternary structure of the HBs particle for both a good anti-HBs response and an improved T-cell response. SHBs particles have been used as immunogenic carriers for other epitopes (130), but HBc particles are more immunogenic and thus preferable for this purpose (see below).

C. PreS2 as a Vaccine Component

Immunization of chimpanzees using a conjugate of preS2 [14–32] peptide with keyhole limpet hemocyanine protected the animals against experimental HBV infection (69). A mixture of rabbit antibodies against preS2 [1–24] peptide with HBV was no longer infectious (62). Immunization with the complete preS2 [1–55] peptide without protein carrier also induced protective immunity (70). It is not exactly known by which mechanism anti-preS2 protects. Anti-preS2 [1–24] most likely interferes with albumin binding and, possibly, with the preS2 glycopeptide binding to a hypothetical liver lectin; anti-preS2 [14–32] could only block albumin binding. Furthermore, it cannot be completely excluded that T-cell immunity was essential for the immunity in the experiments of Itoh (69) or Emini (70). If proteolysis of preS2 next to the S domain is indeed an important step in the infection process, antibodies against the carboxy-terminal part of preS2 may be also protective, but subtype differences would be quite prominent.

D. Immunogenicity of preS2

Conflicting results have been reported regarding the immunogenicity of preS2-containing vaccines. In inbred mice preS2 did not only induce anti-preS2 but also could circumvent immunogenetically determined nonresponsiveness to SHBs antigen (131). However, immunization of primates or humans resulted in a different outcome. An HBs particle vaccine containing preS2 expressed in Chinese Hamster Ovary cells induced anti-preS2, but was on a whole not more immunogenic in humans than was a plasma-derived vaccine from the same producer, which contained only traces of preS (132). A Belgian vaccine producer reported that a yeast-derived MHBs was very immunogenic in mice but less effective than a yeast-derived SHBs vaccine in humans or primates (72). In contrast, an American vaccine producer found that a similar type of MHBs vaccine was also superior to their yeast-derived SHBs vaccine in humans (133). Kuroda et al. (134) even defined a protective anti-preS2 level in humans which was regularly surpassed after vaccination with their MHBs vaccine from yeast.

The binding of human serum albumin may have some negative effect on immunogenicity in humans, which would not be observed in rodents because only human or primate serum albumin is bound. The presence of the glycan is also not desirable because it may mask important T- and B-cell epitopes. PreS2 in a mixture of MHBs and SHBs as in natural HBs particles would be preferable. However, MHBs is highly sensitive to proteolysis. Due to this, particles expressed only by the MHBs gene will still expose many SHBs epitopes.

E. PreS1 Epitopes as Vaccine Components

There are several reasons to include parts of the preS1 domain into an optimized hepatitis B vaccine. Neurath et al. (62) have shown that antibodies against preS1 [12–47] peptide neutralize infectivity of HBV for chimpanzees. Direct immunization with such a peptide was also protective (63). In contrast to the preS2 domain, addition of the preS1 domain enhances the immunogenicity of HBs particles dramatically not only in mice but also in humans. Ferrari et al. (135) found in recipients of a plasma-derived vaccine that most HBs-inducible T-helper cell clones were specific for preS1 although the vaccine contained only traces of preS1. A preS1 [1–50]-containing HBs particle was able to induce an anti-preS1 and an anti-SHBs response in nonresponders to a conventional SHBs vaccine (136). Plasma-derived vaccines were able to induce detectable anti-preS1 responses, although these vaccines contained no detectable or only traces of preS1 (137). Furthermore, this anti-preS1 competed with the monoclonal antibody MA 18/7, which is directed against the preS1 attachment site.

PreS1 antigen is enriched in HB virions and HBs filaments, but is diminished in 20-nm particles. In case of an inoculation, less anti-preS1 antibody would be consumed by noninfectious HBs particles than would be in the case with anti-SHBs or anti-preS2.

Addition of complete LHBs to an HBs particle vaccine seems to be impractical. A high proportion of LHBs prevents particle assembly. Thus, certain regions of the LHBs gene were deleted for expression as a yeast-derived vaccine component to facilitate particle formation (72). In a L cell–derived experimental vaccine, some of the SHBs molecules carried the 50 amino-terminal preS1 amino acids instead of their own sequence (136). Both vaccines have been used in a small number of human recipients with very good success.

F. Protective Immunity by HBc/e Protein

Immunization of chimpanzees with natural liver-derived core particles (138), with recombinant core particles (139), or with proteolytically degraded core protein exposing HBe antigenicity (140) rendered them partial immunity against a challenge with infectious virus. The experiment has been reproduced with woodchuck HB core particles (141).

It appears that anti-HBc cannot be the protective factor, because it is present in high titers in HBV carriers without suppressing chronic infection. Anti-HBe could be a protective factor because it would neutralize HBeAg. If HBeAg is indeed a tolerogen for HBc/e-specific T-cell immunity, its neutralization would not allow establishment of an ongoing HBV replication. Particulate HBeAg, as produced by carboxy-terminal truncation of HBc protein in bacteria, is a better antigen than soluble HBe protein (43). The major protective mechanism is probably priming of HBc/e-specific T-helper cells. Such priming allows for a rapid anti-HBs response in mice injected with HBV particles (142). It would be very interesting to confirm the validity of this concept in an animal that can be infected by a hepadnavirus.

G. HBc Particles as Immunogenic Carriers

Core particles are an extremely good immunogen both in experimental animals and in the naturally infected host. One major epitope region is formed by a loop near amino acid 80 of the HBc protein. This native antigenic HBc sequence can be replaced using recombinant DNA techniques by other antigenic sequences, which then also acquire the high immunogenicity of the core particle. PreS epitopes (143) and picornavirus epitopes (144) have been found to be excellent immunogens if inserted into that region. Amino- or carboxy-terminal additions or substitutions in the HBc protein are less suitable. An interesting aspect is that core particles can be efficiently expressed in bacteria. This allows for simple production in vitro or—if a live attenuated bacterial vaccine is used—in vivo (145).

H. HBx—A Possible Vaccine Component?

Since HBx protein is very unlikely to be a structural protein, protective immunity could only be conferred by cytotoxic immune reactions. HBx is, as far as is known, not present on the plasma membrane, and thus HBx-specific CD8 lymphocytes would be the protective agent. HBx-specific T lymphocytes have been found in chronic HBV carriers. This does not exclude a protective effect of such HBx-specific lymphocytes, because in absence of neutralizing antibody a cytotoxic immune reaction can probably not stop persistent infection. Such T lymphocytes may be essential for the control of HBx-induced hepatomas. Protection by T-cell immunity against a nonstructural immediate early protein has been found with mouse cytomegalovirus. Suitability of HBx protein as a vaccine component remains speculative at the moment, but may be worth further investigation.

IX. SUMMARY

Hepatitis B vaccines consisting of SHBs particles as an immunogen have been very efficacious and successful, but further improvement of their T-cell immunogenicity and virus-neutralizing capacity appears possible and desirable. Improved vaccines should require a smaller number of injections, yield a longer duration of protection, leave fewer low responders or nonresponders, and would not allow development of escape mutants when the vaccine is given after exposure. Addition of the preS2 domain and of the amino-terminal part of the preS1 domain to a part of the SHBs molecules within one HBs particle would be the most promising improvement. Combination of such an antigenically enriched HBs particle with HBc/e particles should induce protective immunity even in the most difficult cases by maximal induction of HBV-specific T cells. The suitability of HBx protein as a vaccine component should be studied because, as a viral oncogene and transcription activator, HBx would be an interesting vaccination target. Both HBs and HBc particles have been used as immunogenic carriers for a variety of interesting epitopes. Most promising are HBc particles in which the major HBc/e epitope has been replaced by the peptide of interest.

REFERENCES

1. Germain, R. N. 1991. Antigen presentation—the second class story. Nature 353:605–607.
2. McLachlan, A. 1992. Molecular Biology of Hepatitis B viruses. CRC Press, Boca Raton, FL.
3. Mason, W. S., Seeger, C. 1991. Hepadnaviruses—Molecular Biology and Pathogenesis. Current Topics in Microbiology and Immunology, Vol. 168, Springer, Berlin.

4. Prince, A. M. 1968. An antigen detected in the blood during the incubation period of serum hepatitis. Proc. Natl. Acad. Sci. USA 60:814.

5. Blumberg, B. S., Alter, H. J., Visnich, S. 1965. A "new" antigen in leukemia sera. JAMA 191:541–546.

6. Dane, D. S., Cameron, C. H., Briggs, M. 1970. Virus-like particles in serum from patients with Australia antigen-associated hepatitis. Lancet 1:695–698.

7. Almeida, J. D., Rubenstein, D., Stott, E. J. 1971. New antigen-antibody system in Australia-antigen positive hepatitis. Lancet 2:1225.

8. Robinson, W. S., Clayton, D. A., Greenman, R. L. 1974. DNA of a human hepatitis B virus candidate. J. Virol. 14:384–391.

9. Peterson, D. L. 1981. Isolation and charaterization of the major protein and glycoprotein of hepatitis B surface antigen. J. Biol. Chem. 256:6975–6983.

10. Peterson, D. L., Roberts, J. M., Vyas, G. N. 1977. Partial amino acid sequence of two major component polypeptides of hepatitis surface antigen. Proc. Natl. Acad. Sci. USA 74:1530.

11. Valenzuela, P., Gray, P., Quiroga, M., Zaldivar, J., Goodman, H. M., Rutter, W. J. 1979. Nucleotide sequence of the gene coding for the major protein of hepatitis B virus surface antigen. Nature 280:815–819.

12. Heerman, K-H., Goldmann, I., Schwartz, W., Seyffarth, T., Baumgarten, H., Gerlich, W. H. 1984. Large surface proteins of hepatitis B virus containing the preS sequence. J. Virol. 52:396–402.

13. Galibert, F., Mandart, E., Fitoussi, F., Tiollais, P., Charnay, P. 1979. Nucleotide sequence of hepatitis B virus genome (subtype ayw) cloned in E. coli. Nature 281:646–650.

14. Valenzuela, O., Quiroga, M., Zaldivar, J., Gray, P., Rutter, W. J. 1980. The nucleotide sequence of the hepatitis B viral genome and the identification of the major viral genes. In: Fields, B. N., Jaenisch, R., eds., Animal Virus Genetics, ICN/UCLA Symp. Mol. Cell. Biol., pp. 57–70.

15. Tiollais, P., Charnay, P., Vyas, G. N. 1981. Biology of hepatitis B virus. Science 213:406–409.

16. Stibbe, W., Gerlich, W. H. 1983. Structural relationships between minor and major proteins of hepatitis B surface antigen. J. Virol. 46:626–628.

17. Summers, J., Mason, W. S. 1982. Replication of the genome of a hepatitis B-like virus by reverse transcription of an RNA intermediate. Cell 29:403–415.

18. Gerlich, W. H., Robinson, W. S. 1980. Hepatitis B virus contains protein attached to the 5' terminus of its complete DNA strand. Cell 21:801–809.

19. Schlicht, H. J., Radziwill, G., Schaller, H. 1989. Synthesis and encapsidation of duck hepatitis B virus reverse transcriptase do not require formation of core-polymerase fusion proteins. Cell 56:85–92.

20. Bartenschlager, R., Schaller, H. 1988. The amino-terminal domain of the hepadnaviral P-gene encodes the terminal protein (genome linked protein) believed to prime reverse transcription. EMBO J. 7:4185–4192.

21. Albin, C., Robinson, W. S. 1980. Protein kinase activity in hepatitis B virions. J. Virol. 34:297–302.

22. Gerlich, W. H., Goldmann, U., Müller, R., Stibbe, W., Wolff, W., 1982.

Specificity and localization of the hepatitis B virus-associated protein kinase. J. Virol. 42:761–766.

23. Wu, T-T., Zhou, Z. Y., Judd, A., Cartwright, C. A., Robinson, W. S. 1990. The hepatitis B virus encoded transcriptional trans-activator hbx appears to be a novel protein serine/threonine kinase. Cell 63:687–695.

24. Krone, B., Lenz, A., Heermann, K.-H., Seifer, M., Lu, X., Gerlich, W. S. 1990. Interaction between hepatitis B surface proteins and monomeric human serum albumin. Hepatology 11:1050–1056.

25. Madalinski, K., Burczynska, B., Heermann, K-H., Uy, A., Gerlich, W. H. 1991. Analysis of viral proteins in circulating immune complexes from chronic carriers of hepatitis B virus. Clin. Exp. Immunol. 84:493–500.

26. Eble, B. E., Lingappa, V. R., Ganem, D. 1986. Hepatitis B surface antigen: an unusual secreted protein initially synthesized as a transmembrane polypeptide. Mol. Cell. Biol. 6:1454–1463.

27. Eble, B. E., Lingappa, V. R., Ganem, D. 1990. The N-terminal (preS2) domain of a hepatitis B virus surface glycoprotein translocated across membranes by downstream signal sequences. J. Virol. 64:1414–1419.

28. Eble B. E., Macrae D. R., Lingappa V. R., Ganem D. 1987. Multiple topogenic-sequences determine the transmembrane orientation of hepatitis B surface antigen. Mol. Cell. Biol 7:3591–3601.

29. Bruss, V., Ganem, D. 1991. Mutational analysis of hepatitis B surface antigen particle assembly and secretion. J. Virol. 65:3813–3820.

30. Guerrero, E., Gavilanes, F., Peterson, D. L. 1988. Model for the protein arrangement in HBsAg particles based on physical and chemical studies. In: Viral Hepatitis and Liver Disease, Zuckerman, A. J., ed., Alan R. Liss, pp. 606–613.

31. Heermann, K-H., Gerlich, W. H. 1992. Surface proteins of hepatitis B viruses. In: Molecular Biology of Hepatitis B Virus, McLachlan, A. ed., CRC Press, Boca Raton, FL.

32. Heermann, K-H., Kruse, F., Seifer, M., Gerlich, W. H. 1987. Immunogenicity of the gene S and pre-S domains in hepatitis B virions and HBsAg filaments. Intervirology 28:14–25.

33. Persing, D. H., Varmus, H. E., Ganem, D. 1987. The preS1 protein of hepatitis B virus is acylated at its amino terminus with myristic acid. J. Virol. 61:1672–1677.

34. Simon, K., Lingappa, V., Ganem, D. 1988. Secreted hepatitis B surface antigen polypeptides are derived from a transmembrane precursor. J. Cell. Biol. 107: 2163–2168.

35. Moriarty, A. M., Hoyer, B. H., Shih, J. W. K., Gerin, J. L., Hamer, D. H. 1981. Expression of the hepatitis B virus surface antigen gene in cell culture by using a simian virus 40 vector. Proc. Natl. Acad. Sci. USA 78:2606–2610.

36. McLachlan, A., Milich, D. R., Raney, A. K., Riggs, M. G., Hughes, J. L., Sorge, J., Chisari, F. V. 1987. Expression of hepatitis B virus surface and core antigens: influences of preS and precore sequences. J. Virol. 61:683–692.

37. Persing, D. H., Varmus, H. E., Ganem, D. 1986. Antibodies to preS and X determinants arise during natural infection with ground squirrel hepatitis virus. J. Virol. 60:177–184.

38. Standring, D. N., Ou, J., Rutter, W. J. 1986. Assembly of viral particles in

Xenopus oocytes: presurface antigens regulate secretion of the hepatitis B viral surface envelope particle. Proc. Natl. Acad. Sci. USA 83:9338–9342.

39. Cheng, C., Smith, K., Moss, B. 1986. Hepatitis large surface protein is not secreted but is immunogenic when selectively expressed by recombinant vaccinia virus. J. Virol. 60:337–344.

40. Chisari, F. V., Filippi, P., McLachlan, A., Milich, D. R., Riggs, M., Lee, S., Palmiter, R. D., Pinkert, C. A., Brinster, R. L. 1986. Expression of hepatitis B virus large envelope polypeptide inhibits hepatitis B surface antigen secretion in transgenic mice. J. Virol. 60:880–887.

41. Prange, R., Clemen, A., Streeck, R. E. 1991. Myristilation is involved in intercellular rentention of hepatitis B virus envelope proteins. J. Virol. 65:3919–3923.

42. Kuroki, K., Russnak, R., Ganem, D. 1989. Novel N-terminal amino acid sequence required for retention of a hepatitis B virus glycoprotein in the endoplasmatic reticulum. Mol. Cell. Biol. 9:4459–4466.

43. Korec, E., Gerlich, W. H. 1992. HBc and HBe specificity of monoclonal antibodies against complete and truncated HBc proteins from E. coli. Arch. Virol. Suppl. 4:119–121.

44. Marquardt, O., Heermann, K-H., Seifer, M., Gerlich, W. H. 1987. Cell type specific expression of preS1 antigen and secretion of hepatitis B surface antigen. Postgrad. Med. J. 63:41–50.

45. Dienes, H. P., Gerlich, W. H., Wörsdörfer, M., Gerken, G., Bianchi, L., Hess, G., Meyer zum Büschenfelde, K-H. 1990. Hepatic expression patterns of the large and middle hepatitis B virus surface proteins in viremic and nonviremic chronic hepatitis B. Gastroenterology 88:1–7.

46. Chisari, F. V., Klopchin, K., Moriyama, T., Pasquinelli, C., Dunsford, H. A., Sell, S., Pinkert, C. A., Brinster, R. L., Palmiter, R. D. 1989. Molecular pathogenesis of hepatocellular carcinoma in hepatitis B virus transgenic mice. Cell 59:1145–1156.

47. Bruss, V., Ganem, D. 1991. The role of envelope protein in hepatitis B virus assembly. Proc. Natl. Acad. Sci. USA 88:1059–1063.

48. Ueda, K., Tsurimoto, T., Matsubara, K. 1991. Three envelope proteins of hepatitis B virus: large S, middle S, and major S proteins needed for the formation of Dane particles. J. Virol. 65:3521–3529.

49. Patzer, E. H., Nakamura, G. R., Yaffe, A. 1984. Intracellular transport and secretion of hepatitis B surface antigen in mammalian cells. J. Virol. 51:346–353.

50. Ulrich, P. P., Bhat, R. A., Seto, B., Mack, D., Sninsky, J., Vyas, G. N. 1989. Enzymatic amplification of hepatitis B virus DNA in serum compared to infectivity testing in chimpanzees. J. Infect. Dis. 160:37–43.

51. Bchini, R., Capel, F., Danguet, C., Dubanchet, S., Petit, M. A. 1990. In vitro infection of human hepatoma (HepG2) cells with hepatitis B virus. J. Virol. 64:3025–3030.

52. Gripon, P., Diot, C., Thezem, N., Fourel, I., Loreal, O., Brechot, C., Guguen-Guillouzo, C. 1988. Hepatitis B virus infection of adult human hepatocytes cultured in the presence of dimethyl sulfoxide. J. Virol. 62:4136–4143.

53. Ochiya, T., Tsurimoto, R., Ueda, K., Okubo, K., Shiozawa, M., Matsubara, K.

1989. An in vitro system for infection with hepatitis B virus that uses primary human fetal hepatocytes. Proc. Natl. Acad. Sci. USA 86:1875–1879.

54. Sells, M. A., Chen, M-L., Acs, G. 1987. Production of hepatitis B virus particles in Hep G2 cells transfected with cloned hepatitis B virus DNA. Proc. Natl. Acad. Sci. USA 84:1005–1009.

55. Neurath, A. R., Kent, S. B. H., Strick, N., Parker, K. 1986. Identification and chemical synthesis of a host cell receptor binding site on hepatitis B virus. Cell 46:429–436.

56. Petit, M-A., Dubanchet, S., Capel, F., Voet, P., Dauguet, C., Hauser, P. 1991. HepG2 cell binding activities of different hepatitis B virus isolates: inhibitory effect of anti-HBs and anti-preS1 (21–47). Virology 180:483–491.

57. Pontisso, P., Petit, M. A., Bankowski, M. J., Peeples, M. E. 1989. Human liver plasma membranes contain receptors for the hepatitis B virus pre-S1 region and, via polymerized human serum albumin, for the pre-S2 region. J. Virol. 63:1981–1988.

58. Pontisso, P., Ruvoletto, M. G., Gerlich, W. H., Heermann, K-H., Bardini, R., Alberti, A. 1989. Identification of an attachment site for human liver plasma membranes on hepatitis B virus particles. Virology 173:522–530.

59. Neurath, A. R., Strick, N., Sproul, P., Ralph, H. E., Valinsky, I. 1990. Detection of receptors for hepatitis B virus on cells of extrahepatic origin. Virology 176:448–457.

60. Pontisso, P., Gerlich, W. H., Bassi, N., Alberti, A. 1991. Molecular mimicry of hepatitis B virus. In: Viral Hepatitis and Liver Disease, Hollinger, F. B., Lemon, S. M., Margolis, H. S., eds., Williams & Wilkins, Baltimore, pp. 291–292.

61. Neurath, A. R., Strick, N. 1990. Antigenic mimicry of an immunoglobulin A epitope by a hepatitis B virus cell attachment site. Virology 178:631–634.

62. Neurath, A. R., Seto, B., Strick, N. 1989. Antibodies to synthetic peptides from the pre-S1 sequence of the hepatitis B virus (HBV) envelope *(env)* protein are virus neutralizing and protective. Vaccine 7:234–236.

63. Thornton, G. B., Moriarty, A. M., Milich, D. R., Eichberg, J. W., Purcell, R. H., Gerin, J. L. 1989. Protection of chimpanzees from hepatitis-B virus infection after immunization with synthetic peptides: identification of protective epitopes in the pre-S region. In: Vaccines 89: Modern Approaches to New Vaccines Including Prevention of AIDS, Lerner, R. A., Ginsberg, H., Chanock, R. M., Brown, F., eds. Cold Spring Harbor Laboratory, New York, p. 467.

64. Alberti, A., Cavaletto, D., Chemello, L., Belussi, F., Fattovich, G., Pontisso, P., Milanesi, G., Ruol, A. 1990. Fine specificity of human antibody response to the preS1 domain of hepatitis B virus. Hepatology 12:199–203.

65. Stibbe, W., Gerlich, W. H. 1982. Variable protein composition of hepatitis B surface antigen from different donors. Virology 123:436–442.

66. Machida, A., Kishimoto, S., Ohnuma, H., Baba, K., Ito, Y., Miyamoto, H., Funatsu, G., Oda, K. 1984. A polypeptide containing 55 amino acid residues coded by the preS region of hepatitis B virus deoxyribonucleic acid bears the receptor for polymerized human as well as chimpanzee albumins. Gastroenterology 86:910–918.

67. Trevisan, A., Gudat, F., Guggenheim, R., Krey, G., Dürmüller, V., Luond, G., Duggelin, M., Landmann, J., Rondelli, P., Bianchi, L. 1982. Demonstration of

albumin receptors on isolated human hepatocytes by light and scanning electron microscopy. Hepatology 2:832–839.

68. Neurath, A. R., Kent, S. B. H., Parker, K., Prince, A. M., Strick, N., Brotman, B., Sproul, P. 1986. Antibodies to a synthetic peptide from the preS 120–145 region of the hepatitis B virus envelope are virus-neutralizing. Vaccine 4:35–37.

69. Itoh, Y., Takai, E., Ohnuma, H., Kitajima, K., Tsuda, F., Machida, A., Mishiro, S., Nakamura, T., Miyakawa, Y., Mayumi, M. 1986. A synthetic peptide vaccine involving the product of the pre-S(2) region of hepatitis B virus DNA: protective efficacy in chimpanzees. Proc. Natl. Acad. Sci. USA 83:9174–9178.

70. Emini, E. A., Larson, V., Eichberg, J., Conard, P., Garsky, V. M., Lee, D. R., Ellis, R. W., Miller, W. J., Anderson, C. A., Gerety, R. J. 1989. Protective effect of a synthetic peptide comprising the complete preS2 region of the hepatitis B virus surface protein. J. Med. Virol. 28:7.

71. Yu, M. W., Finlayson, J. S., Shih, J. W. 1985. Interaction between various polymerized human albumins and hepatitis B surface antigen. J. Virol. 55:736–743.

72. De Wilde, M., Rutgers, T., Cabezon, T., Hauser, P., Van Opstal, O., Harford, N., et al. 1991. PreS-containing HBsAg particles from *Saccharomyces cerevisiae*: production, antigenicity and immunogenicity. In: Viral Hepatitis and Liver Disease, Hollinger, F. B., Lemon, S. M., Margolis, H. S., eds., Williams & Wilkins, Baltimore, pp. 732–736.

73. Heermann, K-H., Waldeck, F., Gerlich, W. H. 1988. Interaction between native human serum and the pre-S2 domain of hepatitis B virus surface antigen. In: Viral Hepatitis and Liver Disease, Zuckerman, A. J., ed., Alan R. Liss, Inc., New York, pp. 697–700.

74. Budkowska, A., Riottot, M. M., Dubreuil, P., Lazizi, Y., Brechot, C., Sobczak, E., Petit, M. A., Pillot, J. 1986. Monoclonal antibody recognizing pre-S(2) epitope of hepatitis B virus: characterization of pre-S(2) epitope and anti-preS(2) antibody. J. Med. Virol. 20:111–125.

75. Komai, K., Peeples, M. E., 1990. Physiology and function of the Vero cell receptor for the hepatitis B small S protein. Virology 177:332–338.

76. Leenders, W. H., Glansbeek, H. L., Bruin, W. C. C., Yap, S-H. 1990. Binding of the major and large HBsAg to human hepatocytes and liver plasma membranes: putative external and internal receptors for infection and secretion of hepatitis B virus. Hepatology 12:141–147.

77. Carman, W. F., Zanetti, A. R., Karayiannis, P., Waters, J., Manzillo, G., Tanzi, E., Zuckerman, A. J., Thomas, H. C. 1990. Vaccine-induced escape mutant of hepatitis B virus. Lancet 336:325–329.

78. Prince, A. M., Ikram, H., Hopp, T. P. 1982. Hepatitis B virus vaccine: identification of HBsAg/a and HBsAg/d but not HBsAg/y subtype antigenic determinants on a synthetic immunogenic peptide. Proc. Natl. Acad. Sci. USA 79:579–582.

79. Peterson, D. L., Paul, D. A., Lam, J., Tribby, I., Achord, D. T. 1984. Antigenic structure of hepatitis B surface antigen: identification of the "d" subtype determinant by chemical modification and use of monoclonal antibodies. J. Immunol. 132:920.

80. Okamoto, H., Tsuda, F., Sakugawa, H., Sastrosoewignijo, R. I., Imai, M., Miyakawa, Y., Mayumi, M. 1988. Typing hepatitis B virus by homology in

nucleotide sequence: comparison of surface antigen subtypes. J. Gen. Virol. 69:2575.

81. Mimms, L. T., Floreani, M., Tyner, I., Whitters, E., Rosenlof, R., Wray, L., Goetze, A., Sarin, V., Eble, K. 1990. Discrimination of hepatitis B virus (HBV) subtypes using monoclonal antibodies to preS1 and preS2 domains of the viral envelope. Virology 176:604–619.

82. Schlicht, H. J., Kuhn, C., Guhr, B., Mattaliano, R. J., Schaller, H. 1987. Biochemical and immunological characterization of the duck hepatitis B virus envelope proteins. J. Virol. 61:2280–2285.

83. Chang, C., Enders, G., Sprengel, R., Peters, N., Varmus, H. E., Ganem, D. 1987. Expression of the precore region of an avian hepatitis B virus is not required for viral replication. J. Virol. 61:3322–3325.

84. Mack, D. H., Block, W., Nath, N., Sninsky, J. J. 1988. Hepatitis B virus particles contain a polypeptide encoded by the largest open reading frame: a putative reverse transcriptase. J. Virol. 62:4786–4790.

85. Bavand, M., Feitelson, M., Laub, O. 1989. The hepatitis B virus-associated reverse transcriptase is encoded by the viral pol gene. J. Virol. 63:1019–1021.

86. Hirsch, R., Lavine, J., Chang, L., Varmus, H., Ganem, D. 1990. Polymerase gene products of hepatitis B virus are required for genomic RNA packaging as well as for reverse transcription. Nature 344:522–555.

87. Junker-Niepmann, M., Bartenschlager, R., Schaller, H. 1990. A short cis-acting sequence is required for hepatitis B virus pregenome encapsidation and sufficient for packing of foreign RNA. EMBO J. 9:3389–3396.

88. Köchel, H. G., Kann, M., Thomssen, R. 1991. Identification of a binding site in the hepatitis B virus RNA pregenome for the viral *pol* gene product. Virology 182:94–101.

89. Melegari, M., Bruss, V., Gerlich, W. H. 1991. The arginine-rich carboxy-terminal domain is necessary for RNA packaging by hepatitis B core protein. In: Viral Hepatitis and Liver Disease, Hollinger, F. B., Lemon, S. M., Margolis, H. S., eds., Williams & Wilkins, Baltimore, pp. 164–168.

90. Birnbaum, N., Nassal, M. 1990. Hepatitis B virus nucleocapsid assembly: Primary structure requirements in the core protein. J. Virol. 64:3319–3330.

91. Gallina, A., Bonelli, F., Zentilin, L., Rindi, G., Muttini, M., Milanesi, G. 1989. A recombinant hepatitis B core antigen polypeptide with the protamine-like domain deleted self-assembles into capsid particles but fails to bind nucleic acids. J. Virol. 63:4645–4652.

92. Uy, A., Bruss, V., Gerlich, W. H., Köchel, H. G., Thomssen, R. 1986. Pre-core sequence of hepatitis B virus inducing e-antigen and membrane association of the viral core protein. Virology 155:89–96.

93. Machida, A., Ohnuma, H., Tsuda, F., Yoshikawa, A., Hoshi, Y., Tanaka, T., Kishimoto, S., Akahane Y., Miyakawa, Y., Mayumi, M. 1991. Phosphorylation in the carboxyl-terminal domain of the capsid protein of hepatitis B virus: evaluation with a monoclonal antibody. J. Virol. 65:6024–6030.

94. Seeger, C., Summers, J., Mason, W. S. 1991. Viral DNA synthesis. In: Current Topics in Microbiology and Immunology 168, Hepadnaviruses, Mason, W. S., Seeger, C., eds., Springer, Berlin.

95. Jean-Jean, O., Levrero, M., Will, H., Perricaudet, M., Rossignol, J. M. 1989. Expression mechanism of the hepatitis B virus (HBV) C gene and biosynthesis of HBe antigen. Virology 170:99–106.

96. Möller, B., Hopf, U., Stemerowicz, R., Henze, G., Gelderblom, H. 1989. HBcAg expressed on the surface of circulating Dane particles in patients hepatitis B virus infection without evidence of anti-HBc formation. Hepatology 10:179–185.

97. Possehl, C., Repp, R., Heermann, K-H., Uy, A., Thomssen, R., Gerlich, W. H. 1992. Absence of free vore antigen in anti-HBc negative viremic hepatitis B carriers. Arch. Virol. Suppl. 4:39–41.

98. Whitten, T. M., Quats, A. T., Schloemer, R. H. 1991. Identification of the hepatitis B factor that inhibits expression of the beta interferon gene. J. Virol. 65:4599–4704.

99. Foster, G. R., Ackrill, A. M., Goldin, R. D., Kerr, I. M., Thomas, H. C., Stark, G. R. 1991. Expression of the terminal protein region of hepatitis B virus inhibits cellular responses to interferons α and γ and double-stranded RNA. Proc. Natl. Acad. Sci. USA 88:2888–2992.

100. Magnius, L. O., Espmark, J. A. 1972. New specificities in Australian antigen positive sera distinct from the Le Bouvier determinants. J. Immunol. 109:1017–1021.

101. Ou, J., Laub, O., Rutter, W. J. 1986. Hepatitis B virus gene function: the precore targets the core antigen to cellular membranes and causes the secretion of the antigen. Proc. Natl. Acad. Sci. USA 83:1578–1582.

102. Bruss, V., Gerlich, W. H. 1988. Formation of transmembranous hepatitis B e-antigen by cotranslational in vitro processing of the viral protein. Virology 163:268–275.

103. Standring, D. N., Ou, J-H., Masiarz, F. R., Rutter, W. J. 1988. A signal peptide encoded within the precore region of hepatitis B virus directs the secretion of a heterogeneous population of e antigens in Xenopus oocytes. Proc. Natl. Acad. Sci. USA 85:8405–8409.

104. Takahashi, K., Machida, A., Funatsu, G., Nomura M., Usuda, S. Aoyagi, S., Tachibana, K., Miyamoto, H., Imai, M., Nakamura, R., Miyakawa, Y., Mayumi, M. 1983. Immunochemical structure of hepatitis B e antigen in the serum. J. Immunol. 130:2903–2907.

105. Seifer, M., Heermann, K. H., Gerlich, W. H. 1990. Expression pattern of the hepatitis B virus genome in transfected mouse fibroblasts. Virology 179:287–299.

106. Garcia, P., Ou, J., Rutter, W. J., Walter, P. 1988. Targeting of protein of hepatitis B virus to the endoplasmic reticulum membrane: after signal peptide cleavage translocation can be aborted and the product released into the cytoplasm. Cell Biol. 106:1093–1104.

107. Ou, J-H., Yeh, C-T., Yen, T. S. B. 1989. Transport of hepatitis B virus precore protein into the nucleus after cleavage of its signal peptide. J. Virol. 63:5238–5243.

108. Schlicht, H. J., Schaller, H. 1989. The secretory core protein of human hepatitis B virus is expressed on the cell surface. J. Virol. 63:5399–5404.

109. Schlicht, H. J., Wasenauer, G. 1991. The quaternary structure, antigenicity and

aggregational behavior of the secretory core protein of human hepatitis B virus are determined by its signal sequence. J. Virol. 65:6817–6825.

110. Brunetto, M. A., Giarin, E., Oliveri, F., Chiaberge, E., Baldi, M., Alfarano, A., Serra, A., Saracco, G., Verme, G., Will, H., Bonino, F. 1991. Wild-type and e antigen deficient hepatitis B viruses and course of chronic hepatitis. Proc. Natl. Acad. Sci. USA 88:1186–1190.

111. Bertoletti, A., Ferrari, C., Fiaccadori, F., Penna, A., Margolskee, R., Schlicht, H. J., Fowler, P., Guilhot, S., Chisari, F. 1991. HLA class I-restricted human cytotoxic T cells recognize endogenously synthesized hepatitis B virus nucleocapsid antigen. Proc. Natl. Acad. Sci. USA 88:10445–10449.

112. Milich, D. R., Jones, J. E., Hughes, J. L., Price, J., Raney, A. K., McLachlan, A. 1990. Is a function of the secreted hepatitis B e antigen to induce immunologic tolerance in utero? Proc. Natl. Acad. Sci. USA 87:6599–6603.

113. Hu, K-Q., Vierling J. M., Siddiqui, A. 1990. Transactivation of HLA-DR gene by hepatitis B X gene product. Proc. Natl. Acad. Sci. USA 87:7140–7144.

114. Yaginuma, K., Shirakata, Y., Kobayashi, M., Koike, K. 1987. Hepatitis B virus (HBV) particles are produced in a cell culture system by transient expression of transfected HBV DNA. Proc. Natl. Acad. Sci. USA 84:2678–2682.

115. Twu, J. S., Robinson, W. S. 1989. Hepatitis B virus X gene can transactivate heterologous viral sequences. Proc. Natl. Acad. Sci. USA 86:2046–2050.

116. Twu, J. S., Schloemer, R. H. 1987. Transcriptional transacting function of hepatitis B virus. J. Virol. 61:3448–3453.

117. Zahm, P., Hofschneider, P. H., Koshy, R. 1988. The HBV X-ORF encodes a transactivator: a potential factor in viral hepatocarcinogenesis. Oncogene 3:169–177.

118. Maguire, H. F., Hoeffler, J. P., Siddiqui, A. 1991. HBV X protein alters the DNA binding specificity of CREB and ATF-2 by protein-protein interactions. Science 252:842–844.

119. Wollersheim, M., Debelka, U., Hofschneider, P. H. 1988. A transactivating function encoded in the hepatitis B virus X gene is conserved in the integrated state. Oncogene 3:545–554.

120. Kim, C-M., Koike, K., Saito, I., Miyamura, T., Jay, G. 1991. HBx gene of hepatitis B virus induces liver cancer in transgenic mice. Nature 351:317–320.

121. Höhne, M., Schaefer, S., Seifer, M., Feitelson, M. A., Paul, D., Gerlich, W. H. 1990. Malignant transformation of immortalized transgenic hepatocytes after transfection with hepatitis B virus DNA. EMBO J. 9:1137–1145.

122. Seifer, M., Höhne, M., Schaefer, S., Gerlich, W. H. 1991. Malignant transformation of immortalized cells by hepatitis B virus DNA. In: Viral Hepatitis and Liver Disease, Hollinger, F. B., Lemon, S. M., Margolis, H. S., eds., Williams & Wilkins, Baltimore, pp. 586–588.

123. Seifer, M., Höhne, M., Schaefer, S., Gerlich, W. H. 1992. In vitro-tumorigenicity of hepatitis B virus DNA and HBx protein. J. Hepatol. 13(Suppl. 4):S61–S65.

124. Iwarson, S., Tabor, E., Thomas, H. C., Goodall, A., Waters, J., Snoy, P., Shih, J. W., Gerety, R. J. 1985. Neutralization of hepatitis B virus infectivity by a murine monoclonal antibody: an experimental study in the chimpanzee. J. Med. Virol. 16:89–96.

125. Hauser, P., Thomas, H. C., Water, J., Simoen, E., Voet, P., DeWilde, M., Stephenne, J., Pétre, J. 1988. Induction of neutralizing antibodies in chimpanzees and humans by a recombinant yeast-derived hepatitis B surface antigen particle. In: Viral Hepatitis and Liver Disease, Zuckerman, A. J., ed., Alan R. Liss, p. 1031–1037.

126. Poovorawan, Y., Sanpavat, S., Pongpunlert, W., et al. 1990. Comparison of a recombinant DNA hepatitis vaccine alone or in combination with hepatitis B immune globulin for the prevention of perinatal acquisition of hepatitis B carriage. Vaccine 1990:556.

127. Iwarson, S., Wahl, M., Ruttimann, E., Snoy, P., Seto, B., Gerety, R. J. 1988. Successful postexposure vaccination against hepatitis B in chimpanzees. J. Med. Virol. 25:433–439.

128. Wahl, M., Iwarson, S., Snoy, P., Gerety, R. H. 1989. Failure of hepatitis B immune globulin to protect against experimental infection in chimpanzees. J. Hepatol. 9:198–203.

129. Celis, E., Kato, I., Miller, R. W. 1985. Regulation of the human immune response to HBsAg: effects of antibodies and antigen conformation in the stimulation of helper T cells by HBsAg. Hepatology 5:744–751.

130. Delpeyroux, F., Peilon, N., Blondel, B., Crainic, R., Streek, R. E. 1988. Presentation and immunogenicity of the hepatitis B surface antigen and poliovirus neutralization antigen on mixed empty envelope particles. J. Virol. 62:1836–1839.

131. Milich, D. R., McLachlan, A., Chisari, F. V., Nakamura, T., Thornton, G. B. 1986. Two distinct but overlapping antibody binding sites in the pre-S(2) region of HBsAg localized within 11 continuous residues. J. Immunol. 137:2703–2710.

132. Tron, F., Degos, F., Bréchot, C., Courouce, A-M., Goudeau, A., Marie, F-N., Adamowicz, P., Saliou, P., Laplanche, A., Benhamou, J-P., Girard, M. 1989. Randomized dose range study of a recombinant hepatitis B vaccine produced in mammalian cells and containing the S and preS2 sequences. J. Inf. Dis. 160:199–203.

133. Miskovsky, E., Gershman, K., Clements, M. L., Cupps, T., Calandra, G., Hesley, T., et al. 1991. Comparative safety and immunogenicity of yeast recombinant hepatitis B vaccines containing S and pre-S2+S antigens. Vaccine 9:346–350.

134. Kuroda, S., Fujisawa, Y., Iino, S., Akahane, Y., Suzuki, H. 1991. Induction of protection level of anti-pre-S2 antibodies in humans immunized with a novel hepatitis B vaccine consisting of M (pre-S2 + S) protein particles (a third generation vaccine). Vaccine 9:163–169.

135. Ferrari, C., Penna, A., Bertoletti, A., Cavalli, A., Valli, A., Schianchi, C., Fiaccadori, F. 1989. The preS1 antigen of hepatitis B virus is highly immunogenic at the T cell level in man. J. Clin. Invest. 84:1314–1319.

136. Thoma, H. A., Hemmerling, A. E., Koller, E., Kapfer, G. 1991. Does PreS2 have the same effect in improving the HBV immune response as PreS1? In: Viral Hepatitis and Liver Disease, Hollinger, F. B., Lemon, S. M., Margolis, H. S., eds., Williams & Wilkins, Baltimore, pp. 736–741.

137. Deepen, R., Heermann, K-H., Uy, A., Thomssen, R., Gerlich, W. H. 1990. Assay of preS epitopes and preS1 antibody in hepatitis B virus carriers and immune persons. Med. Microbiol. Immunol. 179:49–60.

138. Iwarson, S., Tabor, E., Thomas, H. C., Snoy, P., Gerety, R. J. 1985. Protection against hepatitis B virus infection by immunization with hepatitis B core antigen. Gastroenterology 88:763.

139. Murray, K., Bruce, S. A., Hinnen, A., Wingfield, P., van Erd P. M.C.A., de Reus, A., Schellekens, H. 1984. Hepatitis B virus antigens made in microbial cells immunise against viral infection. EMBO J. 3:645–651.

140. Murray, K., Bruce, S. A., Wingfield, P., van Erd, P., de Reus, A., Schellekens, H. 1987. Protective immunisation against hepatitis B with an internal antigen of the virus. J. Med. Virol. 23:101.

141. Fuchs, K., Schödel, D, Manneck, K., Neckermann, G., Will, H., Roggendorf, M. 1991. Protection from infection with woodchuck hepatitis virus (WHV) by immunization with recombinant core protein of WHV and HBV. In: Viral Hepatitis and Liver Disease, Hollinger, F. B., Lemon, S. M., Margolis, H. S., eds., Williams & Wilkins, Baltimore, pp. 267–270.

142. Milich, D. R., McLachlan, A., Thornton, G. B., Hughes, J. L. 1987. Antibody production to the nucleocapsid and envelope of hepatitis B virus primed by a single synthetic T cell site. Nature 329:547–549.

143. Schödel, F., Moriarty, A. M., Peterson, D. L., Zheng, J., Hughes, J. L., Will, H., et al. 1992. The position of heterologous epitopes inserted in hepatitis B virus core particles determines their immunogenicity. J. Virol. 66:106–114.

144. Brown, A. L., Francis, M. J., Hastings, G. Z., Parry, N. R., Barnett, P. V., Rowlands, D. J., Clarke, B. E. 1991. Foreign epitopes in immunodominant regions of hepatitis B core particles are highly immunogenic and conformationally restricted. Vaccine 9:595–601.

145. Schödel, F. 1990. Oral vaccination using recombinant bacteria. Semin. Immunol. 2:341–349.

4

Survey of Licensed Hepatitis B Vaccines and Their Production Processes

Robert D. Sitrin, D. Eugene Wampler, and Ronald W. Ellis

Merck Research Laboratories,
West Point, Pennsylvania

I. INTRODUCTION

Hepatitis B vaccine first became available for routine use in 1981 with the licensure of a plasma-derived vaccine (HEPTAVAX B®, Merck Sharp & Dohme) in the United States. By the mid-1980s, this and other plasma-derived vaccines became available worldwide. The production process for this vaccine (reviewed in Chapter 2 of this volume) was state-of-the-art and unique to any vaccine at that time, given that the biological source material was highly infectious for hepatitis B. Despite its excellent efficacy and safety profile in millions of individuals worldwide, acceptance of the vaccine was slow. The process used was rather cumbersome and time-consuming, with a manufacturing cycle of as long as one year. Furthermore, availability of suitably qualified donors of HBsAg-containing plasma has limited the production of vaccine for use worldwide. Therefore, a need was recognized for a second-generation hepatitis B vaccine. This need was fulfilled beginning in 1986 by the licensure of recombinant DNA (rDNA)–derived vaccines, which rendered the plasma-derived vaccines generally obsolete. Nevertheless, plasma-derived vaccines are still available in many countries of the world (Table 1). However, it is likely that production and distribution of these plasma-derived vaccines will be discontinued during the 1990s, as was the plasma-derived vaccine in the United States in the late 1980s.

As shown in Table 1, all of the vaccines produced today can be classified by

Table 1 Survey of Commercially Available Hepatitis B Vaccines

Trade name of vaccine	Source	Manufacturer	Where licensed
ENGERIX B®	yeast	SmithKline Beecham	United States, E.E.C.[d], other Europe, Far East[e], other worldwide[f]
RECOMBIVAX HB[®a]/H-B-VAX II[®b]	yeast	Merck	United States, E.E.C.[d], Japan, other Europe, other worldwide[f]
BIMMUGEN®	yeast	Kaketsuken	Japan, Far East
EICHI-BI-WAI®	yeast	Green Cross	Japan
HEPRECOMB®	yeast	Berna	Switzerland, Colombia
GENHEVAC B®	mammalian[c]	Pasteur-Merieux	France, Argentina
r-HB VACCINE®	mammalian[c]	Mitsubishi	Japan
HEVAC B®	plasma	Pasteur-Merieux	E.E.C.[d], Far East[e], other[g]
HB VACCINE MIDORI®	plasma	Green Cross (Japan)	Japan
HEPAVAX B®	plasma	Green Cross (Korea)	Far East[e]
HB VACCINE-HOKKEN®	plasma	Kitasato	Japan
HEPACCINE B®	plasma	Cheil Sugar	Far East[e], other[g]

[a]Trade name in United States only.
[b]Trade name elsewhere in the world.
[c]Chinese hamster ovary cells.
[d]Generally available throughout European Economic Community.
[e]Excluding Japan.
[f]Available in Canada, other developed countries, and many developing countries.
[g]Available in many developing countries.

the nature of the antigen source: plasma, yeast, or mammalian cell culture. Subsequent purification strategies follow in part from this choice of antigen source. This chapter will focus on the two major technology improvements that have led to second-generation hepatitis B vaccines: the use of recombinant organisms for antigen production and the application of more efficient processes for its isolation and purification. As background on the development of this modern purification technology, some discussion of early purification work is presented.

II. USE OF RECOMBINANT DNA TECHNOLOGY FOR ANTIGEN EXPRESSION

A. Overview of Alternative Expression Systems

Research toward alternative sources for second-generation hepatitis B vaccines began in the late 1970s as restrictions on the routine laboratory use of rDNA technology were relaxed. This work culminated in the early 1980s with the identification of the HBV S gene, which encodes the surface antigen (HBsAg), and with the expression in yeast and mammalian cells of the recombinant S gene as 22-nm HBsAg particles, as reviewed in Chapter 3. Both yeast-derived and mammalian cell–derived [Chinese hamster ovary (CHO) cells] recombinant vaccines were developed and licensed during the 1980s. Both recombinant vaccines are effective at eliciting high titers of protective anti-HBs antibodies in vaccinees. However, processes based on recombinant yeast generally have been more productive. Also, there was originally less concern for the perceived safety of residual DNA in the yeast-derived compared to mammalian-derived product (1), although adequate DNA clearance can be readily demonstrated for both processes. As a result, most of the second-generation hepatitis B vaccine supplied worldwide is derived from recombinant strains of bakers' yeast, *Saccharomyces cerevisiae*.

The major hepatitis B vaccines available worldwide are listed in Table 1. Two yeast-derived vaccines (ENGERIX B® and RECOMBIVAX HB®/H-B-VAX II®) are licensed in most countries. Three other yeast-derived and two mammalian cell–derived vaccines are licensed in a few countries. All licensed recombinant vaccines consist of the 226-amino-acid S gene product (major surface protein) of HBV, except for GENHEVAC B®, which consists of the 281-amino-acid PreS2 + S gene product (the middle surface protein) (see Chapter 3).

B. Expression in Yeast

The yeast expression systems for HBsAg are similar and typical of systems commonly used for *S. cerevisiae* (2–5). Expression systems use plasmids containing part or all of the yeast 2-μm sequences, which enable amplification to multiple copies, often as high as 100–200 copies per cell (6). Such plasmids are autonomously replicating DNA molecules in the yeast nucleus and contain genes that select for plasmid retention in appropriate host strains, such as the *LEU2* gene for selection in leucine-deficient (leu⁻) strains (7). The expression cassette consists of a strong yeast-derived transcriptional promoter, the HBV S gene and a yeast-derived transcriptional termination sequence. The promoters used include both constitutively active ones, which express HBsAg throughout the fermentation of recombinant yeast (8), as well as inducible ones for which expression of the HBsAg is initiated only upon addition of an inducer [e.g., galactose for the *GAL*1 promoter (9)] or depletion of a medium component [e.g., phosphate for the *PHO*5 promoter (10)]. In addition, the plasmid contains elements that enable their construction and amplification in *Escherichia coli*. The structure of a typical yeast expression plasmid for HBsAg is shown in Figure 1A.

C. Expression in Mammalian Cells

The mammalian expression systems for HBsAg (11) are conceptually similar in design to those used in yeast. The expression cassette consists of a strong mammalian cell-derived transcriptional promoter, the HBV S gene (r-HB VACCINE) or the PreS2 + S gene (GENHEVAC B), and mammalian transcriptional termination sequences. The plasmids also contain a sequence for amplification to multiple copies, in these cases the gene for dihydrofolate reductase (DHFR), which will amplify in dhfr⁻ CHO cells (12) in the presence of the drug methotrexate (13). Similar to yeast, these plasmids also contain appropriate *E. coli* sequences (Fig. 1B). However, the plasmid integrates randomly into the mammalian host cell chromosome, in which configuration it is amplified to multiple copies, often as high as 100 (14).

III. STRATEGIES FOR HBsAg PURIFICATION

A. Particle Assembly

Purifying HBsAg from any source offers a significant process challenge quite different from that of other recombinant proteins because the desired product is not a simple 24-kilodalton (kD) polypeptide but rather a complex of polypeptides assembled with host-derived lipids into 22-nm spherical particles, each containing about 100 polypeptides (Fig. 2). Fortunately, this complex assembly is carried out by the producing cell (yeast, mammalian, or infected carrier liver cells) as the polypeptide is expressed. For yeast, this is evident from the fact that intact particles can be detected in fresh lysates by a radioimmunoassay that is specific for assembled antigen as well as by sucrose gradient centrifugation (2,15). Although in the yeast lysate the particle is only loosely held together by hydrophobic interaction, during purification intermolecular disulfide bonds form

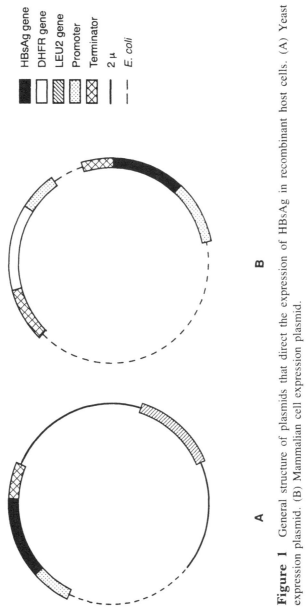

Figure 1 General structure of plasmids that direct the expression of HBsAg in recombinant host cells. (A) Yeast expression plasmid. (B) Mammalian cell expression plasmid.

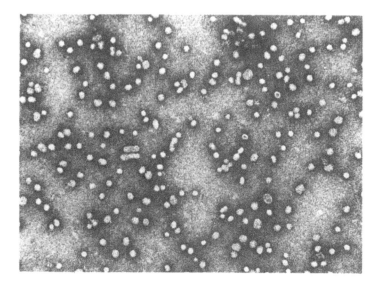

Figure 2 Electron micrograph of hepatitis B vaccine antigen derived from recombinant yeast (×130,000).

which effectively cross-link and fuse the structure into the discrete particle. The particles secreted by mammalian cells or isolated from serum are completely cross-linked at the start of the purification process and can be subjected to more robust conditions. Attempts to purify the constituent 24-kD polypeptide and reconstitute the antigen particle have been unsuccessful (16,17). This also explains the inability to use *E. coli* as an expression system for HBsAg, as the polypeptide fails to assembly into a particle in vivo and instead suffers metabolic degradation.

B.   Analytical Procedures

Before discussing the purfication procedures that have been developed, it is prudent to mention the in-process assays that are essential for monitoring the purification process, especially during the process-development stages. Since the amount of antigen in the starting menstrum (plasma, yeast lysate, or mammalian cell culture fluid) is only about 1% of the total protein, direct analysis can be done only with antibody-based assays in either an enzyme-linked immunosorbent assay (ELISA) or radioimmunoassay (RIA) format. High performance liquid chromatography [HPLC (18)] and sodium dodecyl sulfate–polyacrylamide gel electrophoresis (SDS-PAGE) methods are not specific enough to detect the antigen in very crude preparations. Immunoblot (Western) analysis is also applicable, but this is a very laborious test and at best is only semi-quantitative. Of course HPLC and SDS-PAGE may be used to monitoring purification at later stages, when the antigen is the primary component of the feed-stream. The published HPLC technique (18) as shown in Figure 3 is a size exclusion assay for the intact particle, whereas the SDS-PAGE analysis examines the 24-kD polypeptide. A reversed-phase HPLC analysis on the particle or polypeptide has not yet been reported. Recently the use of capillary zonal electrophoresis has been described to monitor the purification of HBsAg (19).

C.   Early Approaches to HBsAg Purification

Early attempts to prepare vaccines from serum helped to define the basic biochemical properties of HBsAg, which included its heat stability, large size and density, adsorption affinity onto colloidal silica, and chromatographic behavior. Many of these general principles have been incorporated into purification schemes for HBsAg from recombinant sources.

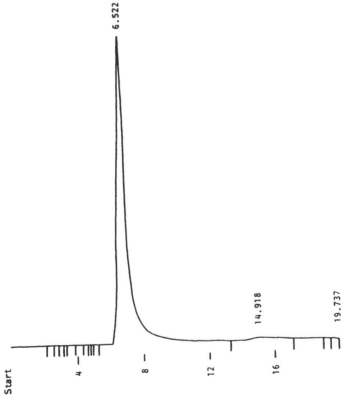

Figure 3   HPLC assay for HBsAg. A 20 - μg sample injected onto a TSK G3000 SW column eluted with phosphate buffer saline, monitored by UV. HBsAg peak is at 6.522 minutes. (From Ref. 18 with permission.)

1. Heat Stability

The first vaccine to be used against hepatitis B infection (20) was used to protect institutionalized children at the Willowbrook State School where hepatitis B was endemic. To prepare this vaccine, Krugman took a sample of human serum known to be infectious for hepatitis B, diluted it 10-fold with distilled water and boiled it for one minute. Although noninfectious, it was surprisingly antigenic. This "primitive" method of heat-inactivating the virus in antigen-containing plasma has been further developed by Prince at the New York Blood Center and has been used as an industrial scale process in the Netherlands and Korea (see below). This purification by differential thermal stability is pasteurizing with relatively little purification, similar to a process used to pasteurize albumin.

2. Size and Density

In the late 1960s and early 1970s, Gerin exploited the unusual size and density of the HBsAg particle to develop a purification process based on centrifugation (21,22). Since the infectious virus (Dane particle) contains DNA, it is considerably more dense than the HBsAg particle, and at the same time, because of its lipid component, the antigen is less dense ($\rho = 1.20$ g/ml) than most plasma proteins. Thus, the desired antigen can be largely separated from the infectious component and most other plasma proteins by equilibrium (isopycnic) centrifugation in a cesium chloride or sodium bromide gradient. Although the procedures are developed from equilibrium experiments, in the manufacturing situation the centrifugation is not held long enough to achieve true density equilibrium. At the same time, HBsAg has a larger sedimentation coefficient than most plasma proteins, and additional separation is accomplished by rate-zonal centrifugation in a sucrose gradient. The combination of isopycnic and rate-zonal centrifugation has developed into the predominant process for purifying HBsAg from human plasma.

3. Adsorption to Aerosil

While developing methods for stabilizing human serum, Stephan introduced the use of Aerosil (fused silica) to adsorb lipoproteins (23,24). Siebke et al. (25) applied this idea to the adsorption of HBsAg as an approach to removing the HBV from donated plasma. Finally, Pillot et al. (26) and Duimel and Krijnen (27) refined the method, including elution with borate buffer at elevated pH, for the particular purpose of purifying HBsAg. Based on our own studies, HBsAg appears to adsorb by a mixed mechanism, with the very specific elution conditions causing a change on the silica surface resulting in elution of the antigen by ion repulsion (28).

4. General Chromatographic Behavior

Chromatographic methods are common in biochemical purification schemes. Because of the large size of the HBsAg particle, size exclusion chromatography was a natural choice and was used in some of the early processes. Unfortunately, on a manufacturing scale a very large column is needed except at the final stages of the process when the sample size is small. Ion exchange chromatography has also been tried (Wampler and Harder, unpublished experiments) but, perhaps because of charge heterogeneity, gradient elution spreads the antigen over a wide region with poor resolution from other components.

5. Immunoaffinity Chromatography

By the mid-1970s, several laboratories were using immunoaffinity chromatography to isolate HBsAg (29–31). Houwen used two columns, the first containing guinea pig anti-HBs attached to Sepharose eluted with 3 M NaSCN and the second containing rabbit anti-human serum antibodies designed to remove residual serum proteins. Antigen was isolated from low titer (titers of 1:64 to 1:128) serum and was sufficiently pure that human serum proteins could not be detected by passive hemagglutination. Immunoaffinity chromatography with a single column was used in some of the early work on yeast-derived HBsAg (32). The antibody in this column was purified from goats that had been immunized with HBsAg isolated from human plasma. The specific anti-HBs antibodies were further purified by passing the goat IgG over an affinity column containing plasma-derived HBsAg. This approach, of using an antigen from one source to prepare antibody for purification of antigen from a different source, ensured that the final affinity column would not contain antibodies to yeast impurities. Although antigen prepared by this method contained no contaminating proteins as measured by conventional methods, it did occasionally give a positive test in sensitive guinea pig anaphylaxis test for goat antibodies. The detection limit of this test was less than 0.001%, but the concern over possible adverse reactions prevented this process from being used to produce commercial vaccine.

D. Summary of Purification Strategies

This early work helped to define the properties of the antigen particle so that rational purification processes could be developed that exploited its unique properties, including:

Size—22 nm in diameter, much larger than most biological molecules but smaller than whole cells, suggesting the use of membrane filtration for purification.

Hydrophobicity—suggesting the use of fractional precipitation with ammonium sulfate or polyethylene glycol (PEG) and hydrophobic interaction chromatography.

Heat resistance—although high temperature and extended time (e.g., 60°C for 60 hours) were originally used to inactivate HBV in plasma fractions, milder conditions can be used to purify the antigen. This approach forms the basis for the Krugman and Prince procedures.

Protease resistance—the HBsAg particle is resistant to pepsin treatment at pH 2, allowing the use of pepsin to degrade contaminants.

Density—because of the high lipid content, the HBsAg particle has density of about 1.20 g/ml vs. typical protein densities of 1.35 g/ml (33).

Biochemical structure—like all biological products, the HBsAg particle can be recognized by biological ligands using antibodies, plant lectins (34), or polymerized human albumin (35).

E.   Vaccines Derived from Human Plasma

1.   Merck Process

The first commercial processes for manufacturing hepatitis B vaccine were based on Gerin's centrifugation procedure. In the Merck process described in detail in Chapter 1, after plasma is converted to serum, the precentrifugation steps (ammonium sulfate fractionation and ultrafiltration) reduced the process volume so that more material can be processed through the cumbersome, labor-intensive, centrifugation steps. The remaining steps (pepsin, urea treatment, and ultrafiltration) are designed to remove minor contaminants, particularly albumin, and, along with formaldehyde treatment, to inactivate any bloodborne pathogens that might be in the product (see Chapter 1).

2.   Institut Pasteur

The process developed by the Institut Pasteur (36) is also based on centrifugation. In this case, however, fractional precipitation is done with PEG in place of ammonium sulfate (Fig. 4). Also, each centrifugation step is performed twice instead of once with concentration by ultrafiltration between the centrifugation steps.

3.   New York Blood Center

The New York Blood Center has developed a process that uses heat instead of chemical or enzymatic inactivation (37). The strategy here is to avoid "harsh" treatment that might reduce antigenic potency. As before, the steps preceding centrifugation serve to reduce volume, in this case from 100 to 0.3 liters. The fractional precipitation with PEG was again used but with the addition of an hydroxyapatite step. This same basic process has been used to prepare vaccine in the Netherlands (38) and by the Green Cross Corporation in Korea (39).

F.   Purification from Yeast

Although prior experience existed for purification of HBsAg from human plasma, significant purification process development needed to be carried out in order to obtain material from recombinant yeast where the product is intracellular, membrane bound, and present as a relatively minor constituent (<5%)

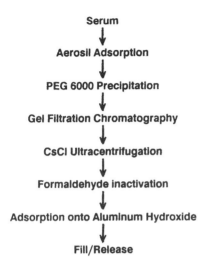

Serum
↓
Aerosil Adsorption
↓
PEG 6000 Precipitation
↓
Gel Filtration Chromatography
↓
CsCl Ultracentrifugation
↓
Formaldehyde inactivation
↓
Adsorption onto Aluminum Hydroxide
↓
Fill/Release

Figure 4 Purification scheme for Institut Pasteur serum-derived vaccine.

among yeast proteins, nucleic acids, and lipids. Whereas the focus of vaccine production from serum is on inactivation of viral contaminants, the emphasis in the purification strategy for isolation from yeast and cell culture is to remove the host cell and media constituents. Although some purification steps such as hydrophobic interaction, size exclusion, and ion exchange chromatography are similar to those used for recombinant proteins in general, several unique technologies such as ultrafiltration and ultracentrifugation have been employed because of the large size and unique density of the antigen particle.

IV. CURRENT MANUFACTURING PROCESSES

A. Antigen Production

1. Seed Lot System

The manufacturing process for recombinant vaccines begins with the creation of a Master Cell Bank. Following transformation of yeast or mammalian cells with the HBsAg expression plasmid, recombinant cells expressing HBsAg are identified and expanded. These cells are then taken through one or two rounds of single-cell cloning, and a clone with the best combination of HBsAg expression levels and stability of HBsAg expression in fermentation scale-up is selected. The selected clone is explanded in cell number to a point where the cells can be aliquoted in parallel to a number of vials (typically 25–100), which are stored frozen, usually at –70°C or colder. These vials are referred to as the *Master Cell Bank*. Subsequently, cells in one or more vials are expanded to a point where they are aliquoted in parallel to a larger number of vials (typically 100–500), which also are frozen. These vials are referred to as the *Manufacturer's Working Cell Bank*. Cells cultivated from one or more of these vials are used as the uniform source of all production cultures. When a given working cell bank is exhausted, another is prepared from one or more vials of the Master Cell Bank. This seed-lot system, used for the manufacture of all biological products, assures the genetic identity and consistency of each production lot. The characterization and control of the master and working cell banks and their scale-up to production cultures are outlined in Chapter 5. A recombinant yeast clone is expanded directly to the Master Cell Bank without any special manipulation. However, CHO cells, which are maintained as an attached cell line in cell culture, are grown most efficiently and productively in suspension in large fermenters. Therefore, the cells are brought to the stage of single-cell cloning as attached cells, then are adapted to grow in suspension culture. Once this adaptation is complete, the cells are preserved in the Master Cell Bank.

2. Production

Production cultures of yeast or mammalian cells producing HBsAg are initiated by thawing one or more vials of the working cell bank for each production run. Yeast cells are initially cultivated on agar plates or in small shake flasks, then transferred to larger shake flasks, small fermentors, and then to the final fermentor. The precise steps used during the culture scale-up phase vary among manufacturers, although the final production fermentor is typically in the range of 1000 liters. The growth medium may be either chemically complex, semi-defined, or chemically defined in nature. The medium may be defined according to the auxotrophies of the host strain and may be deficient in leucine to maintain selective pressure on the leu^+ plasmid in a leu^- host strain (other selection systems also may be used). An inducer, e.g., galactose, may be added to the final fermentor to induce expression from a regulatable promoter. Analogously, recombinant mammalian cells are cultivated initially in small T-flasks, then in larger T-flasks or roller bottles, then either in a small fermentor for inoculation to the final production fermentor or directly into the final production fermentor, which may be of the same scale as production fermentors for yeast. The fermentors are usually of the stirred tank design, which maintain the CHO cells in suspension during production.

The production fermentation may last from several days to 1–2 weeks, depending on the scale and cell inoculum size that achieve maximal HBsAg productivity. Since HBsAg accumulates within recombinant yeast cells, the final production fermentor is harvested, and the cells are separated from the medium by filtration or centrifugation and washed. Cells may then be stored frozen or immediately lysed for HBsAg purification. In contrast, HBsAg is secreted by recombinant mammalian cells, so that the final batch of growth medium is separated from the cells as the initial stage in HBsAg purification.

B.   Isolation/Purification

A variety of the previously described technologies have been used to prepare HBsAg for commercial use. Because of the relatively low dosage level and modest scale of production, the licensed processes are based by and large on the original laboratory procedures first used to prepare vaccine for clinical trials. Table 2 is a summary of process steps used in the various commercial vaccines. The purification processes for three of the major vaccines will be described in further detail below.

1.   RECOMBIVAX HB/H-B-VAX II

The purification scheme used for RECOMBIVAX HB is shown in Figure 5 (15). The cells are separated from the fermentation broth by microfiltration and lysed by passing through a high-pressure homogenizer to release the antigen. To prevent proteolytic degradation of the protein in the antigen particle, phenyl-methylsulfonyl fluoride is added to the cell suspension just before lysis. Prior to removing the cell debris, the antigen is solubilized by adding a Triton X-100 detergent. The crude lysate is clarified by microfiltration using 0.2-μm hollow

Table 2 Summary of Manufacturing Steps Used in Industrial-Scale Manufacturing Processes

	Manufacturer					
	Plasma-derived			Recombinant-DNA-derived		
Process step	Merck	Pasteur	New York Blood Center	Merck	SK/RIT	Pasteur-Merieux
Heating			+			+
Isopycnic centrifugation	+	+	+			+
Rate-zonal centrifugation	+	+				
$(NH_4)_2SO_4$ fractionation	+					+
PEG fractionation		+	+			+
Ultrafiltration	+	+		+	+	
Chromatography						
Size exclusion		+			+	+
Anion exchange					+	
Hydrophobic interaction				+		
Adsorption to Silica				+		+
8 M Urea	+					
Formaldehyde treatment	+	+		+		+

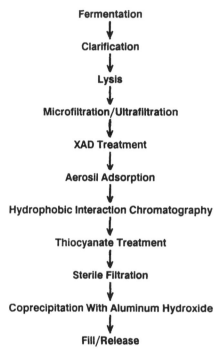

Figure 5   Purification scheme for RECOMBIVAX HB.

fiber cartridges, which pass the antigen into the filtrate along with most of the low molecular weight host cell constituents, leaving debris and unbroken cells in the retentate, which is discarded. This filtrate is concentrated and further purified by ultrafiltration with a 100-kD molecular weight cutoff hollow fiber system, which retains the antigen but allows the lower molecular weight host constituents to pass through. The use of the micro- and ultra filtration sandwiching technique provides an effective purification step, which can be readily carried out in contained equipment and takes advantage of the unusual size of the antigen particle as compared to yeast cell wall debris and soluble proteins (40).

Residual Triton X-100 is removed by adsorption onto polystyrene beads (XAD-4) and antigen is isolated from the lysate by adsorption onto colloidal silica (Aerosil). After the appropriate washes, antigen is eluted from the silica by treatment with warm borate buffer. Recent studies from our laboratories (28) have shown that antigen adsorbs to bare silica by a mixed mode and is specifically eluted by a chemical interaction between the silica surface and borate ion. After a final polishing purification step by hydrophobic interaction chromatography on butyl agarose, the purified antigen is treated with thiocyanate to complete disulfide cross-linking, and the diafiltered product is sterilized by filtration through an 0.22-μm membrane. Formulation of the antigen into a vaccine is carried out by coprecipitation with aluminum hydroxide.

The final hepatitis B vaccine antigen is a purified preparation of 22-nm lipoprotein particles containing S polypeptides (see Fig. 2). Each particle is composed of about 100 polypeptides intercalated with host cell lipids. The S protein expressed in yeast is a 24-kD nonglycosylated polypeptide (2,16). Purity of the final product is confirmed by SDS-PAGE analysis as well as SDS-HPLC analysis for residual yeast protein, both of which show a protein purity of >99% (41). Identity is confirmed by SDS-PAGE as well as by AUSRIA assay. Concentration for dosage determination is measured by Lowry protein with potency confirmed by EIA and mouse potency tests. The released bulks are filled aseptically and released in final dosage form after appropriate testing for pH, sterility, safety, potency, etc.

2. ENGERIX B

The other major commercially available hepatitis B vaccine, ENGERIX B, is also produced in yeast and is structurally and chemically similar to RECOM-BIVAX HB. Its reported purification scheme, shown in Figure 6, is taken from recent publications (18,42). Yeast cells are disrupted in a bead mill, antigen is extracted with a detergent, presumably Tween-80 (43), and debris removed by centrifugation. The clarified product is concentrated by ultrafiltration and purified by size exclusion chromatography followed by anion exchange chromatography to remove nucleic acids and further purified by isopycnic ultracentrifugation in a CsCl gradient followed by a desalting step (43). The final bulk product is sterile filtered and adsorbed onto alumina. Purity is judged on the basis of HPLC analysis as well as SDS-PAGE with Coomassie staining and is reported to be >98%. Identity and potency are confirmed by animal models as well as response to monoclonal antibodies.

3. GENHEVAC B

The purification process for GENHEVAC B has not been published, although an early description of a research-scale purification has been described (44). A pilot-scale process developed by Pharmacia LKB Biotechnology AB and the China National Center for Biotechnology Development was published (45). The process involves three column chromatography steps, butyl Sepharose, anion exchange, and SEC, and results in a product that is free of DNA and calf serum proteins. Recovery is about 40% over an approximately 800-fold purification. The principal innovation is the use of a new type of butyl Sepharose column matrix.

The S protein expressed in mammalian cells (46) is a mixture of 24-kD nonglycosylated and 27-kD glycosylated species (ca. 4 : 1 ratio), the latter with a

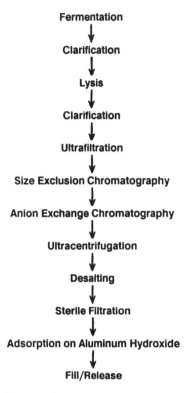

Figure 6 Purification scheme for ENGERIX B.

single N-linked glycan at amino acid residue 146 in the 226-amino-acid polypeptide (47). The PreS2 + S protein expressed in CHO cells is a mixture of 36-kD diglycosylated (amino acid residues 4 and 201) PreS2 + S polypeptides and 27-kD and 24-kD S polypeptides (11).

V. EVOLVING PROCESS TECHNOLOGIES

In spite of their proven safety and efficacy, hepatitis B vaccines have seen use mainly in at-risk populations, primarily health care professionals in developed countries. With the low dosage level and limited demand, production capacity to date has not been strained. Because of the highly regulated environment for biological products, original isolation schemes developed in the laboratory frequently became the basis for the licensed manufacturing process. With the recent CDC recommendations for universal pediatric vaccination in the United States and the potential for increased use in developing countries where much of endemic hepatitis B disease is found, the application of newer more scalable production and purification technologies should be considered to meet world-wide needs. The future will no doubt see the use of more highly regulated expression systems to enhance productivity along with the application of newer chromatographic techniques to enhance the scalability of purification schemes.

REFERENCES

1. R. W. Ellis and R. J. Gerety, Key issues in the selection of an expression system for vaccine antigens, *J. Med. Virol. 31*: 54 (1990).
2. P. Valenzuela, A. Medina, W. J. Rutter, G. Ammerer, and B. D. Hall, Synthesis and assembly of hepatitis B virus surface antigen particles in yeast, *Nature (London) 298*: 347 (1982).
3. W. N. Burnette, B. Samal, J. Browne, and G. A. Ritter, Properties and relative immunogenicity of various preparations of recombinant DNA-derived hepatitis B surface antigen, *Dev. Biol. Stand. 599*: 113 (1983).
4. M. DeWilde, T. Cabezon, H. Harford, T. Rutgers, E. Simoen, and F. van Wijnendaele, Production in yeast of hepatitis B surface antigen by R-DNA technology, *Dev. Biol. Stand. 59*: 99 (1983).
5. R. A. Hitzemann, C. Y. Chen, F. E. Hagie, E. J. Patzer, C.-C. Liu, D. A. Estell, J. V. Miller, A. Yaffe, D. G. Kleid, A. D. Levinson, and H. Opperman, Expression of hepatitis B virus surface antigen in yeast, *Nucl. Acids Res. 11*: 2745 (1983).
6. M. Jayaram, Y.-Y. Li, and J. R. Broach, The yeast plasmid in 2 micron circle encodes components required for its high-copy propagation, *Cell 34*: 95 (1983).
7. E. Erhart and C. P. Hollenberg, The presence of a defective *LEU*2 gene in 2 micron DNA recombinant plasmids is responsible for curing and high copy number, *J. Bacteriol. 156*: 628 (1983).
8. S. Rosenberg, D. Coit, and P. Tekamp-Olson, Glyceraldehyde-3-phosphate dehydrogenase-derived expression cassettes for constitutive synthesis of heterologous proteins, *Methods Enzymol. 185*: 341 (1990).
9. C. G. Goff, D. T. Mopir, T. Kohns, T. C. Gravius, R. A. Smith, E. Yamasaki, and A. Taunton-Rigby, Expression of calf prochymosin in *Saccharomyces cerevisiae*, *Gene 27*: 35 (1984).
10. R. A. Kramer, T. M. DeChiara, M. D. Schaber, and S. Hilliker, Regulated expression of a human interferon gene in yeast: Control by phosphate concentration or temperature, *Proc. Natl. Acad. Sci. USA 81*: 367 (1984).
11. M-L. Michel, P. Pontisso, E. Solczak, Y. Malpiece, R. E. Streeck, and P. Tiollais, Synthesis in animal cells of hepatitis B surface antigen particles carrying a receptor for polymerized human serum albumin, *Proc. Natl. Acad. Sci. USA 81*: 7708 (1984).
12. G. Urlaub and L. A. Chasin, Isolation of Chinese hamster cell mutants deficient in dihydrofolate reductase activity, *Proc. Natl. Acad. Sci. USA 77*: 4216 (1980).
13. G. Ringold, B. Dieckmann, and F. Lee, Coexpression and amplification of dihydrofolate reductase cDNA and *Escherichia coli* xGPRT gene in Chinese hamster ovary cells, *J. Mol. Appl. Genet. 1*: 165 (1981).
14. R. T. Schimke, Gene amplification in cultured cells, *J. Biol. Chem. 263*: 5989 (1988).

15. D. E. Wampler, E. D. Lehman, J. Boger, W. J. McAleer, and E. M. Scolnick, Multiple chemical forms of hepatitis B surface antigen produced in yeast, *Proc. Nat. Acad. Sci. USA 82*: 6830 (1985).

16. J. Skelly, C. R. Howard and A. J. Zuckerman, Hepatitis B polypeptide vaccine preparation in micelle form, *Nature 290*: 51 (1981).

17. W. N. Burnette, B. Samal, J. Browne, and G. A. Ritter, Properties and relative immunogenicity of various preparation of recombinant DNA-derived hepatitis B surface antigen, *Dev. Biol. Stand. 59*: 113 (1985).

18. J. Stephenne, Development and production aspects of a recombinant yeast-derived hepatitis B vaccine, *Vaccine 8* (Suppl): S69 (1990).

19. W. M. Hurni and W. J. Miller, Analysis of a vaccine purification process by capillary electrophoresis, *J. Chromatogr. 559*: 337 (1991).

20. S. Krugman, J. P. Giles, and J. Hammond, Viral hepatitis, Type B (MS-2) strain) Studies on active immunization, *J. Am. Med. Assoc. 217*: 41 (1971).

21. J. L. Gerin, R. H. Purcell, M. D. Hoggan, P. V. Holland, and R. M. Chanock, Biophysical properties of Australia antigen, *J. Virol. 4*: 763 (1969).

22. J. L. Gerin, P. V. Holland, and R. H. Purcell, Australia antigen: large-scale purification from human serum and biochemical studies of its proteins, *J. Virol. 7*: 569 (1971).

23. W. Stephan and L. Roka, Adsorption of lipoproteiden, *Zeit. Clin. Chem. Clin. Biochem. 6*: 186 (1968).

24. W. Stephan, Hepatitis-free and stable human serum for intravenous therapy, *Vox Sang. 20*: 442 (1971).

25. J. C. Siebke, E. Kjeldsberg, and T. Traavik, On the adsorption of Australia antigen to a colloidal silica and some possible applications, *Acta Pathol. Microbiol. Scan. sect B, 80*: 935 (1972).

26. J. Pillot, S. Goueffon and R. G. Keros, Optimal conditions for elution of hepatitis B antigen after adsorption onto colloidal silica, *J. Clin. Microbiol. 4*: 205 (1976).

27. W. J. Duimel and H. W. Krijnen, Adsorption and elution of HBsAg from Aerosil, *Vox Sang. 23*: 249 (1972).

28. W. Sanford, D. Kubek, and R. D. Sitrin, Silica chromatography for the purification of recombinant hepatitis B PreS2 + S surface antigen, *Abstr. Am. Inst. Chem. Eng.* 1991 Meeting, Abstract 275i (1991).

29. A. R. Neurath, A. M. Prince, and A. Lippin, Hepatitis B antigen: Antigenic sites related to human serum proteins revealed by affinity chromatography, *Proc. Natl. Acad. Sci. USA 71*: 2663 (1974).

30. S. E. Charm and B. L. Wong, An immunoadsorbent process for removing hepatitis antigen from blood and plasma, *Biotechnol. Bioeng. 16*: 593 (1974).

31. B. Houwen, A. Goudeau, and J. Dankert, Isolation of hepatitis B surface antigen by affinity chromatography on antibody-coated immunoadsorbents, *J. Immunol. Methods 8*: 185 (1975).

32. D. E. Wampler, E. B. Buynak, B. J. Harder, A. C. Herman, M. R. Hilleman, W. J. McAleer, and E. M. Scolnick, Hepatitis B vaccine purification by immunoaffinity chromatography, *Modern Approaches to Vaccines* (R. Chanock and R. Lerner, eds.), Cold Spring Harbor Laboratories, Cold Spring Harbor, New York, p. 251 (1984).

33. P. M. Kaplan, E. Ford, R. H. Purcell, and J. L. Gerin, Demonstration of sub-populations of Dane particles, *J. Virol. 17*: 885 (1976).

34. M. Einarsson, L. Kaplan, and G. Utter, Purification of hepatitis B surface antigen by affinity chromatography, *Vox Sang. 35*: 224 (1978).

35. A. Machida, S. Kishimoto, H. Ohnuma, H. Miyamoto, K. Baba, K. Oda, T. Nakamura, Y. Miyakawa, and M. Mayumi, A. hepatitis b surface antigen polypeptide (p31) with the receptor for polymerized human as well as chimpanzee albumins, *Gastroenterology 85*: 268 (1983).

36. F. Barin, M. Andre, A. Goudeau, P. Coursager, and P. Maupas, Large scale purification of hepatitis B surface antigen (HBsAg), *Ann. Microbiol. 129B*: 87 (1978).

37. W. K. Chung, H. S. Sun, K. W. Chung, B. S. Kim, B. K. Min, and A. M. Prince, Safety and immunogenicity of a new heat-inactivated hepatitis B virus vaccine in adult recipients, *Vaccine 5*: 175 (1987).

38. P. N. Lelie, H. W. Reesink, J. Niessen, B. Brotman, and A. M. Prince, Inactivation of 10 exp 15 chimpanzee-infectious doses of hepatitis B virus during preparation of a heat inactivated hepatitis B vaccine, *J. Med. Virol. 23*: 289 (1987).

39. K. Shiraki, Clinical trials of HBSIG and hepatitis B vaccine (Green Cross) for the prevention of mother-to-infant infection of HBV, *Viral and Hepatitis B Infection* (S. Lam, C. Lai and E. Yeoh eds.), World Scientific Company, Singapore, p. 189 (1984).

40. D. J. Kubek, W. V. Sanford, and R. D. Sitrin, Macroporous ultrafiltration of recombinant hepatitis B PreS2 + S antigen, 201st American Chemical Society Meeting, New York City, Spring 1991, abstract I&EC 0047 (1991).

41. R. Mancinelli, W. Milller, A. Wolfe, W. Hurni, and J. McCauley, Estimation of residual yeast protein in recombinant hepatitis B vaccine, Ninth International Symposium on HPLC of Proteins, Peptides and Polynucleotides, Philadelphia, Abstract No. 806, (1989).

42. J. Petre, F. Van Wijnendaele, B. De Neys, K. Conrath, O. Van Opstal, P. Hauser, T. Rutgers, T. Cabezon, C. Capiau, N. Hartford, M. De Wilde, J. Stephene, S. Carr, H. Hemling, and J. Swadesh, Development of a hepatitis B vaccine from transformed yeast cells, *Postgrad. Med. J. 63* (Suppl 2): 73 (1987).

43. F. Van Wijnendaele and G. Simonet, Method for the isolation and purification of hepatitis B surface antigen using polysorbate, U.S. Patent 4,649,192 (1987).

44. M. L. Michel and P. Tiollais, Synthesis of hepatitis B surface antigen particles containing the Pre-S region expression product, *Proceedings of 8th International Biotechnology Symposium* (G. Durand, L. Bobichon and J. Florent, eds.), Societe Francaise de Microbiologiey, Paris, p. 725 (1988).

45. M. Belew, M. Yafang, L. Bin, J. Berglof, and J-C. Janson, Purification of recombinant hepatitis B surface antigen produced by transformed chinese hamster ovary (CHO) cell line grown in culture, *Bioseparations 1*: 397 (1991).

46. C-C. Liu, D. Yansura, and A. D. Levinson, Direct expression of hepatitis B surface antigen in monkey cells from an SV40 vector, *DNA 1*: 213 (1982).

47. K. H. Heerman, V. Goldman, W. Schwartz, T. Seyffarth, H. Baumgarten, and W. H. Gerlich. Large surface proteins of hepatitis B virus containing the pre-S sequence, *J. Virol. 52*: 396 (1984).

5

Quality Control of Hepatitis B Vaccine

Victor P. Grachev and David I. Magrath

*World Health Organization,
Geneva, Switzerland*

I. INTRODUCTION

Viral hepatitis is a major public health problem occurring endemically in all parts of the world. There is substantial evidence that hepatitis B may progress to chronic liver disease, including chronic persistent hepatitis, chronic active (aggressive) hepatitis, and cirrhosis. In some regions of the world, delta virus coinfection and superinfection have been associated with a high morbidity and mortality in hepatitis B–positive individuals.

Because of the urgent need for hepatitis B vaccine, particularly for groups that are at increased risk of acquiring infection (1), World Health Organization *Requirements for Hepatitis B Vaccine Prepared from Plasma* were formulated in 1980 (2) and revised in 1984 and 1987 (3, 4). The *Requirements for Hepatitis B Vaccines Made by Recombinant DNA Techniques* were formulated in 1986 (5) and revised in 1988 (6). In this chapter we present the basis of the WHO requirements for hepatitis B vaccines manufactured from plasma (Chapter 2) and made by recombinant DNA techniques (Chapter 4) that are offered as a basis for national legislation.

II. GENERAL CONSIDERATIONS

A number of laboratories have extracted HBsAg from plasma obtained from antigenemic carriers of hepatitis B and vaccines of varying degrees of purity and technological complexity have been prepared.

Source plasma could contain infectious agents possessing a wide range of physicochemical and biological characteristics and various degrees of susceptibility or resistance to different modes of inactivation. Consequently, to ensure as far as possible the safety of hepatitis B vaccines, it is important that, in addition to separation and purification, a procedure or procedures that will inactivate all infectious agents possibly present in human blood should be included in the vaccine manufacturing process. Whatever the procedure used, it is universally expected that the vaccines will be safe (i.e., free from demonstrable virus and other microbial agents), potent (i.e., capable of eliciting antibody against the virus in animals and in humans by the administration of a standardized dose of antigen), and efficacious (i.e., protective against the disease).

Consistency of vaccine production, including uniformity of composition and potency of the final product and effectiveness of virus inactivation procedures applied during manufacture, is most readily achieved for highly purified materials. Consequently, it is desirable that the manufacturing procedure adopted enables a high degree of purification of HBsAg to be reliably achieved.

Studies in chimpanzees showed the efficacy of several vaccines in preventing hepatitis B, and cross-protection studies showed that subtypes are not of major importance in vaccine composition (4), and subsequent experience with these vaccines has confirmed efficacy in humans.

More recently, advances in molecular genetics and nucleic acid chemistry have made it possible to identify genes coding for biologically active substances, to analyze them in detail, to transfer them within and between organisms, and to obtain gene expression under controlled conditions with efficient synthesis of the encoded product. A gene that codes for a specific product can be isolated and propagated by insertion into a suitable vector with the aid of highly specific restriction endonuclease enzymes, which cleave the vector DNA at predetermined sites, and ligases, which join the gene insert to the vector. The vector can then be introduced into host organisms, and individual clones that carry the desired gene can be selected and propagated in mass culture.

The requirements that follow apply to the control and testing of hepatitis B vaccines and have been formulated to take account of the scale-up required for commercial production. Particular emphasis is placed on introducing "in-process" control, which has been highly effective for other bacterial and viral vaccines, rather than relying entirely on tests on the end products.

A detailed description of how the product is made should be given. For vaccines made by recombinant DNA techniques, evidence should be presented that the HBsAg possesses the characteristics of an immunogen that protects against hepatitis B virus (HBV).

Rigorous identification and characterization of recombinant DNA–derived vaccines is required. The ways in which these products differ chemically, structurally, biologically, or immunobiologically from the naturally occurring antigen must be fully documented. Such differences could arise during processing at the genetic or posttranslational level or during purification. Differences between batches of the product may result from genetic instability during serial cultivation. Microbial contamination during fermentation may occur, and tests for contaminants must be thorough.

Special attention should be given to purity because:

1. Unwanted gene products may be co-expressed unexpectedly with the HBsAg, for example, if transcription is initiated at several sites, or if changes occur during culture that effect transcription, initiation, or termination processes or favor the expression of other genes in the vector or the host cell.

2. Biologically active extraneous components such as DNA, proteins, and endogenous retroviruses derived from the host-cell system may be found in the final product; agents used in the purification process (column matrices, antibodies) may give rise to specific contaminants in the final product.

The product arising from the recombinant system must be shown to elicit specific antibody responses to HBsAg in laboratory animals, including a nonhuman primate species. HBsAg of diverse subtypes should be used to characterize the specificity of the response fully. One approach to evaluating the protective potential of recombinant DNA–derived vaccines in human beings is through immunization and challenge studies in chimpanzees.

The vaccine should reliably induce antibody responses to HBsAg in human recipients. The frequency and titer of the antibody responses should be approximately equivalent to those induced by plasma-derived vaccines that fulfill WHO requirements (4). The aim of immunogenicity studies in human subjects should be to define the quantity of antigen and number of doses required to elicit reliable antibody responses to HBsAg. The titer, duration, and quality of the responses should be clearly defined. The relationship between the antigenicity of the product in in vitro tests, in mouse immunogenicity tests, and in human beings should be established. Studies in human subjects should be designed to provide information on the frequency and severity of any local and systemic adverse reactions to vaccination. Vaccine recipients in such studies should be representative of the intended target group of immunization in terms of age and risk.

III.   GENERAL MANUFACTURING REQUIREMENTS

The general manufacturing requirements contained in the revised *Requirements for Biological Substances No. 1* (7) shall apply to establishments manufacturing hepatitis B vaccine, with the addition of the following directives.

Production areas shall be decontaminated before they are used for the manufacture of hepatitis B vaccine. Completely separate areas shall be used for the separation and inactivation steps. All separation and inactivation steps for plasma-derived vaccines shall be carried out in closed systems and closely monitored.

Hepatitis B vaccine shall be produced by staff who have not handled animals or infectious microorganisms in the same working day. The staff shall consist of persons who have been examined medically and have been found to be healthy and not to be carriers of hepatitis B.

No cultures of microorganisms or eukaryotic cells other than those approved by the national control authority shall be introduced into or handled in the production area at any time during manufacture of the vaccine.

Persons not directly concerned with the production processes, other than official representatives of the national control authority, shall not be permitted to enter the production area.

Particular attention is drawn to the recommendations contained in Part A, section 1 of the revised *Requirements for Biological Substances No. 1* (7, p. 13) regarding the training and experience of persons in charge of production and testing and of those assigned to various positions of responsibility in the manufacturing establishment, and to the registration of such personnel with the national control authority.

The preparation of hepatitis B vaccine made by recombinant DNA techniques shall be based strictly on the cell seed lot system. A description of the system used should be provided, including the number of vials of seed available and details of their storage. Particular attention should be paid to the stability of the expression vector and to the plasmid copy number in the seed stock under conditions of storage and recovery.

Full details of the cell cultures process used in manufacture should be provided to the national control authority, with particular reference to tests to monitor microbial contamination in the cell cultures vessels. Information on the sensitivity of methods of detecting such contamination and the frequency of testing should be provided, together with criteria for the rejection of contaminated materials.

The yield of HBsAg shall be monitored during the course of individual production runs of hepatitis B vaccine made by recombinant DNA techniques. Criteria, based on yield, for the acceptance of culture harvests for further processing into vaccine shall be defined, and consistency of production shall be established by testing at least five consecutive lots prepared by the same procedures.

IV. HEPATITIS B VACCINE PREPARED FROM PLASMA

Separated viral coat proteins containing hepatitis B lead to the production of protective antibodies, thus it is possible to use purified, noninfectious 22-nm spherical HBsAg particles, or subunits derived from the surface antigen, as vaccines (8). However, the preparation of such vaccines for use in humans from human viral antigens obtained from the plasma of persistent carriers of hepatitis B antigens demands special consideration, particularly since human blood and plasma may harbor infectious agents, including human immunodeficiency virus (HIV). Particular attention, therefore, must be given during the production and quality control of such vaccines to selecting the donors of the plasma, to the process of separation of the antigen, and to inactivation to ensure that any potential infectious agents that may still be present after the purification of the antigen have been inactivated.

A. Factors that Ensure Quality and Safety of the Vaccine

1. The Collection of Blood and Plasma

Source materials for further processing are obtained from donations of blood or plasma. The medical criteria for accepting donors, in other words, the criteria relating to the safety, purity, potency, and efficacy of the final products, must be the same as those for donors of whole blood components collected by plasmapheresis (9), except that the donors must be antigenemic and need not meet the exclusions relating to hepatitis. Only plasma from donors who are seronegative in appropriate tests for HIV shall be used (10).

The physical fitness of a donor shall be determined by a licensed physician or a person under the direct supervision of a licensed physician. The WHO requirements (4) recommend that donors shall be asymptomatic persons of either sex between the ages of 18 and 65 years, except that the findings in liver function tests may exceed normal limits provided that the values obtained are stable. Before each donation, questions shall be asked to determine that the donor is asymptomatic and has not suffered, or is not suffering, from any serious illness including malignant disease, diabetes, epilepsy, hypertension, renal disease, and malaria. In compliance with WHO requirements (4), national health authorities shall develop policies designed to prevent the transmission of other infectious diseases based on the prevalence of these diseases in the donor population and the susceptibility of recipients to the same diseases.

2. Tests on Single-Donation Plasma and Plasma Pools

Each single-donation plasma, whether obtained from whole blood or by plasmapheresis, shall be tested for HBsAg content by a method approved by the national control authority. Only acceptable plasma shall be included in a plasma pool. A sample of each plasma pool shall be tested for sterility according to the requirements in Part A, section 5 of the revised *Requirements for Biological Substances No. 6* (11, p. 48). In addition, each plasma pool shall be tested for extraneous viruses, including tests in adult and suckling mice, tests in embryonated eggs, and tests in cell cultures.

The plasma pool passes the test if at least 80% of the original inoculated mice survive the observation period and if no mice show evidence of infection with adventitious transmissible agents attributable to the plasma pool. The plasma pool passes the tests in embryonated eggs and in cell cultures if there is no evidence of the presence of any adventitious agents attributable to the plasma pool.

3.   Concentration, Purification, and Inactivation

Each plasma pool shall be subjected to procedures that concentrate and purify HBsAg consistently and result in the inactivation of residual HBV and any extraneous agent that may be present in human blood. The methods used shall remove the bulk of extraneous substances and inactivate infectious agents so that the resultant purified product is safe when administered to humans. In some countries the required HBsAg content of vaccines is not less than 95% of total protein content of the finished vaccine, and the national control authority shall review data to identify protein impurities to show that they do not compromise the safety of the product.

In accordance with WHO requirements (4), the national control authority shall approve the methods used for concentration and purification of HBsAg and for inactivation of HBV and other potential contaminating agents. The national control authority shall ensure that the production process, including purification and particularly inactivation, is reproducible and will give rise to consecutive lots that do not differ with respect to safety.

When new processes for HBV vaccine manufactured from human plasma are introduced, the efficiency of HBV DNA removal at each step during the purification process shall be validated. For validation of the removal of HBV DNA, DNA hybridization assays can be used, and chimpanzee studies may be carried out to validate the inactivation process. In assessing the efficiency of a procedure or procedures for the inactivation, the national control authority shall take into consideration data demonstrating the ability of each method to inactivate infectious agents that may be found in human blood.

Procedures that have been successfully used for the preparation of HBsAg vaccine include concentration with ammonium sulfate and polyethylene glycol and purification by zonal centrifugation, followed by inactivation by chemical or heat treatment. The following methods have been used for preparing plasma-derived vaccines: pepsin, 1 μg/ml at pH 2.0 held at 37°C for 18 hours; urea, 8 mol/l held at 37°C for 4 hours; and formalin 1:4000 (1:10,000 formaldehyde) at 37°C for 3 days (11).

A second method involves the separation of the HBsAg, including isopyknic zonal centrifugation through cesium chloride, followed by treatment with 1:4000 formalin (1:10,000 formaldehyde) at 30°C for 48 hours (4). Yet another method includes three isopyknic zonal centrifugation steps with KBr and rate zonal centrifugation through sucrose followed by heat treatment of the HBsAg at 60°C for 10 hours and treatment with 1:2000 formalin (1:5000 formaldehyde) at 37°C for 4 days (12).

Lelie et al. (13) suggested using differential precipitation with polyethylene glycol and ultracentrifugation, followed by heat inactivation for 90 S at 103°C. After adsorption to aluminum phosphate, the product is heated for 10 hours at 65°C.

Chung et al. (14) used differential precipitations with polyethylene glycol, selective adsorption on hydroxylapatite, and isopycnic centrifugation in KB followed by two heating steps under defined conditions: first at 102°C for 20 S, then at 65°C for 10 hours.

4. Tests on Purified, Inactivated HBsAg Batches

A sample of each batch shall be tested for sterility according to the requirements in Part A, section 5 of the revised *Requirements for Biological Substances No. 6* (15, p. 48). After purification, the protein content shall be measured for both total protein and HBsAg-specific protein. The latter shall be compared with that of a suitable reference preparation.

The content of HBsAg shall be determined by a serological test in comparison with a suitable reference preparation. It is important that the method of production give a reproducible content of HBsAg. The lower limit of concentration permitted shall be determined by the national control authority. The concentration of HBsAg shall be related to the total protein.

The presence of blood group substances and other blood proteins, including liver-specific membrane proteins, shall be tested by methods such as hemagglutination approved by the national control authority. Other extraneous proteins can be tested for by immunoelectrophoresis, agar gel diffusion, radioimmunoassay, ELISA, and polyacrylamide gel electrophoresis. The preparation shall be free from detectable blood group substances. The permitted concentration of non-HBsAg proteins present in the vaccine shall be determined by the national control authority. The preparation shall be free from HBV DNA, as determined by a sensitive hybridization assay approved by the national control authority.

Test for purity of HBsAg shall be made by polyacrylamide gel electrophoresis (PAGE). In reduced preparations there should be two bands shown by PAGE, one at 22,000–23,000 and another at 28,000–30,000 relative molecular mass. However, additional HBV-specified or non-HBV-specified bands may also be present. The national control authority shall determine the electrophoretic pattern permitted as a demonstration of purity.

Finally, a test shall be made for the presence of any potentially hazardous reagent, including inactivating reagents, that may have been used during the manufacture of the HBsAg. The method used and the permitted concentration shall be approved by the national control authority.

5. Final Aqueous Bulk

The final aqueous bulk consists of one or more purified, concentrated HBsAg batches that have passed the above-mentioned tests. The national control authority shall determine whether initial lots of vaccine shall be tested for the presence of infectious HBV in chimpanzees, and the test shall be approved by them.

If a chimpanzee safety test is used, the first five consecutive lots prepared by the same production procedures shall be tested in chimpanzees that shall have been under observation for at least 6 months before inoculation and shown to be free from HBV infection, past or present, as shown by sensitive techniques (negative tests for HBsAg, anti-HBS, and anti-HBc). These five lots shall be tested individually without pooling.

If these five lots pass this test, safety testing of subsequent lots in chimpanzees may be discontinued. If an established manufacturing process is altered or the same process transferred under controlled conditions from one manufacturer to another after initial safety validation in chimpanzees, the national control authority may elect to reduce the number of chimpanzee safety tests required for the new production lots to fewer than five.

A satisfactory test involves two chimpanzees. One animal shall receive one human dose, and the other shall receive 10 human doses by intravenous injection.

During the observation period of 6 months after inoculation, the tests shall include the following: weekly determination of alanine aminotransferase (ALT), which shall remain normal for each individual chimpanzee; any abnormal finding shall be demonstrated to be unrelated to viral hepatitis; weekly determinations of the markers of HBV infection, using sensitive serological methods; antibody assays for HIV before inoculation and 4 and 6 months after inoculation; weekly weight determinations and daily checks of general health; biopsies for light microscopic examination to search for evidence of hepatitis taken monthly and at any time that the chimpanzees show any abnormality.

Aqueous bulks that fail the test shall not be used to prepare vaccine for use in humans. In such cases it shall be considered that the consistency has not been established, and a further five consecutive lots must be tested. The reasons for failing the test shall be investigated and reported to the national control authority. In addition, the final aqueous bulk shall be tested for bacterial and mycotic sterility, for the quantity of HBsAg, and for pyrogenicity.

The sterility test shall be performed according to the requirements in Part A, section 5.2 of the revised *Requirements for Biological Substances No. 6* (15, p. 49).

The quantity of HBsAg compared with the total protein in the final aqueous bulk shall be determined by a quantitative serological procedure in comparison with a suitable reference reagent. The lower limit of HBsAg and limit of total protein per human dose shall be approved by the national control authority.

Each final bulk shall be tested for pyrogenicity by a suitable test, which shall be approved by the national control authority.

6. Final Bulk

The final bulk can contain an adjuvant. In this case, the adjuvant and the concentration used shall be approved by the national control authority. If aluminum salts are used, the concentration of aluminum shall not exceed 1.25 mg per single human dose.

In some countries the alum used as an adjuvant is formed in the presence of the HBsAg, whereas in others preformed alum salts are added to the acqueous bulk. Where preformed aluminum adjuvants are used, it may not be possible to resolubilize the aluminum compound, and the testing for purity and concentration of the HBsAg in the final bulk may not be possible. In addition, tests for completeness of adsorption to adjuvant, for sterility, and for concentration of preservative shall be performed on the final bulk or on material in the final container.

The requirements concerning filling and containers in Part A, section 4 of the revised *Requirements for Biological Substances No. 1* (7, p. 16) shall apply. Studies should be conducted to ensure that the material of which the container is made does not adversely affect the HBsAg under the recommended conditions of storage.

7. Quality and Safety Tests on Final Product

The final lot shall be tested for sterility, innocuity, the presence of preservative, the content of adjuvant, pyrogenicity, as well as potency and identity to demonstrate compliance with the WHO *Requirements for Hepatitis B Vaccine Prepared from Plasma* (4).

As regards potency and identity test, an appropriate quantitative potency assay and identity test shall be performed on each final lot irrespective of how many filling lots are made. The vaccine potency shall be compared with that of the international reference reagent. The potency shall be measured in terms of quantity of vaccine giving an antibody response in 50% of the animals. The national control authority shall determine the lower limit of potency.

B. Conclusion

Since initial licensure in 1981, plasma-derived hepatitis B vaccines have enjoyed ever-expanding use on a worldwide scale. While vaccines of only two manufacturers were initially licensed, there were, by 1987, more than 12 commercial producers globally, and by the end of 1986 approximately 30 million doses of vaccine had been marketed (16). Experience with vaccines made according to these requirements has been excellent. They have been shown to be potent (17) highly efficacious (21–24) with an impressive safety record (18–20), and these vaccines, as currently purified and inactivated, have not transmitted and are not capable of transmitting HIV (16).

V. HEPATITIS B VACCINE PREPARED BY RECOMBINANT DNA TECHNIQUES

Vaccine formulations containing purified recombinant DNA–derived HBsAg materials have been shown to be immunogenic in mice, chimpanzees and other monkeys, and human beings, with antigenic potencies similar to those of vaccine made from plasma-derived antigen (5,6). General requirements, such as tests for potency, purity, toxicity, pyrogenicity, and sterility, apply as much to hepatitis B vaccine made by recombinant DNA methods as to those derived from human plasma. Certain tests are required on every production batch of vaccine, whereas others are required only to establish the validity, acceptability and consistency of a given manufacturing process. The general production precautions formulated in Part A, section 3 of the revised *Requirements for Biological Substances No. 1* (7, p. 15) apply to the manufacture of hepatitis B vaccine.

A. Factors Ensuring Quality and Safety of the Vaccine

1. Strategy for Cloning and Expressing the Gene

A full description of the biological characteristics of the host cell and expression vectors used in production should be given. This should include the details of: potential retroviruslike particles in and genetic markers of the host cell; the construction, genetics, and structure of the expression vector; and the origin and identification of the gene that is being cloned. The physiological measures used to promote and control the expression of the cloned gene in host cell should be described in detail (6).

It is particularly important to have data that demonstrate the stability of the expression system during storage of the Manufacturer's Working Cell Bank (MWCB) and beyond the passage level used for production. Any instability of the expression system occurring in the seed culture or after a production-scale run, for example, involving rearrangements, deletions, or insertions of nucleotides, must be documented. Unstable preparations must not be used until approval to continue use has been obtained from the national control authority. It is desirable that the nucleotide sequence of the gene insert and of adjacent segments of the vector and restriction-enzyme mapping of the vector containing the gene insert be provided by the manufacturer.

Methods that have been used to ascertain that the composition of the recombinant polypeptide is identical to the natural one include amino-acid composition, carboxy- and amino-terminal sequence analysis of the surface antigen protein, and peptide mapping by mass spectroscopy (25).

2. Purification Procedures

The methods used to purify the HBsAg from culture harvests should be fully described and in accordance with WHO requirements (5,6). The capacity of each step of the purification procedure to remove and/or inactivate substances other than HBsAg derived from the host cell or culture medium, including, in particular, virus particles, proteins, and nucleic acids, shall be evaluated. If individual contaminants are difficult to monitor, the results of pilot-scale studies to follow the removal of deliberately added contaminants at appropriate stages of purification will provide valuable information.

If antibodies are used in the purification procedures, their origins and characteristics should be fully described. The degree of purity of monoclonal antibodies produced from hybridoma cell lines and the criteria for freedom from cell-derived DNA and murine viruses should conform to the regulations laid down by the national control authority.

3. Characterization of Gene Products (HBsAg)

The morphological characteristics of the HBsAg particles and degree of aggregation should be established by electron microscopy and by physicochemical methods, for example, by gradient centrifugation. In addition, the protein, lipid, nucleic acid, and carbohydrate contents should be measured.

An ultraviolet absorption spectrum should be recorded. The protein composition should be established by techniques such as sodium dodecyl sulfate–polyacrylamide gel electrophoresis (SDS-PAGE) under reducing conditions (6). The bands should be identified by sensitive staining techniques and, where possible, by specific antibodies to confirm the presence of the expected products of the HBV envelope gene. The identity of the protein should be established by partial N-terminal and C-terminal sequence analysis.

The recombinant DNA–derived vaccine should be shown to induce antibody responses in humans comparable to those elicited by plasma-derived vaccines that have proved effective in the field. In accordance with WHO requirements (6), the antibodies induced by the vaccine in human beings should be titrated and characterized with respect to their activities against relevant determinants of the HBV envelope, for example, group and subtype determinants.

Data on the consistency of yield between runs and during individual production runs shall be provided, and the national control authority shall approve the criteria for an acceptable production run.

4. Manufacturer's Working Cell Bank

The production of a hepatitis B vaccine prepared by recombinant DNA techniques, as well as other vaccines manufactured using continuous cell lines, is based on the cell seed system (26). The cells shall have been characterized as specified under the *Requirements for Continuous Cell Lines Used for Biological Production* (27), shown to be sterile (15), and approved by the national control authority.

The characteristics of the cell seed (host cell in combination with the expression vector system) shall be fully described, and information given on the absence of extraneous agents and on genetic homogeneity. The nucleotide sequence of the HBsAg gene insert and its flanking regions shall be specified where relevant. A peptide map and/or terminal amino acid sequence of the gene products shall be obtained (6).

Cells of the MWCB must be maintained in a frozen state that allows recovery of viable cells such that the genotype and phenotype are unaltered and consistent with the unmodified host and unmodified recombinant DNA vector.

5. Production of Cell Cultures

In accordance with WHO requirements (6), only cell cultures derived from the MWCB shall be used for production. Production cell cultures shall be grown under conditions agreed with the national control authority. These conditions shall include details of the culture system use, the cell doubling time, the number of subcultures or the duration of the period of subcultivation permitted, and the incubation temperature. Cell culture shall be monitored for freedom from microbial contamination.

If serum is used for the propagation of cells for vaccine production, it shall be tested by methods approved by the national control authority, to demonstrate freedom from bacteria, fungi, viruses, and mycoplasmas, according to WHO requirements (2, p. 49), as well as freedom from pathogens of the species of origin of the serum. Antibiotics of the β-lactam type shall not be used at any stage in the production (6).

6. Single Harvests and Purification

Single Harvests In accordance with WHO requirements (6), the yield of HBsAg from each single harvest shall be shown to be within the limits approved by the national control authority. Microbial contamination in the cell culture vessels shall be monitored during and at the end of the production runs.

A sample of cells that are representative of each harvest must be tested to confirm that the recombinant phenotype has been retained. The method used shall be approved by the national control authority.

Purification The antigen must be purified before adsorption onto an adjuvant. The purification procedure can be applied to a single harvest, a part of a single harvest, or a pool of single harvests. The number of single harvests that may be pooled shall be fixed by the national control authority. Adequate purification may require several purification steps based on different principles. This will minimize the possibility of copurification of extraneous cellular materials. The method used for the purification of the HBsAg should be validated and approved by the national control authority.

The experience of several manufacturers has shown that it is possible to produce batches in which HBsAg accounts for at least 95% of the total protein. One suitable method of analyzing the proportion of potential contaminant proteins in the total protein of the product is separation of the proteins by polyacrylamide gel electrophoresis under both nonreducing and reducing denaturing conditions (6). But purity, expressed as a percentage, will depend on the method of measurement used; with high performance liquid chromatography, purity for a recombinant yeast–derived hepatitis B vaccine was estimated as virtually 100% (25). Polyacrylamide gel electrophoresis and Coomassie blue staining of the bulk vaccine samples has consistently yielded purity figures ranging from 98 to 99% on routine lots (25). In other words, a pure bulk vaccine could be obtained with an antigen content exceeding 98% purity in terms of protein content and a DNA level of <10 pg per vaccine dose as measured by a sensitive DNA/DNA hybridization technique.

Tests for Protein and Other Components of the Vaccine In compliance with WHO requirements (6), the total protein content of the vaccine should be determined. It could be done by measuring absorbance at 280 nm by the micro-Kjeldahl method, the Lowry technique, or another suitable method. Lipid and carbohydrate contents may also provide useful information.

Tests shall be made for the presence of any potentially hazardous agent used in manufacture, such as serum in the medium for the production of cell cultures or a monoclonal antibody, used for immunological affinity chromatography to purify HBsAg. The concentration of animal serum in the vaccine shall be not more than 1 μl per liter of vaccine (6). The methods used and the permitted concentrations of antibody shall be approved by the national control authority.

Determination of HBsAg Content In accordance with WHO requirements (6), the HBsAg content of the purified preparation shall be determined using an appropriate method such as radioimmunoassay (ELISA), single radial immunodiffusion, and rocket electrophoresis in which the purified preparation is compared with a known standard. Analysis of the results by the parallel-line method has been found suitable for most of these techniques.

Antigenic Identity Molecular and immunochemical identity tests shall be made for the molecular characteristics of the HBsAg gene product by SDS-PAGE under reducing denaturing conditions (25). The gene products shall be shown to possess antigenic determinants characteristic of HBsAg by means of tests with monoclonal antibodies or other antibodies of defined specificity directed against epitopes of HBsAg known to be relevant to the protective efficacy of the vaccine. Such tests shall be approved by the national control authority, which may require the presence of pre-S antigen that can be detected by SDS-PAGE.

Other Tests If the HBsAg has been treated with formaldehyde and/or other inactivated agents, then material shall be tested for the presence of free formaldehyde and/or other agents. The method used and the permitted concentration shall be approved by the national control authority (6). Each batch of HBsAg shall be tested for sterility according to WHO requirements (15).

7. Final Bulk

Final bulk consists of one or more purified HBsAg batches that have passed the above tests. The maximum number of batches that may be pooled should be approved by the national control authority.

In accordance with WHO requirements (6), the final aqueous bulk should contain at least 90% of the total protein as HBsAg, and the lower limit of the ratio of HBsAg to total protein shall be approved by the national control authority. The protein load should be specified so as to ensure that the assay is of reasonable sensitivity.

The amount of residual cell or plasmid DNA in each batch of vaccine should be determined by sensitive methods, which must be validated and approved by the national control authority. But the WHO Study Group on Biologicals concluded that, based on the experimental data available, the probability of risk associated with heterogenous contaminating DNA in a product derived from continuous cell lines is so small as to be negligible when the amount of such DNA is 100 pg or less in a single dose given parenterally (28). The final bulk shall be tested for presence of preservative for the content of adjuvant and for sterility as described for plasma-derived vaccine (see Sec. IV.A.6).

8. Quality and Safety Tests on Final Product

The final lot shall be tested for sterility, inocuity, pyrogenicity, the presence of preservative, content of adjuvant, potency, and identity according to the rules for plasma-derived vaccine (see Sec. IV.A.7).

B. Conclusion

DNA recombinant technologies in human vaccine development received their first application in the production of hepatitis B vaccines in 1984–1985. Two manufacturers of yeast-derived hepatitis B vaccines were licensed in 1986, and licensure of additional yeast-derived vaccines is expected in the next several years (16). More recently, mammalian cells have been used to express hepatitis B vaccine antigens (29–32). Such a vaccine is manufactured and licensed in one country (France). Licensure of other vaccines is to be expected in the next 2–3 years. Recombinant DNA vaccine is safe, highly immunogenic (33–35), and efficacious (36,37). Thus, it can be concluded that hepatitis B vaccines made by recombinant DNA techniques as described are safe, highly immunogenic, and efficacious preparations.

REFERENCES

1. World Health Organization, *Advances in Viral Hepatitis*, *Report of the WHO Expert Committee on Viral Hepatitis*, Technical Report Series No. 602, Geneva, pp. 1–62 (1977).

2. World Health Organization, *Requirements for Hepatitis B Vaccine*, Technical Report Series No. 658, Annex, 4, pp. 131–156 (1981).

3. World Health Organization, *Requirements for Hepatitis B Vaccine Prepared from Plasma* (revised 1984), Technical Report Series No. 725, Geneva, Annex 3, pp. 70–101 (1985).

4. World Health Organization, *Requirements for Hepatitis B Vaccine Prepared from Plasma*. Technical Report Series No. 771, Geneva, Annex 8, pp. 181–207 (1988).

5. World Health Organization, *Requirements for Hepatitis B Vaccines Made by Recombinant DNA Techniques in Yeast* (*Requirements for Biological Substances No. 39*), Technical Report Series No. 760, Geneva, Annex 6, pp. 106–138 (1987).

6. World Health Organization, *Requirements for Hepatitis B Vaccines Made by Recombinant DNA Techniques* (*Requirements for Biological Substances No. 45*), Technical Report Series No. 786, Geneva, Annex 2, pp. 38–71 (1989).

7. World Health Organization, *General Requirements for Manufacturing Establishments and Control Laboratories* (*Requirements for Biological Substances No. 1*), Technical Report Series No. 323, Geneva, Annex 1, pp. 11–22 (1966).

8. World Health Organization, *Report of a WHO Meeting on Hepatitis B Vaccines Produced by Recombinant DNA Techniques*, Technical Report Series No. 760, Geneva, Annex 5, pp. 87–105 (1987).

9. World Health Organization, *Requirements for the Collection, Processing and Quality Control of Blood, Blood Components, and Plasma Derivatives* (*Requirements for Biological Substances No. 27*) (revised 1988), Technical Report Series No. 786, Geneva, Annex 4, p. 104 (1989).

10. Weekly epidemiological record, WHO, Geneva, No. 18, pp. 138–140 (1986).

11. J. Krugman, Hepatitis B vaccine, *Vaccines* (J. Plotkin and E. Mortimer), W.B. Saunders Company, Philadelphia, pp. 458–473 (1988).

12. T. Novak, E. Luchmore, L. W. Cummins, and J. Hilfenhaus, Inactivation of hepatitis B virus in human plasma protein derivatives by pasteurization, *Proceedings of the 1990 International Symposium on Viral Hepatitis and Liver Disease*, Houston, TX, p. 108 (1990).

13. P. N. Lelie, J. Niessen, P. J. Ochlers, W. P. Zeislemader, and H. W. Reesink, Heat treatment and addition of anti-HBs antibodies potentiate the immunogenicity of a plasma-derived HBsAg vaccine, *Viral Hepatitis and Liver Disease* (A. J. Zuckerman, ed.), Alan R. Liss Inc., New York, pp. 1009–1013 (1988).

14. K. C. Whan, Y. C. Kyu, S. S. Kyu, et al., Safety, immunogenicity and efficacy of a new heat-inactivated hepatitis B vaccine in the newborn, *Viral Hepatitis and Liver Disease* (A. J. Zuckerman, ed.), Alan R. Liss Inc., New York, p. 1014 (1988).

15. World Health Organization, *General Requirements for the Sterility of Biological Substances* (*Requirements for Biological Substances No. 6*) (revised 1973), Technical Report Series No. 530, Geneva, Annexes 4 and 5, pp. 40–63 (1973).

16. J. E. Maynard, M. A. Kane, M. J. Alter, and J. C. Hadler, Control of hepatitis B by immunization: Global perspectives, *Viral Hepatitis and Liver Disease* (A. J. Zuckerman, ed.), Alan R. Liss Inc., New York, p. 967 (1988).

17. J. T. Hsieh, T. L. Chen, R. I. Yang, et al., National control testing on plasma-derived hepatitis B vaccine in Taiwan, *Proceedings of International Symposium on Viral Hepatitis and Liver Disease*, Houston, TX, p. 104 (1990).

18. R. A. Coates, M. L. Halliday, J. G. Rankin, et al., Immunogenicity and safety of yeast-derived recombinant DNA hepatitis B vaccine in health care workers, *Viral Hepatitis and Liver Disease* (A. J. Zuckerman, ed.), Alan R. Liss Inc., New York, pp. 1038–1042 (1988).

19. Progress in the control of viral hepatitis, *WHO Bull.*, Geneva, 66: 443 (1988).

20. L. Y. Hwang, C. Y. Lee, and R. P. Beasley, Five year follow-up of HBV vaccination with plasma-derived vaccine in neonates—evaluation of immunogenicity and efficacy against perinatal transmission, *Proceedings of International Symposium on Viral Hepatitis and Liver Disease*, Houston, TX, p. 107 (1990).

21. A. M. Couronce, A. Laplance, E. Benham, and P. Jugers, Long-term efficacy of hepatitis B vaccination in health adults, *Viral Hepatitis and Liver Disease* (A. J. Zuckerman, ed.), Alan R. Liss Inc., New York, pp. 1002–1005 (1988).

22. S. C. Hadler, P. Coleman, P. O'Malley, et al., Evaluation of long-term protection by hepatitis B vaccine in homosexual men followed for 7 to 9 years, *Proceedings of International Symposium on Viral Hepatitis and Liver Disease*, Houston, TX, p. 107 (1990).

23. R. Wainwright, B. McMahon, and L. Bulkow, Protection provided by hepatitis B vaccine in Yupik eskimo population—7 years results, *Proceedings of International Symposium on Viral Hepatitis and Liver Disease*, Houston, TX, p. 107 (1990).

24. D. Abiteboul and B. Gouaille, B hepatitis vaccination in public hospitals, *Proceedings of International Symposium on Viral Hepatitis and Liver Disease*, Houston, TX, p. 108 (1990).

25. J. Stephenne, Development and production aspects of a recombinant yeast-derived hepatitis B vaccine, *Vaccine*, 8: S69 (1990).

26. V. P. Grachev, World Health Organization attitude concerning the use of continuous cell lines as substrate for production of human virus vaccines, *Viral Vaccines* (A. Mizrahi, ed.), John Wiley, New York, p. 43 (1990).

27. World Health Organization, *Requirements for Continuous Cell Lines Used for Biological Production* (*Requirements for Biological Substances No. 37*), Technical Report Series No. 745, Geneva, Annex 3, pp. 93–107 (1987).

28. World Health Organization, *Acceptability of Cell Substrates for Production of Biologicals*, Technical Report Series No. 747, Geneva, pp. 1–29 (1987).

29. P. Tiollais and M. Michel, Synthesis in CHO cells of hepatitis B surface antigen

particles containing the pre-S2 region expression product, *Viral Infections* (W. Margel et al., eds.), M.M.V. Medizin Verlag, Munich, p. 75 (1986).

30. T. Lee, J. Inokoshi, M. Namiki, et al., Production of hepatitis B virus surface antigen containing pre-S1 and pre-S2 domains by Chinese hamster ovary cells, *Arch. Virol. 106*: 151 (1989).

31. A. Caputo, G. Barbanti-Brodano, P. Reschiglian, et al., Expression of hepatitis B surface antigen in human cells by a recombinant BK virus DNA vector, *J. Gen. Virol., 69*: 459 (1988).

32. H, Samanta and B. Youn, Expression of hepatitis B virus surface antigen containing the pre-S region in mammalian cell culture system, *Vaccine, 7*: 69 (1989).

33. J. C. F. Fonseca, M. J. Castejon, A. L. O. Cesario, M. Barone, and L. U. Brazil, Immunogenicity of a recombinant DNA hepatitis B vaccine in children living in the Amazon basin, Brazil, *Proceedings of International Symposium on Viral Hepatitis and Liver Disease*, Houston, TX, p. 110 (1990).

34. P. Dentico, C. Manno, M. Carbone, et al., Safety and efficacy of a yeast-derived hepatitis B vaccine in haemodialysis patients, *Proceedings of International Symposium on Viral Hepatitis and Liver Disease*, Houston, TX, p. 111 (1990).

35. V. Perez, O. Fay, H. Tanno, F. Villamil, et al., Comparison of the immunogenicity and reactogenicity of a recombinant DNA yeast-derived hepatitis B vaccine in patient with chronic non-B liver diseases and healthy controls, *Proceedings of International Symposium on Viral Hepatitis and Liver Disease*, Houston, TX, p. 111 (1990).

36. C. Goilav, H. Prinsen, A. Safary, et al., Four year follow-up with yeast-derived hepatitis B vaccine (YDV), *Proceedings of International Symposium on Viral Hepatitis and Liver Disease*, Houston, TX, p. 112 (1990).

37. N. Scheiermann, M. Gesemann, C. Maurer, F. Andre, and A. Safary, Immunization with a recombinant hepatitis B vaccine (Engerix B)—5 year follow-up results, *Proceedings of International Symposium on Viral Hepatitis and Liver Disease*, Houston, TX, p. 112 (1990).

6

Serological Assays

William J. Miller

Merck Research Laboratories,
West Point, Pennsylvania

I. INTRODUCTION

During the last 25 years there has been an explosion in hepatitis B research following the discovery of Australian antigen (1), its identification as the hepatitis B virus (HBV) surface membrane antigen (HBsAg) (2), and the dissociation of the causative agents of hepatitis B and hepatitis A (3). This has led to the appearance of more than 50,000 publications in the HBV field. The Australia antigen is overproduced in the serum of chronically infected individuals. The development of assays to measure HBsAg and its antibodies followed by measurements of the remaining HBV markers made it possible to detect HBV in its various stages of infection and culminated in the development of vaccines to prevent this disease. It is now possible to measure 12 HBV-related antigens, antibodies, and DNA present during the course of acute or chronic infection or after resolution of infection.

An important factor aiding researchers in the development of hepatitis B vaccines has been the commercialization of diagnostic assay kits. Because the primary use of these kits is the detection of hepatitis B antigens and antibodies for diagnosing human infections, they require Food and Drug Administration licensure. A procedure involving extensive validation studies, including "clinical trials," demonstrated the utility of these kits for detection of disease-related antigens or antibodies. The manufacturer must be able to produce a product that consistently performs to the same level of sensitivity, specificity, and quality.

The licensing process may involve more than one year of validation studies following final kit development. As a result, the licensed kits represent an important resource that allows the efficient scientific development of important hepatitis B vaccines. This chapter will describe the measurement of many of these various markers, especially as they relate to the development of vaccines.

II. TYPES OF IMMUNOLOGICAL ASSAYS

Assay that measure the binding of antigens to antibodies were described at the end of the nineteenth century. Due to their specificity and subsequent analytical quantitative capability, these have been continually improved and modified. Table 1 lists some of these methods and corresponding levels of sensitivity. There has been a 10,000-fold increase in assay sensitivity to the present state-of-the-art-radioimmunoassay (RIA) and enzyme-linked immunosorbent assay (ELISA or EIA) methods, which detect antibody and antigen concentrations as low as 0.5 ng/ml.

III. DISCUSSION OF MASS VS. AFFINITY

The majority of the assays described in this chapter and presently in use to measure antibodies to HBV antigens are solid-phase based, the detection being highly dependent upon the affinity or avidity of the antibody being determined. The affinity constant is a measurement of the strength of binding of an antibody to a single distinct antigen, while avidity is defined as the net overall binding of a plurality of antibodies to a complex antigen with more than one antibody-binding domain. These constants will be described more fully later in this chapter. In general, antibodies having low binding constants will not survive the extensive high-shear washing procedures of the single-layer ELISA and RIA assays and will not be detected. However, these antibodies are likely to be detected in

Table 1 Sensitivity of Assays to Measure Antibodies

Method (acronym)	Estimated sensitivity of detection (ng/ml)
Immunodiffusion (ID)	5000–10,000
Counter immunoelectrophoresis (CIEP)	1000–2,000
Complement fixation (CF)	200–400
Immune adherence hemagglutination assay (IAHA)	100–200
Passive hemagglutination assay (PHA)	5–20
Competitive radioimmunoassays	2.5–5.0
Enzyme-linked immunosorbent assay (ELISA)	1.0–2.0
Direct radioimmunoassay (RIA)	0.5–1.0

classical serology assays such as ID, CIEP, CF, IAHA, and PHA (see Table 1). In the case of some of the methods, antigen-antibody lattices are formed to create large precipitating aggregates, enabling a more accurate measurement of the total mass of antibody present in a serum independent of binding constants. In the CF and IAHA methods, complement (C') co-binding leads to a more stable antigen-antibody complex, making it more difficult for low-affinity antibodies to dissociate from an antigen and, in effect, increasing the apparent affinity/avidity constants.

The dichotomy between assays measuring total mass vs. affinity-/avidity-dependent methods raises the question of the determination of protective antibody levels in human serum containing C'. Although the most sensitive ELISAs and RIAs do not use C' and would tend to report a serum having a high concentration of low affinity antibody as negative, it may well be that such a serum is in fact functionally protective. However, the present correlates of protective level of antibody to HBsAg (anti-HBs) based upon RIA and ELISA measurements do appear to be valid (4), and these concentrations of high affinity/avidity antibodies are well below the level of sensitivity of detection of mass-detecting serological assays (see Table 1).

IV. THE HBV VIRION

The HBV virion has four major components: its genomic DNA, the core capsid (HBcAg), a viral polymerase, and HBsAg (Table 2) (see also Chapter 3). The negatively charged phosphates of the DNA associate ionically with the HBcAg polypeptides through its arginine-lysine–rich, carboxy-terminal, 35-amino-acid sequences. The HBcAg is surrounded by a cell-derived phospholipid, which intercalates the hydrophobic HBsAg, thus binding the HBsAg to the HBcAg. At present, the vaccines commercially available to prevent hepatitis B are based upon the immune response to HBsAg. In the virus, the HBsAg membrane component has been shown to consist of six polypeptides described in Table 2 and discussed in Section VII.A. As indicated, native HBsAg is composed mostly of the S polypeptide and its glycosylated form. It contains lesser amounts of PreS2+S and Pre-S1+PreS2+S in their mono- and diglycosylated forms. HBsAg produced in liver cells is present in the blood of HBV-infected persons as a separate noninfectious lipoprotein particle free of HBcAg and DNA. Components of HBsAg, derived either from the plasma of infected persons or from genetically engineered microorganisms or cell lines containing the HBV gene for surface antigen, are the basis of all available hepatitis B vaccines.

V. HEPATITIS B SEROLOGICAL ASSAYS

The most commonly performed serological assays used to diagnose HBV infection, to assess the prognosis or to track convalescence, as well as to aid in HBV

Table 2 Components of the Hepatitis B Virus

HBV component	Function	Common name	Size
Membrane antigen	Coats viral core	HBsAg	20-nm lipoprotein particle composed of *ca.* 100 polypeptides of S, PreS2+S, and Pre-S1+PreS2+S.
S		Major or small protein, S antigen	Occurs as 24-kD polypeptide and 27-kD monoglycosylated form.
PreS2+S		PreS2+S, middle protein, M protein	Occurs as 31-kD monoglycosylated and 34-kD di-glycosylated forms.
PreS1+PreS2+S	Attachment of virus to susceptible host cell	PreS1+PreS2+S, large protein	Occurs as 42-kD monoglycosylated and 45-kD di-glycosylated forms.
Phospholipid	Outer envelope of virus into which membrane antigen is intercalated	Lipid	Mixture of cell-derived phospholipids, primarily ether-linked phosphocholine.
HBcAg	Viral core capsid surrounds and bonds to viral DNA	HBcAg, capsid protein, core antigen	28-nm assembly of *ca.* 100 core polypeptides 21 kD in size.
DNA	Carries genetic information to make all HBV components	ds DNA, HBV DNA	2100 kD, 3.2 kbp in size occurs as partially double-stranded DNA.
DNA polymerase	Enzyme synthesizes DNA on a single-stranded template	DNA polymerase	70 kD.
HBV virion	Complete virus composed of all above components	Dane particle, HBV, hepatitis B virus	42-nm particle

vaccine development are shown in Table 3. Listed are the description of the method, sensitivity, utility, and a commercial name of one test manufacturer.

VI. USE OF SEROLOGICAL ASSAYS

The serological assays shown in Table 3 can be used to diagnose acute and convalescent stages of hepatitis B infection. These assays have also been invaluable in the development of vaccines. For the latter use, the appearance of antibodies to surface antigen components indicates immunity resulting from vaccination or possible coincident disease during the conduct of a vaccine clinical trial. In the case of a natural infection, HBV replication in the liver sometimes is accompanied by the detection of HBsAg and its PreS1 and PreS2 antigens. The PreS1+PreS2+S and PreS2+S polypeptides are assembled into the 22-nm HBsAg particle and may be transiently detected at the time of HBsAg detection. Since these polypeptides represent only approximately 10% of the total HBsAg mass, their detection is more difficult. In the 1- to 2-month interval following infection, viral DNA, HBcAg, and HBeAg (an unassembled, secreted form of HBcAg that lacks a 35-amino-acid segment at the C-terminal end) also may be detected. Generally, the more severe the disease, the more easily these antigens can be detected. During this interval it is also possible to detect the viral DNA polymerase in serum pellets, which remains associated within the DNA-containing core. As the infection proceeds to convalescence, antibody to the three HBsAg membrane components, (S, PreS2+S, and PreS1+PreS2+S) can be found. Antibody markers become more apparent in severe disease, while anti-HBs may be the only antibody detected in a mild disease. Likewise, antibodies to HBcAg and HBeAg are usually detected at this time, and HBV DNA and DNA polymerase disappear. An important marker of recent infection is the appearance of IgM antibodies to the HBcAg. In approximately 5–10% of cases of hepatitis B in adults, infection proceeds to the chronic state. In this case, HBsAg levels generally rise several orders of magnitude higher than those at onset, reflecting the extensiveness of liver involvement in the infection; PreS1 and PreS2 antigens are detected more easily as well. The HBV DNA is detected continuously, while anti-HBc levels rise to remarkably high levels (2–4 orders of magnitude higher than those found in convalescence). In the chronic carrier state HBeAg and anti-HBe are important prognostic markers. If HBeAg is present, active disease is present and convalescence is not in the offing, while seroconversion to anti-HBe is usually a favorable long-range prognostic marker.

In the case of vaccine development, it has been shown that anti-HBs levels correlate with immunity, so that this is the most important of the assays. Assays for HBsAg are important to quantitation of the actual vaccine antigen during manufacture and formulation. However, finding HBsAg in sera of vaccinees more than one month after vaccine administration is a marker of infection and

Table 3   Hepatitis B Serological Assays

Name of marker Molecule measured	Common name(s)	How measurement is made	Name of licensed commercial test	Estimated limit of sensitivity	Utility
Hepatitis B surface antigen	HBsAg	Sandwich RIA or EIA	AUSRIA	0.5–1 ng/ml	Diagnose hepatitis B; assay HBsAg vaccines
Antibody to HBsAg	anti-HBs, HBsAb, anti-S	Sandwich RIA or EIA	AUSAB	0.5–1 ng/ml	Diagnose convalescence from disease; measure seroconversion to vaccine
Antibody to core antigen (HBcAg)	anti-HBc, HBcAb	Competition of labeled anti-HBc and test serum for HBcAg	CORAB	2.5–5 ng/ml	Identifies past hepatitis B disease and convalescence
IgM antibody to HBcAg	anti-HBc IgM HBcAb-M	Human IgG capture assay	CORAB-M	>0.1% of total IgM	Measures current hepatitis B disease
Hepatitis B e antigen	HBeAg	Sandwich RIA using anti-HBe as the first and third layers	HBeAg	0.5–1 ng/ml	Indicates active disease and worse prognosis in carriers
Antibody to HBeAg	anti-HBe, HBeAb	Neutralization followed by a sandwich assay	anti-HBe	10 ng/ml	May be seen in active or past disease or optimistic prognosis in carriers
Antibody to PreS2 antigen	anti-PreS2	Second antibody RIA or competitive RIA	none	unknown	Unclear in disease and vaccine
Antibody to PreS1	anti-PreS1	Immunoblot or blocking EIA	none	unknown	Unclear in disease
T-cell response	CMI	Blastogenesis	none	unknown	Possibly important to protection

probable vaccine failure. Measurement of antibody to HBcAg is a very important marker to the conduct of a successful vaccine trial. Since HBcAg is absent from all current commercial vaccines, the appearance of this antibody is taken as evidence of concurrent HBV infection, which is confirmable by detection of the IgM isotype of anti-HBc (5). Measurements of anti-PreS2 and anti-PreS1 are still being evaluated as to their importance to vaccine protection, especially regarding a possible cell-mediated immune response.

VII.   SURFACE MARKER ASSAYS

A.   HBsAg

The HBsAg particle is composed of six types of polypeptides (6,7), 100 of which assemble about a phospholipid core through hydrophobic sequences in the S polypeptide to create a particle 22 nm in diameter. This particle is composed of approximately 90–95% S polypeptide and 5–10% of the PreS1+PreS2+S and PreS2+S polypeptides and presents a number of three-dimensional conformational epitopes called the *a* epitope or antigen. It is the most antigenic and immunogenic domain of HBsAg and elicits protective antibody. Since all known HBV types present *a* epitopes, anti-*a* antibodies are group-common protective. The surface-disposed portions of the *a* antigen lie in the S polypeptide, map to amino acids 124–147 (8), and include two disulfide loops. During the course of evolution, single amino acid mutations have occurred in the HBsAg sequence. These mutations usually have been found outside the disulfide loop regions of the *a* epitope and were first observed by immunodiffusion pattern spurs of nonidentity. These small differences were catalogued and referred to as subtypes (9). The first subtypes were named *d* or *y* and were mutually exclusive, so that HBsAg positive sera were subtypes as *ad* or *ay*. A subsequent additional set of mutually exclusive subspecificities were further noted by the same technique (10) and named *w* and *r*. This led to the further subtyping of HBsAg as *adw*, *adr*, *ayw*, or *ayr*. Sequencing has now shown that there are as many as 50 mutations in the 389 amino acids in surface proteins. This appears to be a random mutational variation with no absolute consensus sequence relating to subtype. The immunodiffusion-determined subtyping likely recognizes a predominance of the amino acids in the *d* subtype, but could contain one-third of the sequence of the *y* subtype. These mutations appear to survive as long as the integrity of the HBV persists. However, these subspecificities appear to have little or no immunological relevance to either convalescence or protection. More recently, however, a single amino acid mutation was reported (11) in the *a* epitope of the S antigen. This change occurred at amino acid 145 in which glycine was replaced with arginine. This mutation replaces an uncharged amino acid with a positively charged one, which may lead to an alteration in the recognition by anti-HBs antibody of the new mutated *a* epitope. This mutation appears to have led to a HBV break-through infection seemingly induced by vaccination with the HBsAg vaccine. The incidence and importance of this mutation remains unknown (Chapter 18).

In the late 1970s vaccines were developed by purifying 22-nm HBsAg particles from the plasma of hepatitis B chronic carriers (12,13). The plasma-derived vaccines (PDV) were shown to elicit anti-HBs and shown (14,15) to afford close to 100% protection to vaccinees. Importantly, it was shown that following administration of PDV of the HBsAg *ad* subtype, chimpanzees and then humans were protected from HBV *ay* challenge (16,17). The *ad* subtype HBsAg protected medical staff in which 81% of the hepatitis B contacts were of the *ay* subtype. These results demonstrated the group-protective nature of antibody to the *a* epitope.

1. AUSRIA Assay

The *a* epitope and antibody raised to it are the basis for the most common hepatitis B assay in use, the AUSRIA® (Abbott Labs, N. Chicago, IL). The AUSRIA® consists of a solid-phase polystyrene bead to which is passively adsorbed purified guinea pig anti-HBsAg. Serum to be assayed for HBsAg is incubated with these beads, and the bead is then washed with water. To the bead is added ^{125}I-labeled purified human anti-HBs. HBsAg present in the serum will bind to the bead and be detected in a sandwich-type direct RIA using the labeled anti-HBs. The assay primarily detects the *a* epitope on HBsAg particles and is sensitive to approximately 0.5 ng HBsAg/ml. This assay is used mostly to screen blood donors, and a positive test is presumptive of disease. As indicated above, it also has been applied in assessing the purification and quantitation of HBsAg vaccines.

2. HBsAg Subtyping

HBsAg subtype was originally determined by an immunodiffusion assay (9), which required approximately 10–50 μg HBsAg/ml, 2 to 3 orders of magnitude higher than found in most sera. This led to the development of a sensitive RIA (18) in which either monospecific anti-*d* or anti-y anti-HBs was added to HBsAg-containing serum and incubated. The mixture then is assayed in an AUSAB® test for residual anti-HBs. For example, if an HBsAg-containing serum absorbed the monospecific-anti-*d* antibody, it would be concluded that the HBsAg was a *d* subtype and would be designated *ad*. A correspondingly sensitive RIA for subtypes *w* and *r* has not been developed to date.

B. Anti-HBs Assays

1. Anti-HBs Antibodies

Anti-HBs of the *a* epitope are most sensitively measured in the AUSAB® RIA. This assay also has the capability to measure anti-*d* and anti-y as well. The

AUSAB® test consists of a bead to which a mixture of *ad* and *ay* subtypes of purified HBsAg is passively adsorbed. Serum or plasma anti-HBs binds to the bead with HBsAg. After washing, the bead is incubated with ^{125}I-labeled HBsAg (*ad* + *ay*), which completes a three-layer sandwich if anti-HBs is present in the sample. The test can detect antibody concentration as low as 0.5–1.0 ng/ml. These antibodies also can be measured using an ELISA such as the AUSAB® EIA. The RIA is slightly more sensitive and allows for greater flexibility in incubation times. However, there exists a potential hazard in the use and disposal of radioisotopes. ELISAs, although slightly less sensitive, do not have the radiation exposure and disposal problems of RIAs and have been gaining wider acceptance.

In order to universalize anti-HBs measurements, the World Health Organization (WHO) established a standard hepatitis B immune globulin (HBIG) prepared from high-titered anti-HBs serum pools. This standard was defined to contain 100,000 milli-International Units (mIU) anti-HBs/ml and, when measured in the AUSAB® assay, gave a linear response upon dilution into the range of 2–100 mIU/ml. It subsequently has been shown in retrospective studies following administration of a HBsAg vaccine (4) that anti-HBs levels ≥10 mIU/ml are protective. Therefore, all vaccine manufacturers quantitate the immunogenicity of their vaccine by determining its capability to raise anti-HBs titers to ≥10 mIU/ml. Most current vaccines elicit levels of >1000 mIU/ml in a majority of persons following a three-dose regimen of vaccine.

2. Anti-HBs Isotypes

The measurement of isotype switching from IgM to IgG is an important feature of a normal immune response to vaccination as well as natural infection. The AUSAB® assay can measure both isotypes of anti-HBs, but these need to be separated prior to making the measurement. This is done most conveniently by a rate-zonal centrifugal separation of a 0.5-ml serum sample through a 4.5-ml linear 5–25% sucrose density gradient at $50,000 \times g$ for 2 hr (J. Gerin, personal communication). After centrifugation is complete, 0.5-ml fractions are collected from the bottom of the tube and directly assayed for anti-HBs. The system is calibrated using known human IgM and IgG and measuring their location in the gradient using immunodiffusion with anti-human IgM and IgG antibodies. Using this technique a study of anti-HBs isotype switching was performed following administration of PDV or recombinant yeast-derived vaccine (YDV). One month after the first dose, the major detectable isotype was IgM, at 2 months most was IgG, and at 3 months IgM was not detectable (19).

3. Anti-HBs Subtype Assays

Based on the known protective efficacy of anti-*a*–directed anti-HBs, it is essential to know that a vaccine elicits this antibody and to follow its persistence. A method was developed by Hoofnagle et al. (18) to measure anti-*a*, anti-*d*, and anti-*y* antibodies. This method was modified (W. J. Miller, unpublished) to quantitate subtypes. Anti-HBs test serum is diluted to contain approximately 200 mIU/ml (~40 ng anti-HBs/ml), and 0.1 ml is mixed in duplicate with 0.1 ml of HBsAg (ad) (200 μg HBsAg/ml) or 0.1 ml of subtype HBsAg (ay) (200 μg HBsAg/ml) or 0.1 ml of normal human serum. The test also includes known anti-*ad* antibody and anti-*ay* antibody and positive and negative controls. All samples are incubated for 2 hours at room temperature, a bead from the Ausab® kit is added, and any free anti-HBs is bound to the bead following a 16-hour incubation at room temperature. After washing, the beads are incubated with radiolabeled HBsAg for 4 hours at room temperature. The washed beads are counted. The percentages of anti-*a* and anti-*d* antibody can be calculated, as in Table 4.

The interpretation of these results is that serum 1 is an *ad* subtype response; since the HBsAg (*ay*) adsorbed 79.8% of the total anti-HBs, which is the amount

Table 4

Condition	CPM		
	Serum 1	Serum 2	Serum 3
Normal human serum (NHS) added	10,417	8,072	14,392
HBsAg (*ad*) added	122	686	119
HBsAg (*ay*) added	2,195	150	138
Negative kit control (NKC)	108	108	108
Positive kit control	13,890	13,890	13,890

For *Serum 1*:

$$\% \text{ blocking with HBsAg } (ad) = 100 - \frac{(\text{CPM HBsAG } ad) - (\text{CPM NKC})}{(\text{CPM NHS}) - (\text{CPM NKC})} \times 100$$

$$= 100 - \frac{129 - 108}{10,417 - 108} \times 100$$

$$= 100 - 0.2\%$$

$$= 99.8\%$$

$$\% \text{blocking with HBsAg } (ay) = 100 - \frac{(\text{CPM HBsAG } ay) - (\text{CPM NKC})}{(\text{CPM NHS}) - (\text{CPM NKC})} \times 100$$

$$= 79.8\%$$

of anti-*a*, 99.8–79.8% or 20% of the anti-HBs is anti-*d*. In order to validate the quantitative capacity of this procedure, various proportions of known anti-*a* and anti-*d* monoclonal antibodies (MAb) were prepared and measured in this test (Table 5). The recoveries of anti-*a* and anti-*d* Mabs are very close to theoretical, especially at the extremes of 100% anti-*a* or anti-*d*, and show the validity of this method. Typically, *ca.* 65% of the anti-HBs antibodies are to the anti-*a* specificity one month after the first vaccine dose, which increases to ≥90% after the third month.

4.   Anti-HBs Affinity and Avidity Determination

The measurement of the binding constant of a MAb or polyclonal antibody to a single distinct antigen is called an *affinity constant*. If the measurement of the binding constant of a polyclonal antibody to an antigen with more than one binding site is performed, the resulting derived net binding value of all antibodies to all antigens is called an *avidity constant*. The measurement of the affinity constant is a precise value, while the avidity constant is an imprecise average value but may better approximate the extent of actual in vivo viral neutralization.

The affinity constant to a synthetic cyclic peptide (amino acid residues 139–147) of S polypeptide or to a HBsAg-derived gp27/p24 polypeptide complex antigen was measured for anti-HBs in human serum (20) using a procedure of Stanley et al. (21). The method involved incubating the test serum with a range of ^{125}I-labeled antigen concentrations at 4°C for 1 hour followed by the addition of an equal volume of saturated ammonium sulfate (for synthetic peptides) or 3.5% polyethylene glycol (for gp27/p24). Following centrifugation the amount of antigen in the pellet and supernatant is determined and the affinity constant determined (22). In an evaluation of the affinity constants of 25 human

Table 5 Validation of A Subtyping Assay for Hepatitis B Antibody

Theoretical % anti-*a*/% anti-*d*[a]	Found % anti-*a*/% anti-*d*[b]
0/100	0/100
40/60	30/69
64/36	52/48
80/20	70/29
85/15	89/11
100/0	100/0

[a]Known mixtures of anti-*a* and anti-*d* monoclonal antibodies to HBsAg were prepared in normal human serum.

[b]These are the % anti-*a* and % anti-*d* anti-HBs antibody concentrations found using this subtyping assay.

sera from PDV and YDV vaccinees (20), the average of PDV-induced antibodies to the cyclic peptide was 40×10^6 l/M and 37×10^6 l/M for the YDV sera. Likewise, the average affinity constants of the PDV sera to the gp27/p24 complex was 27×10^6 l/M and 33×10^6 l/M for the YDV sera. The avidity constants were measured in a group of recipients of the PDV and YDV (19). The method (modified from Refs. 23 and 24) involves the incubation of an appropriately diluted test serum with a constant amount of ^{125}I-HBsAg and a variable amount of unlabeled HBsAg. Following incubation to equilibrium, the antibody-antigen complex is captured using goat antihuman antibody coupled to agarose beads. Following washing and counting of the beads, the data are plotted as amount bound/maximum bound vs. the molar concentration of HBsAg. The avidity constant is 1/HBsAg (molar) at 50% maximum bound and range from $4–8 \times 10^{10}$ l/M for six PDV sera and $1–16 \times 10^{10}$ l/M for six YDV sera.

5. Anti-HBs IgG Subclass Assays

The subclass of the anti-HBs IgG response was measured by Mattila et al. (25) following vaccination with PDV. The method used polystyrene tubes coated with HBsAg to which were added various dilutions of human serum following vaccination. The subclass anti-HBs was measured by the addition first of MAb antihuman subclass IgG and, following incubation and washing, the addition of ^{125}I-labeled rabbit antimouse antibody. The study shows that the early response is nearly 100% IgG1, while the postdose three response indicates that the average IgG1 proportion had decreased to 78% and the IgG2 had risen to 12% with the remainder distributed between IgG3 and IgG4. This pattern of response is similar to that of the natural disease as well as to natural mumps and rubella infections.

C. PreS Antigens

The PreS regions of the HBsAg membrane antigen have come under intensive study in the last 10 years. During the acute phase of hepatitis B infection, the PreS1 and PreS2 antigens have been detected by an ELISA (26,27) from the time of onset of symptoms for up to 8 weeks afterward. There appears to be no prognostic relationship of the presence or clearance of PreS1 and PreS2 antigens in natural disease (28,29). Experimentally, the PreS2 antigen has been implicated in assisting in an anti-HBs response in certain inbred mice unable to respond to HBsAg vaccines containing only the S polypeptide (30), and antibody to PreS2 was shown to be neutralizing (31) in chimpanzees. Immunization of chimpanzees with a synthetic PreS2 peptide was found to be protective (32) to HBV challenge. The PreS1 region has been shown to be implicated in liver cell binding of HBV (33), and amino acids 12–21 induce and elicit a T-cell priming response upon subsequent administration of suboptimal doses of HBsAg in mice (34) leading to the production of anti-HBs conformational *a* epitope antibody. Additionally, anti-PreS1 (aa12–47) antibody was shown to be protective in chimps (35).

1. Anti-PreS2 Assays

Sensitive assays for measuring anti-PreS2 have been reported. In one form of the assay, synthetic PreS2 peptide is adsorbed to a solid phase and used to capture anti-PreS2, which is detected using ^{125}I- or horseradish peroxidase (HPO)– labeled anti-human IgG antibodies (31,36). The second form uses PreS2-containing HBsAg particles adsorbed to a solid phase, and test serum is mixed with either ^{125}I- or HPO-labeled anti-PreS2 MAb and competes for a limited number of PreS2 sites (37,38). Both methods demonstrate the appearance of anti-PreS2 following hepatitis B convalescence. However, when the two assays were used to follow seroconversion to PreS2-containing vaccines, different seroconversion rates were observed. Using the latter assay, approximately threefold higher seroconversion rates were seen than when using the former assay. These differences between the two methods may related to either steric hindrance of anti-PreS2 binding to the PreS2 peptide because of its physical adsorption to the plastic surface or to a difference in folding of the PreS2 peptide compared to the PreS2 sequence on the HBsAg particle of the vaccine.

2. Anti-PreS1 Assays

Two assays have been reported to measure anti-PreS1 antibodies. One assay used a PreS1 (aa 20–120) fusion to the MS2 polymerase from *E. coli* as the antigen (39). This antigen was electrophoresed and, after immunoblotting, was incubated with serial dilutions of chimp or human sera. Anti-PreS1 antibodies were detected using ^{125}I-antihuman IgG antibody or HPO-coupled antihuman IgM. In infected chimpanzees HBsAg appeared 2 weeks before PreS1 antigen, while anti-PreS1 (both IgG and IgM) appeared 2 weeks after PreS1 antigen appearance, and the two coexisted for about 10 weeks until HBsAg and PreS1 simultaneously disappeared. Anti-PreS1 was found in a few acutely infected hepatitis B patients using this assay.

In a second assay to measure anti-PreS1 antibodies (29), test serum was incubated with purified PreS1-containing native HBsAg for 1 hour at 37°C. The mixture was added to a microtiter well previously coated with a MAb to PreS1. The binding of unneutralized HBsAg to the MAb was subsequently detected using HPO-coupled anti-HBs. If binding of the native HBsAg was inhibited by >50%, the test serum was scored as positive for anti-PreS1. Studies using this assay method were more comprehensive than those of Klinkert and involved 58 hepatitis B carriers (4 positive), 54 convalescents (21 positive), and 44 vaccinees of PreS1-containing HBsAg (24 positive) for anti-PreS1. In both the convalescent and vaccinated groups, high anti-HBs levels correlated with a high anti-PreS1 antibody response. In general, it appeared that about 10,000 mIU anti-HBs/ml correlated with 50% inhibition of PreS1 HBsAg binding. The fact that there are about 20–30 a epitopes on a HBsAg particle surface but only about 2–3 PreS1 peptides, coupled with the fact that the HBsAg assay (AUSRIA) is a direct RIA and the PreS1 assay a 5- to 10-fold less sensitive competition assay, may account for the decreased ability to measure anti-PreS1 antibodies using this methodology.

VIII.   T-CELL–MEDIATED IMMUNITY ASSAYS

A more detailed description of the importance of a lymphocyte response to resolution of infection as well as a vaccine-induced white cell response is given elsewhere in this book (Chapter 3). An excellent review by Sylvan (40) supplies the reader a clear view of a complex relatively new field as it relates to prophylaxis. Although anti-HBs in serum was shown to correlate with protection, much data has begun to appear in the literature indicating the involvement of helper T cells and soluble T-cell differentiation factors in the viral recognition and neutralization process.

In a typical assay to measure T-cell help (41), mononuclear cells (PBMC), T-cell–enriched (TCE) fraction, and T-cell–depleted (TCD) fraction are isolated by a combination of Ficoll-hypaque gradient centrifugation and rosetting with treated sheep erythrocytes. The TCE cells are first shown to be free of B cells due to lack of stimulation of anti-HBs using pokeweed mitogen. They are subsequently cultured in replicate wells with several different concentrations of HBsAg and PreS2 peptide antigens. The TCE cells are supplemented with irradiated PBMC cells as a source of antigen-presenting cells. Following 14 days of culturing, the collected supernatants are then assayed by placing them in culture with TCD cells for an additional 10 days. The media of these cultures are then assayed for anti-HBs. Cupps (41) shows that in this system soluble T-cell factors stimulated in TCE cultures by HBsAg and PreS2 antigen are capable of inducing a specific anti-HBs response in the TCD cells from persons remotely infected with HBV. Most interesting was the detection of an anti-S response by TCD cells incubated with culture broths from TCE cells stimulated with the PreS2 peptide, thus perhaps demonstrating an example of a primed memory response, which may be important in anamnestic protection following natural disease or vaccination. These techniques are laborious to perform, control, and, in many cases, the differences are not profound. These determinations are important to understanding immunological memory and to development of potential improved vaccines, which may depend on T-cell help evoked from inclusion of PreS sequences, but presently are not amenable to routine evolution of vaccines.

IX. CORE MARKER ASSAYS

The remaining assays described in this chapter were developed to assess the disease state during HBV infection. The methods are largely validated, licensed procedures and are important to vaccine development in detecting possible concurrent natural infection among clinical vaccinees during efficacy studies. These markers of infection are likewise useful in chimpanzee challenge studies since the present commercial vaccines do not contain any core components. Finally, if future HBV vaccines do intentionally include core proteins, the assays to assess their immunogenicity are in place. However, a possible core-containing future vaccine would compromise the utility of some of these assays such as HBcAg, anti-HBc, HBeAg, and anti-HBe, but the polymerase chain reaction (PCR) assay for DNA, as well as liver function assays such as ALT, will still be available to assess HBV infection among vaccinees.

A. Total Anti-HBc Assay

The most broadly employed assay to measure anti-HBc is a competitive RIA (Corab, Abbott Labs), which involves the incubation of equal volumes of human serum and ^{125}I-labeled anti-HBc with a recombinant HBcAg-coated polystyrene bead. Following overnight incubation, the washed beads are counted. If a test serum is devoid of anti-HBc, it records as a high CPM, and conversely a positive serum records as a low CPM. This competitive configuration usually detects antibody concentrations as low as 5–10 ng/ml. Anti-HBc usually is found along with anti-HBs in sera for 10 years and longer after convalescence from natural infection. This antibody is not detected following vaccination with HBsAg vaccines.

B. Anti-HBc IgM Assay

Specific IgM antibodies are measured most easily using an antihuman IgM capture assay. This type of test depends upon the presence of a sufficient proportion of specific IgM to total IgM so that a signal significantly greater than background can be obtained. In general, the specific IgM will have to be $\geq 0.1\%$ of the total IgM in the serum to allow this method to work. If the ratio is less than 0.1%, then the IgM will have to be separated from the IgG and the specific IgM antibody can be measured in a direct RIA, as is required in the case of anti-HBs IgM. This latter method is quite laborious and error prone. Fortunately, anti-HBc antibodies appear during HBV infection at levels allowing detection in an IgM capture assay. The assays use a solid phase coated with antihuman IgM, which is used to capture IgM antibodies from diluted serum. Following incubation and washing, the solid phase is incubated with HBcAg, which will bind to anti-HBc IgM. Finally, the HBcAg is detected using a labeled anti-HBc antibody to complete the four layers of this assay. A study of 12 infected patients (5) using a commercial assay kit (CORAB-M, Abbott Labs) showed that all sera were anti-HBc IgM–positive for 2 months following illness, with 11 or 12 patients negative at 6 months following onset. This method has been shown to be an excellent marker of ongoing infection, especially since in many cases HBsAg positivity may persist for only a few weeks and may be negative in most serum samples.

C.   Anti-HBe/HBeAg Assays

HBeAg and its antibody occur in serum during HBV infection. HBeAg is the 15-kD polypeptide fragment of HBcAg that lacks the 35 carboxy-terminal arginine-rich amino acids involved in DNA binding (42). It has been found to be present in serum during the acute phase of infection, and appearance of anti-HBe is taken as a sign of convalescence. Recombinant HBeAg has been expressed (43) and used as a reagent in a test capable of sensitively measuring anti-HBe or HBeAg in human serum. The assay configured to measure HBeAg is a direct RIA sandwich method in which an anti-HBe–coated solid phase is incubated in test serum; after incubation and washing, HBeAg is detected using labeled anti-HBe. The assay for anti-HBe (Abbott) involves the addition of a precise amount of recombinant HBeAg to the test serum, then an anti-HBe–coated solid phase is added and a competitive situation ensues. If anti-HBe is present at high levels in the test serum, it combines with the added HBe, which then will not be available to bind to the anti-HBe on the solid phase. The subsequent detection of HBeAg, or lack thereof, using labeled anti-HBe completes the test. Therefore, a low signal indicates high anti-HBe levels in the test serum.

D.   HBV DNA Assays

DNA in HBV was first imputed to be present in infected serum by measuring the activity of the DNA polymerase enzyme present within the virion (44), but this method suffered from insensitivity, requiring a concentration of approximately 10^8 virions/ml to be detected. A hybridization method subsequently was described to detect HBV DNA (45) using a ^{32}P-labeled DNA probe and later using ^{125}I-labeled DNA at high specific activity (46). These assays required 10^6 virions/ml for detection. The PCR assay for HBV DNA was found to be the most sensitive and is now the preferred method (47). This assay was shown to provide a $>10^4$-fold increase over direct slot blot hybridization. The primers used two core sequences, which after amplification were detected by ethidium bromide staining of the agarose gel (PCR-EB) or Southern blot hybridization of the transferred DNA (PCR-SBH). It was found using cloned HBV DNA that the PCR-SBH was 10^3-fold more sensitive than PCR-EB. When these methods were applied to three groups of hepatitis sera [A: patients with chronic hepatitis positive for HBsAg, anti-HBc, and HBeAg; B: patients with chronic hepatitis positive for HBsAg, anti-HBc, and anti-HBe; C: patients with chronic hepatitis (by liver biopsy) positive only for anti-HBs], the data indicated that HBV DNA is still present in sera of all three groups by PCR-SBH in the face of the usual markers associated with convalescence and confirming HBV replication continues after appearance of seroconversion markers. This latter method theoretically needs only two DNA molecules for detection.

X. CONCLUSION

Sensitive assays have been developed to detect the HBV antigens and antibodies associated with the acute, convalescent, chronic carrier, and vaccinated states. These assays have been of immeasurable help in the timely development of protective HBV vaccines. If future vaccines are to contain PreS1 peptides, a simple and sensitive assay needs to be developed. If future vaccine development depends upon the measurement of elicited T-cell responses, assays facilitating these difficult measurements will also be needed. The HBV vaccine model has demonstrated how assays can be used to aid in vaccine development as well as for disease detection. This experience will doubtless have a long-range effect upon the future development of vaccines against other human diseases. The progress in this field during these last 25 years has been monumental.

REFERENCES

1. B. S. Blumberg, H. J. Alter, and S. Visnich, A "new" antigen in leukemia sera, *J. Am. Med. Assoc.*, *191*: 541 (1965).
2. A. M. Prince, An antigen detected in the blood during the incubation period of serum hepatitis, *Proc. Natl. Acad. Sci. USA*, *60*: 814 (1968).
3. S. Krugman, J. P. Giles, and J. Hammond, Infectious hepatitis, *J. Am. Med. Assoc.*, *200*: 365 (1968).
4. Centers for Disease Control, Update on hepatitis B prevention, *Morbid. Mortal. Wkly. Rep.*, *36*: 353 (1987).
5. K. H. Chau, M. P. Hargie, R. H. Decker, I. K. Mushahwar, and L. R. Overby, Serodiagnosis of recent hepatitis B infection by IgM class anti-HBc, *Hepatology*, *3*: 142 (1983).
6. W. Stibbe and W. H. Gerlich, Structural relationships between minor and major proteins of hepatitis B surface antigen, *J. Virol.*, *46*: 626 (1983).
7. K. H. Heermann, U. Goldman, W. Schwartz, T. Seyffarth, H. Baumgartern, and W. H. Gerlich, Large surface proteins of hepatitis B virus containing the pre-S sequence, *J. Virol.*, *52*: 396 (1984).
8. A. M. Prince, H. Ikram, and T. P. Hopp, Hepatitis B virus vaccine: Identification of HBsAg/a and HBsAg/d but not HBsAg/y subtype antigen determinants on a synthetic immunogenic peptide, *Proc. Natl. Acad. Sci. USA*, *79*: 579 (1982).

9. G. L. Le Bouvier, The heterogeneity of Australia antigen, *J. Infect. Dis.*, *123*: 671 (1971).

10. W. H. Bancroft, F. K. Mundon, and P. K. Russell, Detection of additional antigenic determinants of hepatitis B antigen, *J. Immunol.*, *109*: 842 (1972).

11. W. F. Carman, A. R. Zanetti, P. Karayianoris, J. Water, G. Manzilla, E. Tanji, A. J. Zuckerman, and H. C. Thomas, Vaccine-induced escape mutant of hepatitis B virus. *Lancet*, *336*: 325 (1990).

12. M. R. Hilleman, A. U. Bertland, E. B. Buynak, G. P. Lampson, W. J. McAleer, A. A. McLean, R. R. Roehm, and A. A. Tytell, Clinical and laboratory studies of HBsAg vaccine, *Viral Hepatitis* (G. N. Vyas, S. N. Cohen, and R. Schmid, eds.), The Franklin Institute Press, Philadelphia, p. 525 (1978).

13. R. H. Purcell and J. L. Gerin, Hepatitis B vaccines: A status report, *Viral Hepatitis* (G. N. Vyas, S. N. Cohen, and R. Schmid, eds.), The Franklin Institute Press, Philadelphia, p. 491 (1978).

14. W. Szmuness, C. E. Stevens, E. A. Zang, et al., A controlled clinical trial of the efficacy of the hepatitis B vaccine (Heptavax-B). A final report, *Hepatology*, *1*: 377 (1981).

15. D. P. Francis, S. C. Hadler, S. E. Thompson, J. E. Maynard, D. G. Ostrow, N. Altman, E. H. Braff, P. O'Malley, D. Hawkins, F. N. Judson, K. Penley, T. Nylund, G. Christie, F. Meyers, J. N. Moore, Jr., A. Gardner, I. L. Doto, J. H. Miller, et al., The prevention of hepatitis B with vaccine: Report of the Centers for Disease Control multi-center efficacy trial among homosexual men, *Ann. Intern. Med.*, *97*: 362 (1982).

16. B. L. Murphy, J. E. Maynard, and G. L. Le Bouvier, Viral subtypes and cross-protection in hepatitis B virus infections of chimpanzees, *Intervirology*, *3*: 378 (1974).

17. W. Szmuness, C. E. Stevens, E. J. Harley, et al., Hepatitis B vaccine in medical staff of hemodialysis units: Efficacy and subtype cross-protection, *N. Engl. J. Med.*, *307*: 1481 (1982).

18. J. H. Hoofnagle, R. J. Gerety, L. A. Smallwood, and L. F. Barker, Subtyping of hepatitis B surface antigen and antibody by radioimmunoassay, *Gastroenterol.*, *72*: 290. (1977).

19. E. A. Emini, R. W. Ellis, W. J. Miller, W. J. McAleer, E. M. Scolnick, and R. J. Gerety, Production and immunological analysis of recombinant hepatitis B vaccine, *J. Infect.*, *13*: 3 (1986).

20. S. E. Brown, C. R. Howard, A. J. Zuckerman, and M. W. Steward, Determination of the affinity of antibodies to hepatitis B surface antigen in human sera, *J. Immunol. Meth.*, *72*: 41 (1984).

21. C. Stanley, A. M. Lew, and M. W. Steward, The measurement of antibody affinity: A comparison of five techniques utilizing a panel of monoclonal anti-DNP antibodies and the effect of high affinity antibody on the measurement of low-affinity antibody, *J. Immunol. Meth.*, *64*: 119 (1983).

22. M. W. Steward and R. E. Petty, The use of ammonium sulphate globulin precipitation for determination of affinity of anti-protein antibodies in mouse serum, *Immunol.*, *22*: 747 (1972).

23. R. P. Ekins, Radioimmunoassay and saturation analysis, basic principles and theory, *Br. Med. Bull.*, *30*: 3 (1974).

24. F. Celada, Quantitative studies of the adoptive immunological memory in mice, I. An age-dependent barrier to syngeneic transplantation, *J. Exp. Med.*, *124*: 1 (1966).

25. P. S. Mattila, J. Pelkonen, and O. Makela, Proportions of IgG subclasses in antibodies formed during vaccination with hepatitis B surface antigen, *Scand. J. Immunol.*, *24*: 699 (1986).

26. A. Budkowska, M-M. Riottot, P. Dubreuil, Y. Lazizi, C. Brechot, E. Sobczak, M-A. Petit, and J. Pillot, Monoclonal antibody recognizing Pre-S(2) epitope of hepatitis B virus: Characterization of Pre-S(2) epitope and anti-Pre-S(2) antibody, *J. Med. Virol.*, *20*: 111 (1986).

27. G. Gerken, M. Manns, W. H. Gerlich, G. Hess, and K-H. Meyer zum Buschenfelde, Pre-S encoded surface proteins in relation to the major viral surface antigen in acute hepatitis B virus infection, *Gastroenterology*, *92*: 1864 (1987).

28. T. J. M. van Ditzhuijsen, L. P. C. Kuijpers, M. J. Koens, P. J. M. Rijntjes, A. M. van Loon, and S. H. Yap, Hepatitis B Pre-S1 and Pre-S2 proteins: Clinical significance and relation to hepatitis B virus DNA, *J. Med. Virol.*, *32*: 87 (1990).

29. R. Deepen, K.-H. Heermann, A. Uy, R. Thomssen, and W. H. Gerlich, Assay of preS epitopes and preS1 antibody in hepatitis B virus carriers and immune persons, *Med. Microbiol. Immunol.*, *179*: 49 (1990).

30. D. R. Milich, M. K. McNamara, A. McLachlan, G. B. Thornton, and F. V. Chisari, Distinct H-2-linked regulation of T-cell responses to the pre-S and S regions of the same hepatitis B surface antigen polypeptide allows circumvention of nonresponsiveness to the S region, *Proc. Natl. Acad. Sci USA*, *82*: 8168 (1985).

31. A. R. Neurath, S. B. Kent, N. Strick, D. Stark, and P. Sproul, Genetic restriction of immune responsiveness to synthetic peptides corresponding to sequences in the pre-S region of the hepatitis B virus (HBV) envelope gene, *J. Med. Virol.*, *17*: 119 (1985).

32. E. A. Emini, V. Larson, J. Eichberg, *et al.*, Protective effect of a synthetic peptide comprising the complete Pre-S2 region of the hepatitis B virus surface protein, *J. Med. Virol.*, *28*: 7 (1989).

33. A. R. Neurath, S. B. H. Kent, N. Strick, and K. Parker, Identification and chemical synthesis of a host cell receptor binding site on hepatitis B virus, *Cell*, *4*: 429 (1986).

34. D. R. Milich, A. McLachlan, A. Moriarty, *et al.*, A single 10-residue pre-S(1) peptide can prime T cell for antibody production to multiple epitopes within the pre-S(1), pre-S(2) and S regions of HBsAg, *J. Immunol.*, *138*: 4457 (1987).

35. A. R. Neurath, B. Sero, and N. Strick, Antibodies to synthetic peptides from the pre-S1 region of the hepatitis B virus (HBV) envelope (env) protein are virus neutralizing and protective, *Vaccine*, *7*: 234 (1989).

36. M. I. Galan, J. Tomas, M. C. Bernal, F. J. Salmeron, and M. C. Maroto, Evaluation of the pre-S (pre-S(1)Ag/pre-S(2)Ab) system in hepatitis B virus infection, *J. Clin. Pathol.*, *44*: 25 (1991).

37. A. Budkowska, P. Dubreuil, and J. Pillot, Detection of antibodies to pre-S2 encoded epitopes of hepatitis B virus by monoclonal antibody-enzyme immunoassay, *J. Immunol. Meth.*, *102*: 85 (1987).

38. W. M. Hurni, R. R. Roehm, and W. J. Miller, Anti-PreS2 antibody assay for evaluating immune responses among recipients of recombinant hepatitis B PreS2+S vaccine, *J. Med. Virol.*, *30*: 146 (1990).

39. M-Q. Klinkert, L. Theilmann, E. Pfaff, and H. Schaller, Pre-S1 antigens and antibodies early in the course of acute hepatitis B virus infection, *J. Virol.*, *58*: 522 (1986).

40. S. P. E. Sylvan, Cellular immune responses to hepatitis B virus antigens in man, *Liver*, *11*: 1 (1991).

41. T. R. Cupps, J. H. Hoofnagle, R. W. Ellis, W. J. Miller, L. Seeff, A. Guerrera, J. L. Gerin, and S. A. Haas-Smith, *In vitro* immune responses to hepatitis B surface antigen (Pre-S2 and S) following remote infection by hepatitis B virus in humans, *J. Clin. Immunol.*, *9*: 229 (1989).

42. K. Takahashi, A. Machida, G. Funatsu, M. Nomura, S. Usuda, S. Aoyagi, K. Tachibana, H. Miyamoto, M. Imai, T. Nakamura, Y. Miyakawa, and M. Mayumi, Immunochemical structure of hepatitis B e antigen in the serum, *J. Immunol.*, *130*; 2903 (1983).

43. L. Mimms, J. Staller, I. K. Mushahwar, K. S. Spiezia, A. Kapsalis, and P. Andersen, Production, purification, and immunological characterization of a recombinant DNA-derived hepatitis B e antigen, *Viral Hepatitis and Liver Disease* (A. J. Zuckerman, ed.), Alan R. Liss, Inc., New York, p. 248 (1988).

44. P. M. Kaplan, R. L. Greenman, J. L. Gerin, R. H. Purcell, and W. S. Robinson, DNA Polymerase associated with human hepatitis B antigen, *J. Virol.*, *12*: 995 (1973).

45. J. Scotto, M. Hadchouel, C. Hery, J. Yvart, P. Tiollais, and C. Brechot, Detection of hepatitis B virus DNA in serum by a simple spot hybridization technique: Comparison with results for other viral markers, *Hepatology*, *3*: 279 (1983).

46. M. C. Kuhns, A. L. McNamara, C. M. Cabal, R. H. Decker, V. Thiers, C. Brechot, and P. Tiollais, A new assay for the quantitative detection of hepatitis B viral DNA in human serum, *Viral Hepatitis and Liver Disease* (A. J. Zuckerman, ed.), Alan R. Liss, Inc., New York, p. 258 (1988).

47. S. Kaneko, R. H. Miller, S. M. Feinstone, M. Unoura, K. Kobayashi, N. Hattori, and R. H. Purcell, Detection of serum hepatitis B virus DNA in patients with chronic hepatitis using the polymerase chain reaction assay, *Proc. Natl. Acad. Sci. USA*, *86*: 312 (1989).

7

Epidemiology of Hepatitis B Virus Infection

Stephen C. Hadler and Harold S. Margolis

Centers for Disease Control,
Atlanta, Georgia

I. INTRODUCTION

The hepatitis B virus (HBV) is an epidemiologically versatile pathogen able to cause both acute and chronic infections. The latter establishes a reservoir of persons able to transmit the virus and also results in chronic liver disease and primary hepatocellular carcinoma (PHC). Infection is spread relatively efficiently by several pathways, including by direct blood exposure, through homosexual and heterosexual activity, and from mother to infant both at birth and during early childhood. The prevalence of HBV varies widely throughout the world and ranges from a highly endemic disease of infancy and childhood in most of the developing world to a disease of low endemicity in developed countries limited primarily to adults with certain lifestyle-associated, medical, or occupational risk factors.

II. GLOBAL DISTRIBUTION OF HBV INFECTION

The distribution of infection is usually defined by three distinct levels of endemicity (1). These differ in the prevalence of chronic HBV infection, in the overall infection rate, in the usual age at which infection is acquired, and in the predominant modes of disease transmission. In high endemicity areas, 7–20% of persons are chronically infected with HBV, and the majority (>70%) of adults show evidence of prior infection. These regions include most of Asia (except

141

Japan and India), Africa, most of the Middle East, the Amazon basin of South America, most Pacific Island groups, and other specific populations such as Eskimos, Australian aborigines, and Maoris (2–10). Among these populations almost all infections are acquired in infancy or early childhood, and few adults remain susceptible to infection. HBV transmission occurs either during the perinatal period (vertical transmission) from chronically infected mothers to their infants or during the postnatal period (horizontal transmission) from infected mothers, siblings, or other chronically infected individuals inside or outside of the family to susceptible infants and children (11–18). Those who remain susceptible until adolescence may become infected by sexual exposure.

In intermediate-endemicity areas, the prevalence of chronic HBV infection is between 2 and 7%, and 20–50% of adults show evidence of infection. These areas include India, part of the Middle East, western Asia, Japan, eastern and southern Europe, and most of South and Central America (18). Disease transmission patterns are mixed, and transmission occurs in all age groups (newborn, childhood, and adult), but the predominant period of transmission probably occurs among younger children, adolescents, and young adults.

In low-endemicity areas, prevalence of HBV carriage is less than 2%, and prevalence of infection is less than 20% among adults. These areas include the United States, Canada, western Europe, Australia, and New Zealand. Disease transmission occurs primarily among adults. Nevertheless, transmission during the perinatal period and during early childhood provides a significant contribution to the HBV carrier burden.

HBV endemicity is relatively uniform on a regional as well as local level. In high-endemicity areas the prevalence of infection is quite uniform, even at the village level, although some variation occurs and the prevalence of HBsAg carriage may rarely reach 20–30% in some local areas. The widest variations in prevalence of infection occur in intermediate-endemicity areas, where racial and socioeconomic factors may lead to wide differences in risk of infection and to secular changes in infection rates (19). In areas of low endemicity there may reside ethnic or racial groups whose infection rates are dramatically different from the general population. Examples include Eskimo populations in Alaska, Canada, and Greenland (8, 9, 20); the Maoris of New Zealand (10); as well as immigrant populations coming from high- or intermediate-endemicity areas (18, 21). Nonetheless, the general uniformity of risk has greatly simplified the design of immunization strategies to prevent HBV infection and its long-term consequences such as cirrhosis or PHC.

III. MODES AND PATHWAYS OF TRANSMISSION

Because HBV produces a persistent infection, chronically infected individuals serve as the primary virus reservoir. Worldwide, an estimated 300 million persons are HBV carriers, the majority living in Asia and Africa (1). The HBV carrier state, defined as detection of HBsAg in blood over a 6-month interval, usually lasts indefinitely, although prospective studies suggest that 1–2% of such persons may resolve their chronic infection annually (22, 23). The infectivity of HBsAg carriers varies over time and is determined by the concentration of HBV in the blood. Hepatitis B e antigen (HBeAg) has been the most widely used marker of infectivity, although detection of HBV-DNA more precisely quantitates infectivity (24, 25). Early in the course of chronic HBV infection essentially all individuals are HBeAg positive, but they begin to lose HBeAg and infectivity as the HBV genome becomes integrated into the host DNA (26). The age-specific rate of HBeAg positivity varies in each of the endemicity areas, including in areas of high endemicity. In eastern Asia, the proportion of adult chronic HBV carriers who are HBeAg positive ranges from 30 to 40% (1, 2, 11, 13), while in Africa and the Middle East only 5–20% of chronically infected adults are positive (14, 17, 27). Acutely infected persons serve as temporary reservoirs for infection because they have high levels of HBV (HBeAg-positive) in their blood. They are important sources of transmission, particularly in areas of intermediate and low endemicity of infection.

As defined epidemiologically, the major pathways for HBV transmission include parenteral exposure to blood or other infective body fluids, sexual transmission, transmission to infants or young children from contact with an infected person, and transmission from mother to infant at birth. Within this framework, HBV transmission may occur through a wide range of exposures and routes, including those that are readily apparent as well as among those that are relatively obscure.

A.   Blood or Infectious Body Fluids

The primary vehicle for virus transmission is blood or serous fluids from HBV-infected individuals. In chimpanzee infectivity studies, HBV has been shown to circulate at levels above 10^8 virions per ml in HBeAg-positive persons (28, 29). Direct assessment of HBV-DNA levels gives estimates of 10^{10}/ml for HBeAg-positive persons and 10^1–10^7 in anti-HBe–positive persons (30). Body fluids directly derived from blood, such as exudates, pleural and peritoneal fluids, and other fluids from internal body cavities, contain high concentrations of virus that are likely comparable to those found in serum. Semen and saliva have also been consistently shown to contain HBV; however, the concentrations are about 10^3 times lower than in serum of the same individual. HBsAg and HBV-DNA have been detected less consistently in other body fluids such as urine, feces, and breast milk unless they are clearly contaminated with blood (28–35). The lower concentrations of virus in these fluids indicate a proportionally lower likelihood of disease transmission unless there is repeated exposure (36).

Transmission by contact with infected blood or body fluids encompasses the greatest range of pathways, both in high- and low-endemicity areas. Direct parenteral exposure to contaminated blood through transfusion or from serum used as a diluent/medium in vaccines or medications led to the recognition of this virus as a distinct entity from infectious hepatitis or hepatitis A (37, 38). Screening of blood and blood products for HBsAg and elimination of serum as a diluent for vaccines has virtually eliminated this risk in developed countries (39). However, recipients of pooled clotting factor concentrates that have not undergone terminal inactivation have remained at risk of infection because of subdetectable levels of HBsAg. In countries where blood is not systematically screened for HBsAg or where breaks in screening occur, risk of infection remains high (39).

Direct blood exposure through contaminated needles is the common pathway for transmission among parenteral drug users who share needles, their rate of infection being related directly to duration of drug use (40, 41). Contaminated needles have also been implicated in transmission in a variety of other settings, including tattoo parlors, acupuncture, among health-care and public-safety workers who sustain needlesticks, and during medical care in less developed countries where reusable needles and syringes have not been adequately sterilized (42–44). The average amount of blood transferred in needlesticks in the occupational setting (approximately 1 μl) combined with the high concentration of HBV in blood assures a relatively high efficiency of infection, which has been measured at 12–30% (45–47).

B. Sexual Contact

This is a well-documented pathway of HBV transmission in developed countries and likely of great, although less well-documented, importance in high and intermediate endemicity areas. HBV transmission by homosexual contact was recognized in the 1970s, when studies in numerous cities in Europe and the United States showed HBV prevalence of up to 80% in homosexual men—10–20 times higher than in adults in the same populations (48, 49). Detailed studies showed that major risk factors included anal intercourse and large numbers of sexual partners, as well as activities or other diseases associated with anal trauma or mucosal lesions (48–50).

HBV transmission by heterosexual contact was inferred from studies of prostitutes, sexual contacts of HBV carriers, and attendees of clinics for treatment of sexually transmitted diseases (51–55). The prevalence of markers of HBV infection in these groups were three- to fivefold higher than in the general population. In these groups and in the general population in the United States, HBV infection risk has been associated with increasing numbers of sexual partners and with prior syphilis infection (56–60). The strong association with syphilis infection could result from its ulcerative nature, which would increase the efficiency of HBV transmission, or it could be a surrogate marker for other chronic ulcerative genital diseases or for sexual contact with high-risk persons. The most recent studies in the United States have documented that transmission of HBV by heterosexual contact accounts for at least 25% of disease reported among adults, comparable to the disease burden due to parenteral drug use (58).

Studies of postexposure prophylaxis for spouses of acute hepatitis B cases have shown a 15–30% likelihood of disease transmission when no treatment is offered, and that transmission from men to women is approximately threefold more efficient than transmission from women to men (61, 62). From these studies and studies in homosexual men, it is estimated that the risk of HBV transmission through a single unprotected sexual contact between an infected person and susceptible partner is on the order of 1–3%. The clear evidence of sexual transmission in developed countries points to its likely importance in less developed countries. If children reach adolescence still susceptible to HBV infection, they would be more likely to have sexual contact with HBV carriers.

C. Early Childhood Infection

In populations with a high endemicity of infection, early childhood represents a period of high risk of infection and accounts for the majority of all infections. However, the pathways for transmission of the virus that occur during the first 5 years of life, except for perinatal transmission, have not been elucidated. Infections cluster in families with an HBV carrier but also occur in families without another carrier or infected person (12, 14, 17, 18, 21, 63, 64). Epidemiological studies have shown the major determinants of risk to include an HBsAg-positive mother or sibling (17, 21, 63, 64). The possible role of saliva as the pathway for HBV transmission must be considered in these situations that involve intimate nonsexual contact. The roles of semen and vaginal secretions in sexual transmission of HBV are clear; however, it is less clear whether saliva, which contains a similar concentration of virus as semen, plays a significant role in HBV transmission. Studies in chimpanzees have shown that saliva can cause infection if inoculated parenterally, but not when administered by nasal spray, when ingested orally, or when brushed on the gums (28, 29). Nevertheless, transmission by bite has been reported in several situations (32), shared chewing gum has been reported to cause disease transmission (65), and a case-control study in Shanghai showed a significant risk of infection among infants of HBV carrier mothers who premasticated their infant's food. The most likely pathway for HBV transmission in daycare centers in Okinawa has been thought to be saliva (66, 67).

Another possible pathway for transmission of HBV in these settings is through occult blood entering mucous membranes or inapparent transfer through nonintact skin. Transfer of virus through nonintact skin or through mucosal membranes (from splash accidents) has been shown to cause infection, while virus contamination of intact skin is not known to cause infection (29, 30, 68). Environmental sampling has demonstrated virus on surfaces and objects in medical laboratories, hemodialysis units, and dental operatories following treatment of HBV carriers, and HBV has been shown to survive on a surface of room temperature for at least one week in the dried state (69–71). In the hospital setting, an outbreak linked to transmission by computer cards contaminated with blood provides an example of the role fomites may play in disease transmission (72). A much larger outbreak of hepatitis B among participants in orienteering races in Sweden, attributed to scratches by bushes contaminated with blood, shows the potential for spread outside the hospital setting (73). HBV has also been found in skin lesions and wound exudates of chronically infected persons, and environmental sampling in homes with an HBV carrier showed HBsAg on a number of surfaces and objects (33). Environmental contamination and transfer of virus by fomites has been accepted as the primary pathway for disease transmission in hemodialysis units (74, 75). In all household settings where an HBV carrier resides, susceptible contacts are at risk of infection (52, 53), and the pathway of fomite transmission must be considered to be important.

The possibility of disease transmission by insects in tropical areas has been extensively debated. HBV can be detected in bedbugs and mosquitos following a blood meal from an HBV carrier and may persist for up to 2 weeks in the gut of bedbugs (76). Nevertheless, the limited host range for replication of HBV (humans and great apes) is confirmed by lack of evidence of viral replication in these insects (76, 77). Combined with lack of transfer to HBV from the gut to the insect's mouthparts, these studies indicate that hepatitis B is not a vectorborne disease in the classical sense. Transfer of virus into bite wounds could occur mechanically but would not be efficient. Epidemiological data in a few tropical areas have not shown a correlation between intensity of exposure to mosquitos and prevalence of infection.

Another possible pathway of HBV transmission among children in developing countries is person-to-person transmission from infected skin lesions. HBsAg has been detected in exudative lesions of HBV carriers (33) and impetiginous lesions are common in young children in these areas. Shared sleeping areas and crowded living conditions would be postulated to facilitate HBV transmission.

Unfortunately, direct parenteral exposure continues to play a role in HBV transmission. The use of unsterilized needles and syringes for the injection of medications is a common practice in some areas and has been shown to contribute to early childhood infections (44). The transfusion of blood or blood products that have not been screened for HBsAg contribute to HBV infection in children, especially in areas where young children receive blood transfusions for anemia (39).

D. Perinatal Infection

HBV transmission during the perinatal period is a major route of transmission. A central feature is that transmission occurs mainly at the time of birth rather than in utero, making infection amenable to prevention with hepatitis B vaccine and/or hepatitis B immune globulin (HBIG). The other important features are that efficiency of transmission is high and related to presence of HBeAg or HBV-DNA in the mother and that risk of becoming an HBV carrier and having subsequent long-term disease is highest in this subgroup. Infants born to HBsAg⁻, HBeAg-positive mothers have a 60–90% risk of developing HBV infection within 9 months of birth, and 90% of those infected become HBV carriers (11, 78, 79). Among babies born to HBeAg-negative mothers the risk of infection in the first year of life is lower (2–15%) but not negligible (18, 25, 27, 80). Fulminant hepatitis B infection has been reported among infants of such mothers and is possibly due to HBV with mutations in the precore region of the genome (81–83). Infants not infected in the first year of life remain at high risk of horizontal transmission in early childhood from contact with the mother and from other siblings in the household or in the village (12, 17, 21). The relative importance of perinatal HBV transmission varies with HBV endemicity and frequency of HBeAg positivity among HBV carrier mothers. In all parts of the world it is a major contributor (15–40%) to the number of HBV carriers in the population.

IV. REGIONAL PATTERNS OF DISEASE EPIDEMIOLOGY

Four major patterns of disease epidemiology can be defined that segregate by region. In high endemicity areas, there are two patterns; one is characterized by the significant proportion of infections that occur during the perinatal period and is found primarily in Asia, while the other is characterized by early childhood (horizontal) transmission of infection as is primarily seen in Africa. The other two patterns of disease epidemiology are represented by intermediate- and low-endemicity areas, respectively.

A. High-Endemicity Areas

In east and southeast Asian countries, transmission of HBV from mother to infant during the perinatal period is a major determinant of the outcome and epidemiology of HBV infection. In these countries, between 8 and 15% of women of childbearing age are HBV carriers, and 35–50% of these are HBeAg positive (1, 3, 11, 13, 78, 80). This high rate of HBeAg positivity increases the efficiency and rate of HBV transmission from carrier mothers to their newborn infants (13, 78, 80). It is estimated that 3–5% of all infants become HBV carriers and that between 30 and 50% of all chronic HBV infections in these countries result from perinatal disease transmission.

However, perinatal HBV transmission is not the sole determinant of the high rate of HBV infection observed in these areas. Studies have demonstrated that HBV transmission during the first 5 years of life is also frequent and accounts for most of the remaining chronic HBV infections in these countries. Beasley and

Hwang (12) showed a high frequency of postneonatal transmission among children of both HBeAg-positive and HBeAg-negative mothers in Taiwan. It is estimated that 30–50% of infections occur within families, and the importance of intrafamilial HBV transmission has been shown in studies in Taiwan and the Philippines (12, 13, 63, 64). The highest risk of infection was among children of HBsAg-positive mothers, and HBsAg positivity clustered in families. An elevated risk of infection was also associated with children exposed to HBsAg-positive siblings or fathers. These studies have also shown that at least 30% of infections occur in persons not living with an HBsAg-positive family member, suggesting a high rate of extrafamilial disease transmission (63). Studies in Okinawa have shown that extrafamilial transmission may be important in some countries, particularly through contact among young children in daycare centers (66). These patterns of transmission appear to persist when persons from Asia emigrate or become refugees in more developed countries (21, 84, 85). Transmission among older children and adults has not been as well studied in these areas; nevertheless, between 5 and 20% of adults may remain susceptible to infection, and transmission among adults similar to that in developed countries must be presumed to occur.

The relative contribution of perinatal and postneonatal HBV infection to the HBV carrier pool in a country such as China is shown in Figure 1. The assumptions used for each of the outcome determinants (e.g., HBeAg-positive rate, infection rate, chronic infection rate) can be considered representative of Asia. At the end of the first year of life of a birth cohort, almost all chronic HBV infections are attributable to perinatal transmission. However, by the end of 5 years, the contribution of perinatal transmission, while significant, drops to 20% because of the continued high rate of postneonatal infection in children born to HBsAg-negative mothers.

Areas with a high rate of perinatal infection are defined by adult women, likely infected in early childhood, who remain HBeAg positive and are able to transmit infection efficiently to their newborn infants. Although women in other parts of the world, particularly Africa and tropical South America, acquire infection in early childhood, fewer remain HBeAg positive when they reach childbearing age. The reason that Asian women remain HBeAg positive is not fully understood. Possible explanations include a genetic predisposition to remain HBeAg positive, birth spacing that affects clearance of HBeAg (86, 87), or that perinatal infection itself, as opposed to early childhood infection, predisposes to retention of HBeAg positivity (88).

In most other high-HBV-endemicity areas, perinatal HBV transmission occurs but contributes less to the HBV carrier pool than does postneonatal person-to-person (horizontal) transmission to young children. In Africa, South America, the Middle East, and Pacific Islands (1, 4–6, 14, 17, 27), 10% or more of adult women may be HBV carriers, but fewer than 20% are HBeAg positive.

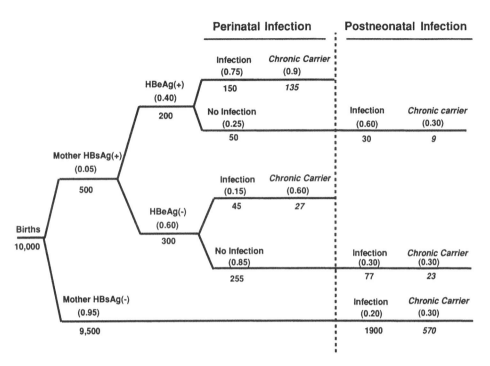

Figure 1 Occurrence of hepatitis B virus infections by 5 years of age in a birth cohort residing in an area of high endemicity of infection that also has a high rate of HBeAg positivity (e.g., China). Outcomes are presented in a decision analytical model. Risk of outcome is indicated above the line; the actual number of persons affected is indicated below the line.

Thus, in these areas, only an estimated 1.5–2% of infants acquire chronic HBV infection from their mothers during the perinatal period, and only 10–20% of all chronic HBV infections result from perinatal transmission. In most of these areas, particularly in Africa, infection is acquired rapidly among young children, so that 80–90% become infected by age 10 years (4, 14, 16, 18, 27). While risk factors are less well defined in these areas, family studies have shown high risks of postneonatal transmission from infected mothers and from infected siblings and lower risks from fathers and other adults (16, 17, 27). Studies in Jordan have shown family size to be directly associated with risk of infection and socioeconomic status to be inversely related to infection (17).

B. Intermediate-Endemicity Areas

In these areas, patterns of disease transmission generally represent a combination of perinatal, childhood, and adult transmission. In these areas, only 2–7% of adult women are HBV carriers and generally fewer than 20% are HBeAg positive; thus only a modest proportion (10–20%) of HBV carriers may be estimated to result from perinatal disease transmission. Transmission in childhood may be inferred from review of age-specific HBV infection prevalence data, while transmission in adulthood generally occurs in the same risk groups as in developed countries of low HBV endemicity. Some areas with intermediate endemicity, particularly Brazil and other parts of tropical South America, show wide variations in HBV prevalence. In Brazil, Surinam, and Trinidad, infection prevalence may vary with race, being highest in those with Asian ancestry, intermediate in black or mestizo groups, and lower in those of European ancestry (6, 89). Indigenous groups in these areas tend to have higher HBV prevalences, comparable to those found in Africa and Asia. Local variations in prevalence may be large in these areas (e.g., Colombia and Brazil), and socioeconomic status is often inversely associated with prevalence. For these reasons, studies to define transmission patterns and to devise control strategies in these areas may of necessity be more complex than in high-HBV-endemicity areas.

C.   Low-Endemicity Areas

Transmission of HBV in these areas has been studied intensively and is defined in greatest detail in the United States. In the United States, data from seroprevalence studies and from surveillance of acute hepatitis cases provide complementary information on disease transmission. Prevalence of chronic infection among adults averages 0.3%, and 5% have had prior HBV infection (59). Incidence data suggest that 300,000 new infections occur annually and that 20,000–30,000 persons become HBV carriers at risk of chronic liver disease and PHC. From national birth data, an estimated 22,000 infants are born to HBV carrier mothers annually, and, prior to national prevention programs, 4–6000 became HBV carriers due to perinatal transmission (18). Perinatal transmission, which accounts for 15–20% of new HBV carriers, occurs primarily in minority groups, with Asians and blacks accounting for 60 and 15% of perinatal transmission, respectively. Thus, perinatal transmission remains important even in this country and its prevention has become the cornerstone of HBV-prevention programs in the United States and in many other low-endemicity areas (90). HBV transmission in childhood is of modest importance in the United States, with children less than 15 years old accounting for only 3% of reported acute hepatitis B cases in 1988. Nevertheless, the chronic disease burden from childhood transmission is manyfold higher, as younger children are more likely to become HBV carriers (18). Pathways of transmission are not clearly defined in this group. Among immigrants from high-endemicity areas and families of adopted children from these areas, household contact with HBV carriers, particularly mothers and siblings, is the most important factor and leads to significant risk of disease (21, 91). Extrafamilial contact has also been implicated in transmission among Asian refugees (21). Transmission has rarely been reported in daycare centers in the United States except when extenuating circumstances such as aggressive behavior (biting) occur (67). Transmission in institutions for the developmentally disabled has diminished with the improvements in conditions and implementation of hepatitis B vaccination programs.

HBV transmission among adolescents and adults accounts for approximately 95% of acute HBV infections in the United States and 70–75% of new chronic HBV infections annually; young adults aged 15–39 years account for 75% of all disease cases (18, 92). Adults may be at risk due to lifestyle (parenteral drug abuse, sexual activity with multiple partners), occupation (health care and public safety), exposure to blood in medical settings (hemodialysis, hemophiliacs receiving pooled donor products), and intimate (household) contact with HBV carriers. In the United States, parenteral drug abuse and heterosexual exposures are the most important risk factors, and each account for about 25% of HBV transmission. Homosexual exposures and occupationally acquired disease account for diminishing proportions of disease (less than 10 and 5%, respectively) due to changing sexual behavior and hepatitis B vaccine use. About 30% of acute disease cases do not have identifiable risk factors, although denial of drug abuse and sexual and household exposure to HBV carriers may account for some of this problem (18, 57, 58).

Thus, sexual transmission and blood exposure through drug abuse remain the major pathways of transmission in this country and in most developed countries in Europe. Risk of infection amoung U.S. adults is higher in certain racial groups, including blacks (two- to fourfold higher risk) and Hispanics (1.5–fold higher risk), compared to whites. In addition, low socioeconomic status is associated with higher risk of infection in both prevalence and incidence data, and HBV, like other STDs and bloodborne diseases, has clearly become a disease of the underclass (57, 58).

Other pathways of disease transmission among adults have varied widely. Nosocomial HBV transmission in hospitals has not been found to account for significant amounts of disease transmission in a recent case-control study in the United States (57), probably due to rigorous standards for sterilization of blood-contaminated equipment and use of disposable needles. In the past, outbreaks of hepatitis B were frequent among patients and staff in hemodialysis units, but transmission has been largely eliminated in the United States (93).

V. CONCLUSION

The availability of safe and effective hepatitis B vaccines makes the prevention of chronic HBV infection and its consequences possible. The epidemiology of the various patterns of HBV infection must be considered in the design of any immunization strategy. The proper timing of immunization must be determined from the regional or local epidemiology with respect to the contribution of perinatal HBV infection to the overall infection rate and must be balanced with the feasibility of vaccine delivery. Within the various modes of HBV transmission and patterns of infection endemicity, there are ample points at which hepatitis B vaccination would interrupt transmission of infection.

REFERENCES

1. J. E. Maynard, Kane, M. A., Hadler, S. C. Global control of hepatitis B through vaccination: Role of hepatitis B vaccine in the expanded program of immunization. *Rev. Inf. Dis. 11*(S3): S574 (1989).
2. M. D. Hu, Schenzle, D., Dienhardt, F., Scheid, R. Epidemiology of hepatitis A and B in the Shanghai area: Prevalence of serum markers. *Am. J. Epidemiol. 120*: 404 (1984).
3. J. L. Sung, and Asian Regional Study Group. Hepatitis B virus eradication strategy for Asia. *Vaccine 8* (Suppl): 96 (1990).
4. F. Barin, Perrin, J., Chotard, J., et al. Cross-sectional and longitudinal epidemiology of hepatitis B in Senegal. *Prog. Med. Virol. 27*: 148 (1981).
5. A. Toukan, Al-Faleh, F., Al-Kandari, et al. Strategy for the control of hepatitis B virus infection in the Middle East and North Africa. *Vaccine 8* (Suppl): 117 (1990).
6. G. Bensabath, Hadler, S. C., Periera Soares, M. C., et al. Epidemiologic and serologic studies of acute viral hepatitis in Brazil's Amazon basin. *PAHO Bull 21*: 16 (1987).
7. D. C. Wong, Purcell, R. H., Rosen, L. Prevalence of antibody to hepatitis A and hepataitis B viruses in selected populations of the South Pacific. *Am. J. Epidemiol. 110*: 227 (1979).
8. M. T. Schreeder, Bender, T. R., McMahon, B. J., et al. Prevalence of hepatitis B in selected Alaskan Eskimo villages. *Am. J. Epidemiol. 118*: 543 (1983).
9. G. Y. Minuk, Nicolle, L. E., Postl, B., et al. Hepatitis virus infection in an isolated Canadian Inuit (Eskimo) population. *J. Med. Virol. 10*: 255 (1982).
10. A. Milne, Allwood, G. K., Moyes, C. D., Pearce, N. E., Lucas, C. R. Prevalence of hepatitis B infections in a multiracial New Zealand community. *N.Z. Med. J. 10*: 529 (1985).
11. C. E. Stevens, Neurath, R. A., Beasley, R. P., Szmuness, W. HBeAg and anti-HBe detection by radioimmunoassay: Correlation with vertical transmission of hepatitis B virus in Taiwan. *J. Med. Virol. 3*: 237 (1979).
12. R. P. Beasley, Hwang, L.-Y. Postnatal infectivity in hepatitis B surface antigen carrier mothers. *J. Infect. Dis. 147*: 185 (1983).
13. A. L. Lingao, Domingo, E. O., West, S., et al. Seroepidemiology of hepatitis B virus in the Philippines. *Am. J. Epidemiol. 123*: 473 (1986).
14. K. C. Hyams, Osman, N. M., Khaled. E. M., Koraa, A. A. E.-W., Imam, I. Z., et al. Maternal infant transmission of hepatitis B in Egypt. *J. Med. Virol. 24*: 191 (1988).

15. A. M. Prince, White, T., Pollock, N., et al. Epidemiology of hepatitis B infection in Liberian infants. *Infect. Immun. 32*: 675 (1981).

16. H. C. Whittle, Inskip, H., Bradley, A. K., Mclaughlan, K., et al. The pattern of childhood hepatitis B infection in two Gambian villages. *J. Infect. Dis. 161*: 1112 (1990).

17. A. U. Toukan, Sharaiha, Z. K., Abu-el-Rob, O. A., et al. The epidemiology of hepatitis B virus among family members in the Middle East. *Am. J. Epidemiol. 132*: 220 (1990).

18. H. S. Margolis, Alter, M. J., Hadler, S. C., Hepatitis B. Evolving epidemiology and implications for control. *Semin. Liver Dis. 11*: 84 (1991).

19. T. Tanaka, Nagai, M., Yoshihara, S., et al. Changing pattern of age-specific seroprevalence of hepatitis B surface antigen and corresponding antibody in Japan. *Am. J. Epidemiol. 124*: 368 (1986).

20. P. Skinhoj, Hart Hansen, J. P., Nielsen, N. H., Mikkelsen, F. Occurrence of cirrhosis and primary liver cancer in an Eskimo population hyperendemically infected with hepatitis B virus. *Am. J. Epidemiol. 108*: 121 (1978).

21. A. L. Franks, Berg, C. J., Kane, M. A., et al. Hepatitis B virus infection among children born in the United States to Southeast Asian refugees. *N. Engl. J. Med. 321*: 1301 (1989).

22. R. E. Sampliner, Hamilton, F. A., Iseri, O. A., et al. The liver histology and frequency of clearance of the hepatitis B surface antigen (HBsAg) in chronic carriers. *Am. J. Med. Sci. 277*: 17 (1979).

23. K. L. Lindsay, Redeker, A. G., Ashcavai, M. Delayed HBsAg clearance in chronic hepatitis B viral infection. *Hepatology 1*: 586 (1981).

24. T. Shikata, Karasawa, T., Abe, K., et al. Hepatitis B e antigen and infectivity of hepatitis B virus. *J. Infect. Dis. 136*: 571 (1977).

25. S. D. Lee, Lo, K. J., Wu, J. C., et al. Prevention of maternal-infant hepatitis B transmission by immunization: The role of serum hepatitis B virus DNA. *Hepatology 6*: 369 (1986).

26. W. S. Robinson, Marion, P. L. Biological features of hepadna viruses. *Viral Hepatitis and Liver Disease* (A. J. Zuckerman, ed.), Alan R. Liss, New York, p. 449 (1988).

27. E. Marinier, Barrois, V., Larouze, B., London, W. T., et al. Lack of perinatal hepatitis B virus infection in Senegal, West Africa. *J. Pediatr. 106*: 843 (1985).

28. H. J. Alter, Purcell, R. H., Gerin, J. L., et al. Transmission of hepatitis B to chimpanzees by hepatitis B surface antigen-positive saliva and semen. *Infect. Immun. 16*: 928 (1977).

29. W. H. Bancroft, Snitbhan, R., Scott, R. M., et al. Transmission of hepatitis B virus to gibbons by exposure to human saliva containing hepatitis B surface antigen. *J. Infect. Dis. 135*: 79 (1977).

30. S. A. Jenison, Lemon, S. M., Baker, L. N., Newbold, J. E. Quantitative analysis of hepatitis B virus DNA in saliva and semen of chronically infected homosexual men. *J. Infect. Dis. 156*: 299 (1987).

31. M. Darani, Gerber, M. Hepatitis B antigen in vaginal secretions. *Lancet 2*: 1008 (1974).

32. T. P. Cancio-Bello, de Medina, M., Shorey, J., et al. An institutional outbreak of hepatitis B related to a human biting carrier. *J. Infect. Dis. 146*: 652 (1982).

33. N. J. Peterson, Barrett, D. H., Bond, W. W., et al. Hepatitis B surface antigen in saliva, impetiginous lesions, and the environment in two remote Alaskan villages. *Appl. Environ. Microbiol. 32*: 572 (1976).

34. D. P. Francis, Favero, M. S., Maynard, J. E. Transmission of hepatitis B virus. *Semin. Liver Dis. 1*: 27 (1981).

35. Men, B-Y, Xu, H-W, Wang, X-L. Hepatitis B surface antigen (HBsAg) in feces of convalescent hepatitis B patients. *Chin. Med. J. 102*: 596 (1989).

36. R. P. Beasley, Stevens, C. E., Shiao, I. S., et al. Evidence against breast feeding as a mechanism for vertical transmission of hepatitis B. *Lancet 2*: 740 (1975).

37. S. Krugman, Giles, J. P., Hammond, J. Infectious hepatitis: Evidence for two distinctive clinical, epidemiological, and immunological types of infection. *J. Am. Med. Assoc. 200*: 95 (1967).

38. L. B. Seeff, Beebe, G. W., Hoofnagle, J. H., et al. A serologic follow-up of the 1942 epidemic of post-vaccination hepatitis in the United States Army. *N. Engl. J. Med. 316*: 965 (1987).

39. Y. Ghendon, Kane, M. A. Assuring a hepatitis B-free blood supply in developing countries. *Viral Hepatitis and Liver Disease* (F. B. Hollinger, Lemon, S. M., Margolis, H. S., eds.), Williams and Wilkins, Baltimore, p. 722 (1991).

40. W. Cates, Warren, J. W. Hepatitis B in Nuremberg, Germany. Epidemiology of a drug-associated epidemic among US Army soldiers. *J. Am. Med. Assoc. 234*: 930 (1975).

41. G. Schatz, Hadler, S., McCarthey, J., Smith, M., Birch, F. Outreach to needle users and sexual contacts: a multi-year, community-wide hepatitis B/delta hepatitis control program in Worcester, Massachusetts. *Progress in Hepatitis B Immunization* (P. Coursaget, Tong, M. J., ed.), John Libbey, London, p. 533 (1990).

42. A. L. Limentani, Elliott, L. M., Noah, N. D., Lamborn, J. K. An outbreak of hepatitis B from tattooing. *Lancet 2*: 86 (1979).

43. G. P. Kent, Brondum, J., Keenlyside, R. A., et al. A large outbreak of acupuncture-associated hepatitis B. *Am. J. Epidemiol. 127*: 591 (1988).

44. Y. C. Ko, Li, S. C., Yen, Y. Y., et al. Horizontal transmission of hepatitis B virus from siblings and intramuscular injection among preschool children in a familial cohort. *Am. J. Epidemiol. 133*: 1015 (1991).

45. G. F. Grady, Lee, V. A., Prince, A. M., et al. Hepatitis B immune globulin for accidental exposures among medical personnel: Final report of a multicenter controlled trial. *J. Infect. Dis. 138*: 625 (1978).

46. L. B. Seeff, Wright, E. L., Zimmerman, J. H., et al. Type B hepatitis after needle-stick exposure: Prevention with hepatitis B immune globulin. Final report of the Veterans Administration cooperative study. *Ann. Int. Med. 88*: 285 (1978).

47. S. C. Hadler, Doto, I. L., Maynard, J. E., et al. Occupational risk of hepatitis B infection in hospital workers. *Infect. Control 6*: 24 (1985).

48. W. Szmuness, Much, I., Prince, A. M., et al. On the role of sexual behavior in the spread of hepatitis B infection. *Ann. Intern. Med. 83*: 489 (1975).

49. M. T. Schreeder, Thompson, S. E., Hadler, S. C., et al. Hepatitis B in homosexual

men: Prevalence of infection and factors related to transmission. *J. Infect. Dis. 146*: 7 (1982).

50. N. Reiner, Judson, F. N., Bond, W. W., et al. Asymptomatic rectal mucosal lesions and hepatitis B surface antigen at sites of sexual contact in homosexual men with persistent hepatitis B virus infection. *Ann. Int. Med. 96*: 170 (1984).

51. W. Kaklamani, Kyriakidou, A., Trichopoulos, D., et al. Hepatitis B serology in Greek prostitutes: Significance of the different serum markers. *J. Hyg. Camb. 84*: 257 (1980).

52. R. H. Bernier, Sampliner, R., Gerety, R., et al. Hepatitis B infection in households of chronic carrier of hepatitis B surface antigen: Factors associated with prevalence of infection. *Am. J. Epidemiol. 116*: 199 (1982).

53. W. Szmuness, Harley, E. J., Prince, A. M. Infrafamilial spread of asymptomatic hepatitis B. *Am. J. Med. Sci. 270*: 293 (1975).

54. M. J. Alter, Margolis, H. S. The emergence of hepatitis B as a sexually transmitted disease. *Med. Clin. North. Am. 74*: 1529 (1990).

55. L. M. Baddour, Bucak, V. A., Somes, G., et al. Risk factors for hepatitis B virus infection in black female attendees of a sexually transmitted disease clinic. *Sex. Transm. Dis. 15*: 174 (1988).

56. M. J. Alter, Ahtone, J., Weisfuse, I., et al. Hepatitis B virus transmission between heterosexuals. *J. Am. Med. Assoc. 256*: 1307 (1986).

57. M. J. Alter, Coleman, P. J., Alexander, W. J., et al. Importance of heterosexual activity in the transmission of hepatitis B and non-A non-B hepatitis. *J. Am. Med. Assoc. 262*: 1201 (1989).

58. M. J. Alter, Hadler, S. C., Margolis, H. S., et al. The changing epidemiology of hepatitis B in the United States and need for alternative vaccination strategies. *J. Am. Med. Assoc. 263*: 1218 (1990).

59. G. M. McQuillan, Townsend, T. R., Fields, H. A., et al. Seroepidemiology of hepatitis B virus infection in the United States. *Am. J. Med. 87* (Suppl 3A): 5 (1989).

60. L. S. Rosenblum, Hadler, S. C., Castro, K. G., et al. Heterosexual transmission of hepatitis B virus in Belle Glade, Fla. *J. Infect. Dis. 161*: 407 (1990).

61. A. G. Redeker, Mosley, J. W., Gocke, D. J., et al. Hepatitis B immune globulin as a prophylactic measure for spouses exposed to acute type B hepatitis. *N. Engl. J. Med. 293*: 1055 (1975).

62. A. Roumeliotou-Karayannis, Papavangelou, G., Tasopoulos, N., et al. Post-exposure active immunoprophylaxis of spouses of acute viral hepatitis B patients. *Vaccine 3*: 31 (1985).

63. S. K. West, Lingao, A. L., Domingo, E. O., Raymundo, D., Caragay, B., and the Liver Study Group. Incidence and prevalence of hepatitis B. A community-based study in the Philippines. *Am. J. Epidemiol. 123*: 681 (1986).

64. R. P. Beasley, Hwang, L.-Y., Lin, C.-C., Leu, M.-L., et al. Incidence of hepatitis B virus infections in preschool children in Taiwan. *J. Infect. Dis. 146*: 198 (1982).

65. A. M. Leichtner, Leclair, J., Goldmann, D. A., Schumacher, R. T., et al. Horizontal nonparenteral spread of hepatitis B among children. *Ann. Intern. Med. 94*: 346 (1981).

66. J. Hayashi, Kashiwagi, S., Normura, H., et al. Hepatitis B virus transmission in nursery schools. *Am. J. Epidemiol. 125*: 492 (1987).

67. C. N. Shapiro, McCaig, L. F., Gensheimer, K. F., et al. Hepatitis B virus transmission between children in day care. *Pediatr. Infect. Dis. J. 8*: 870 (1989).

68. W. W. Bond, Peterson, N. J., Favero, M. S., et al. Transmission of type B viral hepatitis via eye inoculation of a chimpanzee. *J. Clin. Microbiol. 15*: 533 (1982).

69. M. S. Favero, Maynard, J. E., Peterson, N. J., et al. Hepatitis B antigen on environmental surfaces. *Lancet 2*: 1455 (1973).

70. W. W. Bond, Favero, M. S., Peterson, N. J., et al. Survival of hepatitis B virus after drying and storage for 1 week. *Lancet 1*: 550 (1981).

71. J. L. Lauer, VanDuren, N. A., Washburn, J. W., Balfour, H. H. Transmission of hepatitis B virus in clinical laboratory areas. *J. Infect. Dis. 140*: 513 (1979).

72. C. P. Pattison, Boyer, K. P., Maynard, J. E., Kelly, P. C. Epidemic hepatitis in a clinical laboratory: Possible association with computer card handling. *J. Am. Med. Assoc. 230*: 854 (1974).

73. O. Ringertz, Zetterberg, B. Serum hepatitis among Swedish track finders. *N. Engl. J. Med. 276*: 540 (1967).

74. D. R. Snydman, Bryan, J. A., Macon, E. J., et al. Hemodialysis associated hepatitis: Report of an epidemic with further evidence on mechanisms of transmission. *Am. J. Epidemiol. 104*: 563 (1976).

75. M. S. Favero. Dialysis-associated diseases and their control. *Hospital Infections* (J. V. Bennett, Brachman, P. S., eds.), Little, Brown, Boston, pp. 267–284 (1985).

76. P. G. Jupp, McElligott, S. E. Transmission experiments with hepatitis B surface antigen and the common bedbug. *S. Afr. Med. J. 56*: 54 (1979).

77. K. R. Berquist, Maynard, J. E., Francy, D. B., et al. Experimental studies of the transmission of hepatitis B by mosquitos. *Am. J. Trop. Med. Hyg. 25*: 730 (1976).

78. R. P. Beasley, Hwang, L. Y., Lee, G. C. Y., et al. Prevention of perinatally transmitted hepatitis B virus infections with hepatitis B immune globulin and hepatitis B vaccine. *Lancet 2*: 1099 (1983).

79. R. P. Beasley, Hwang, L. Y., Stevens, C. E., et al. Efficacy of hepatitis B immune globulin (HBIG) for prevention of perinatal transmission of the HBV carrier state: Final report of a randomized double-blind, placebo-controlled trial. *Hepatology, 3*: 135 (1983).

80. Z. Y. Xu, Liu, C. B., Francis, D. P., et al. Prevention of perinatal acquisition of hepatitis B virus carriage using vaccine: Preliminary report of a randomized, double-blind placebo-controlled and comparative trial. *Pediatrics 76*: 713 (1985).

81. M. J. Tong. The clinical consequences of perinatal infection of the hepatitis B virus. *Progress in Hepatitis B Immunization* (Coursaget, P., Tong, M. J., eds.), John Libbey Eurotext, Paris, p. 3 (1990).

82. S. Terazawa, Kojima, M., Yamanaka, T., et al. Hepatitis B virus mutants with precore-region defects in two babies with fulminant hepatitis and their mothers positive for antibody to hepatitis B e antigen. *Pediatr. Res. 29*: 5 (1991).

83. D. A. Shafritz. Variants of Hepatitis B virus associated with fulminant liver disease. *N. Engl. J. Med. 324*: 1737 (1991).

84. C. E. Stevens, Toy, P. T., Tong, M. J., et al. Perinatal hepatitis B virus transmission in the United States. Prevention by passive-active immunization. *J. Am. Med. Assoc. 253*: 1740 (1985).

85. S. M. Friedman, De Silva, L. P., Fox, H. E., Bernard, G. Hepatitis B screening in a New York City obstetrics service. *Am. J. Public Health 78*: 308 (1988).

86. H. H. Lin, Chen, P. J., Chen, D. S., Sung, J. L., Yang, K. H., et al. Postpartum subsidence of hepatitis B viral replication in HBeAg-positive carrier mothers. *J. Med. Virol. 29*: 1 (1989).

87. G. C. B. Chan, Yeoh, E. K., Young, B., Chang, W. K., et al. Effect of pregnancy on the hepatitis B carrier state. *Viral Hepatitis and Liver Disease* (F. B. Hollinger, Lemon, S. M., Margolis, H. S., eds), Williams and Wilkins, Baltimore, p. 678 (1991).

88. W. L. M. Alward, McMahon, B. J., Hall, D. B., Heyward, W. L., et al. The long-term serological course of asymptomatic hepatitis B virus carriers and the development of primary hepatocellular carcinoma. *J. Infect. Dis. 151*: 604 (1985).

89. O. H. Fay, Hadler, S. C., Maynard, J. E., Pinheiro, F. Hepatitis in the Americas. *Bull. Pan. Am. Health Org. 19*: 401 (1985).

90. Centers for Disease Control. Hepatitis B virus: A comprehensive strategy for eliminating transmission in the United States through universal childhood vaccination: Recommendations of the Immunization Practices Advisory Committee. *MMWR 40*(No. RR-13): 1 (1991).

91. R. C. Hershow, Hadler, S. C., Kane, M. A. Adoption of children from countries with endemic hepatitis B: Transmission risks and medical issues. *Pediatr. Infect. Dis. J. 6*: 431 (1987).

92. Centers for Disease Control. Hepatitis Surveillance Report No. 53, Atlanta, p. 13 (1990).

93. M. J. Alter, Favero, M. S., Maynard, J. E. Impact of infection control strategies on the incidence of dialysis-associated hepatitis in the United States. *J. Infect. Dis. 153*: 1149 (1986).

8

Scope and Design of Hepatitis B Vaccine Clinical Trials

David J. West

Merck Research Laboratories,
West Point, Pennsylvania

I. INTRODUCTION

Human clinical studies of any investigational vaccine are done to assess its safety, immunogenicity, and protective efficacy. An acceptable vaccine must not pose a significant safety hazard to recipients and should be generally well tolerated. The vaccine should also be highly immunogenic, stimulating the formation of protective antibody in the populations for whom it is intended. Finally, efficacy studies are done to demonstrate that vaccinees actually do experience lower rates of infection and disease than similar, unvaccinated persons.

This chapter begins with a brief review of the regulatory environment in which vaccine clinical studies take place, then traces the structure and findings of studies that were done to establish the safety, immunogenicity, and efficacy of present-day plasma-derived and recombinant hepatitis B vaccines. It concludes with comments on current and future clinical studies needed to extend the applications of existing vaccines and to evaluate new hepatitis B vaccine formulations.

II. REGULATION OF CLINICAL STUDIES

Vaccine clinical studies are regulated by designated national agencies according to the laws of the countries in which they are conducted. A brief summary is given here of the regulations that apply in the United States (1,2).

The U.S. Food and Drug Administration (FDA) has statutory authority to regulate human clinical trials. Within the FDA, biological products, including vaccines, are the responsibility of the Center for Biologics Evaluation and Research (CBER), previously called the Office of Biologics Research and Review (OBRR). CBER is charged with enforcing regulations that apply to clinical studies and to other aspects of the development, manufacture, licensure, and use of vaccines (3).

Before a clinical study may be inititated, the sponsor must submit to the FDA an investigational new drug application (IND). The IND includes (a) a description of the composition, source, and manufacture of the vaccine, (b) methods used to test the vaccine for safety, purity, and potency, (c) a summary of all laboratory and preclinical testing of the vaccine, and (d) a description of the proposed clinical study and the names and qualifications of the clinical investigators. There is a 30-day waiting period following submission of an IND. CBER reviews the IND during this period to ascertain that study participants will not be subjected to unreasonable risks.

Permission for an investigator to receive vaccine and proceed with the clinical study under the IND is contingent upon (a) written approval from a local institutional review board of the proposed study and the consent form that each study participant must sign and (b) completion of a statement of investigator form, which details the investigator's qualifications, summarizes the proposed study, and affirms that certain procedures will be followed in conducting the study.

The clinical testing of an investigational vaccine proceeds through several phases. *Phase I* consists of small studies, usually in healthy subjects, that focus on vaccine safety. *Phase II* studies are larger and are conducted in the populations for whom the vaccine is ultimately intended. Safety continues to be a focus, but the immunogenicity of vaccine administered using various schedules and dosages is also evaluated. *Phase III* encompasses more extensive studies to evaluate safety and immunogenicity as well as the actual protective efficacy of the vaccine. There may not always be a clear demarcation between Phase II and III studies.

Two phases of postlicensure clinical studies are recognized. *Phase IV* studies may be done to actively assess the safety and tolerability of the vaccine in a substantially larger population than could be observed in prelicensure trials. *Phase V* includes studies done with licensed vaccine to support changes in indications for its use (e.g., additions to or revisions in target population, or changes in dosage or schedule).

III. CLINICAL DEVELOPMENT OF PLASMA-DERIVED HEPATITIS B VACCINES

A number of epidemiological and laboratory studies in the early 1970s showed that antibody to HBsAg (anti-HBs) is associated with immunity to hepatitis B (4). Later, immune globulin containing a high titer of anti-HBs was found to protect persons exposed to hepatitis B virus (HBV) (5). Thus, HBsAg was indicated as a key component for a hepatitis B vaccine. No practical in vitro cell culture system existed for producing HBV, but the plasma of persons with chronic HBV infection contains a high multiplicity of HBsAg particles, and this was used as a source of antigen for several hepatitis B vaccines (6–9).

A. Safety

Hepatitis B vaccine should contain only purified subunits of the HBV surface envelope (see also Chapter 1). However, since the plasma of persons with chronic HBV infection contains both virulent HBV particles and noninfective HBsAg particles, protocols were developed to eliminate HBV or any other virus during the purification of HBsAg. Procedures used in the manufacture of various plasma-derived vaccines include differential centrifugation plus treatment with heat (6), formalin (7), heat and formalin (8), or a combination of pepsin at low pH, urea, and formalin (9).

Preclinical studies of susceptible chimpanzees showed that plasma-derived vaccines did not transmit HBV (6,8–10), but human clinical studies were still designed to detect possible vaccine-associated HBV infection. Vaccine recipients were tested for HBsAg and antibody to hepatitis B virus core antigen (anti-HBc). The liver enzyme alanine aminotransferase (ALT) was also measured in most vaccinees. By focusing on healthy individuals at low risk of HBV infection, it was possible to demonstrate convincingly that the plasma-derived vaccines do not transmit HBV.

In addition to serological surveillance, subjects in clinical studies were actively monitored for local injection site reactions or systemic illness following the administration of vaccine. Plasma-derived hepatitis B vaccine proved to be well tolerated. For example, healthy adult vaccinees reported mild transient discomfort at the injection site (pain, soreness, swelling, redness) following only 12–28% of all injections (11–14).

Several studies designed to test the efficacy of vaccine versus alum placebo also afforded an opportunity to assess the reactogenicity of HBsAg apart from other vaccine components. None of the participants in these trials had serious adverse reactions, and the frequencies of minor side effects (e.g., sore arm, fever, fatigue, nausea, joint pain, dizziness, rash, respiratory symptoms) were very similar in recipients of vaccine and placebo, although sore arm was reported somewhat more frequently by persons given vaccine in two of the studies (11–14). These studies also showed that multiple injections of vaccine did not induce hypersensitivity reactions. Subjects received three injections of either vaccine or placebo over a 6-month interval, but the frequencies of local and systemic complaints did not increase with successive injections.

A specific safety issue arose following the licensure of plasma-derived hepatitis B vaccines. With the emergence of AIDS in the early 1980s and the recognition that human immunodeficiency virus (HIV) and HBV are both transmitted in blood, there was concern that hepatitis B vaccine might be contaminated with HIV. Several studies were carried out to address this issue. At the laboratory level, each of the three inactivation steps used in producing one of the plasma-derived vaccines (pepsin at low pH, urea, formalin) was shown capable of inactivating high concentrations of HIV (10^4–10^5 virus particles per milliliter) (15). Furthermore, tests of final containers of vaccine failed to detect any HIV nucleic acid. Studies of vaccinated health-care personnel revealed no seroconversions for antibody to HIV (16,17). Follow-up of homosexual men in a placebo-controlled efficacy trial of vaccine showed that the rate of seroconversion for antibody to HIV among vaccinees did not exceed that among placebo recipients (18).

The sensitivity of Phase I–III clinical studies to detect adverse experiences possibly due to vaccination is limited by the size of the study populations. Typically, data from a few thousand clinical study participants provide the basis for vaccine licensure. Thus, reactions occurring with a frequency less than 10^{-3} may well escape detection. Formal postlicensure studies with active or at least stimulated passive surveillance to assess vaccine safety and tolerability (Phase IV) may involve tens of thousands of vaccinees. However, even these studies have no power to detect very rare events occurring with frequencies on the order of 10^{-5} or less.

An assessment of whether a vaccine may cause very rare reactions requires surveillance of adverse experiences associated with the use of marketed product in large populations. In 1982, the U.S. Centers for Disease Control (CDC), the FDA, and the manufacturer of the plasma-derived hepatitis B vaccine licensed in the United States (Merck & Co., Inc.) created a surveillance system to monitor spontaneous reports of rare neurological adverse experiences associated with receipt of plasma-derived hepatitis B vaccine (19). Passive surveillance of this kind is always subject to underreporting, although serious events are much more likely to be reported than trivial ones. In this case, reporting was stimulated to an unknown degree through a publication in the *Morbidity and Mortality Weekly Report* and through letters to state epidemiologists, CDC immunization senior public health advisors and project directors, and members of the American Hospital Association. A variety of neuropathies were found to occur no more frequently in vaccinees than in unvaccinated members of the population. Guillain-Barré syndrome (GBS) was reported slightly more often than expected, although there was no conclusive evidence of a causal role for the vaccine. The excess GBS case rate potentially attributable to vaccine was only about 0.5/100,000 vaccinees. Thus, vaccination could still be seen as highly beneficial for persons at risk of HBV infection.

B. Immunogenicity

Early studies on the immunogenicity of plasma-derived hepatitis B vaccines were mostly of open design, sometimes with randomization of subjects to two or more vaccine dosages, and generally involved small populations of healthy seronegative adults. Subjects were usually given a series of three or four injections of vaccine. Outcomes of principal interest were the fact and timing of seroconversion for anti-HBs. Blood samples taken prior to the initial vaccination and at various times during and after completion of the series were tested for HBV serological markers, usually by a radioimmunoassay (RIA) procedure.

The initial studies of the vaccine that was subsequently licensed in the United States evaluated the antibody responses of healthy adults to both aqueous and alum-adsorbed formulations using a variety of dosages (5–40 μg HBsAg) and schedules. A series of three 20-μg doses of vaccine administered by intramuscular injection at intervals of 0, 1, and 6 months proved to be optimal and was adopted as the standard adult regimen (9, 20–22). Typically, more than 90% of healthy adult vaccinees developed detectable anti-HBs using this regimen. The studies showed that the first two injections in the series serve to prime the immune response in most vaccinees. While the third dose seroconverts a few hyporesponsive subjects, its main effect is to elicit a secondary antibody response, which generally increases the titer of anti-HBs by a factor of 10 or more.

Seroconversion rate for anti-HBs and the maximal titer of antibody proved to be age dependent, children and young adults being more responsive to a given dosage of vaccine than middle-aged and older adults (21,23). The excellent immune responses of younger individuals permitted adoption of a lower dosage. Ninety-five to 100% of children and adolescents given 5- or 10-μg doses of vaccine developed anti-HBs, and these responders generally developed titers higher than adult responders to the 20-μg dose (24–26). In one study, a dosage of 5 μg even sufficed to seroconvert more than 90% of adults under 30 years of age (23). While the vaccine was immunogenic for neonates, their antibody response was less than that of children and young adults. Ninety-three percent of healthy neonates given 10-μg doses of vaccine within 7 days of birth and at 1 and 6 months developed anti-HBs (27). Consequently, 10 μg was adopted as the standard pediatric dosage of this vaccine.

Clinical studies led to selection of a 40-μg dosage of HBsAg administered at 0, 1, and 6 months for patients with end-stage renal disease receiving hemodialysis. Even with this regimen, seroconversion rates were suboptimal, ranging from as low as 32% in elderly patients up to 86% in young adults (28–30).

Studies of other plasma-derived hepatitis B vaccines have yielded results similar to those obtained with the vaccine licensed in the United States. Yet, while all of the vaccines incorporate HBsAg as the active immunogen, they differ in the purification and inactivation protocols used during manufacture, and these differences do affect the immunopotency of the final vaccine. Thus, a 3-μg dosage of a less purified, heat-treated vaccine (6) and a 5-μg dosage of a more extensively purified, formalin-treated vaccine (31) had potency in healthy adults similar to a 20-μg dosage of a highly purified vaccine made using a three-step purification-inactivation process involving pepsin at low pH, urea, and formalin (9).

C. Efficacy

The protective efficacy of hepatitis B vaccine can be assessed with respect to a variety of outcomes such as the incidence of clinical disease, antigenemia (HBsAg$^+$ with or without other clinical manifestations of infection), or any HBV infection (including benign asymptomatic infection detected only through seroconversion for anti-HBc). Vaccine efficacy (E) is calculated as follows:

$$E(\%) = \left[1 - \left(\frac{\text{incidence}_{\text{vaccinees}}}{\text{incidence}_{\text{controls}}}\right)\right] \times 100$$

Randomized double-blind clinical trials of the efficacy of plasma-derived vaccine versus alum placebo among adults have enrolled homosexual males (11,14,32), patients in dialysis units (30,31,33), and medical staff (12,13,31, 33). Because of the high rates of HBV infection within these groups, it was expected that vaccine efficacy could be demonstrated by following fairly small populations for relatively short periods of time. For example, Szmuness (34), using baseline data on the prevalence of HBV markers and the incidence of new HBV infections in the United States together with information from early studies of vaccine immunogenicity and estimates of loss to follow-up, concluded that reductions in the incidence of clinical hepatitis B or antigenemia of 56–75% in vaccinated male homosexuals, dialysis patients, and dialysis center staff could be detected with samples of 234–736 subjects per treatment group followed for periods of 1–2 years ($\alpha = 0.05$ and $1 - \beta = 0.90$).

Vaccine reduced the incidence of significant HBV infection (infection accompanied by antigenemia with or without ALT elevation) in homosexual males by 80–87% (11,14,32). Among vaccine responders with an anti-HBs titer of ≥ 10 sample ratio units (SRU), the efficacy was as high as 98% (14). Significant reductions of 87–92% in the rate of HBsAg$^+$ hepatitis B infection were observed in two studies of dialysis center staff (12,31). No HBsAg$^+$ infections were observed among vaccinated health-care personnel in two other studies, but low overall infection rates in the study populations precluded demonstration of significant reductions in the incidence of infection among vaccinees (13,33). In two studies of patients receiving hemodialysis, the incidence of significant HBV infection was reduced by 54% and 81%, respectively (31,33). Another study of such patients, in whom the overall incidence of HBV infection was less than expected, failed to demonstrate vaccine efficacy (30).

Infants born to HBV carrier mothers, especially those who are HBsAg$^+$ and HBeAg$^+$, are at very high risk of developing chronic HBV infection. Without prophylaxis, as many as 66–93% of these infants become chronically infected within the first year of life (35–38). Prior to the introduction of hepatitis B vaccine, a clinical study showed that multiple doses of hepatitis B immune globulin (HBIG) given to infants of HBsAg$^+$/HBeAg$^+$ mothers could reduce the incidence of infection by up to 71% (39). Several studies were then done to assess the efficacy of passive-active prophylaxis (HBIG at birth followed by a course of vaccine) in infants of HBsAg$^+$/HBeAg$^+$ carrier mothers. With the risk of infection so high, it was possible to demonstrate efficacy within a year of vaccination with as few as 20–100 subjects. Passive-active prophylaxis was found to reduce the incidence of chronic infection by ≥85% (35,36,40,41).

IV. CLINICAL DEVELOPMENT OF RECOMBINANT HEPATITIS B VACCINES

Even as the first plasma-derived hepatitis B vaccines achieved licensure, efforts were underway to develop an alternate supply of HBsAg. Human plasma was viewed as an unreliable source of antigen that might become scarce and expensive, especially if widespread use of vaccine started to reduce the pool of carriers. This effort received added impetus as concern grew over the perception of blood products as possible vehicles for the transmission of HIV.

By 1983, clinical studies were underway with two investigational hepatitis B vaccines formulated with HBsAg synthesized by genetically engineered strains of the common bakers' yeast, *Saccharomyces cerevisiae*, which contained copies of the HBV gene coding for this antigen (42–44). Those studies are considered here (see also Chapter 4). More recently, recombinant hepatitis B vaccines have also been made with antigen synthesized by transfected mammalian cell lines (45–47).

A. Safety

Vaccines made with HBsAg synthesized by genetically engineered yeast cells carry no risk of contamination with HBV, HIV, or other viruses that may be present in human plasma. The vaccines are highly purified with >98% of the protein present accountable as HBsAg (43,44). Consequently, the safety of these preparations was expected to be excellent. Active surveillance of several thousand healthy adults in clinical studies revealed no serious adverse experiences attributable to vaccination (48,49). Minor local reactions, principally soreness at the injection site, were reported by adult vaccinees following about one-fifth of all injections. Systemic complaints were reported even less often, the most common being mild fatigue or headache. Elevated temperatures at any time during a 3- to 5-day period after injection were reported after only 2–3% of all injections. These elevations showed no tendency to occur in close temporal apposition to injection, and the low overall frequency suggested that the vaccine was not pyrogenic. The frequencies of local reactions and systemic complaints reported by parents of vaccinated children were similar to or less than those reported by vaccinated adults.

While any vaccine has the potential to induce hypersensitivity with the attendant possibility of rare anaphylactic reactions, the yeast-derived hepatitis B vaccines present no unusual hazards in this regard. Like the previous generation of plasma-derived vaccines, they contain neither egg protein nor antibiotics, which have been sources of serious allergic reactions with some other vaccines.

The yeast-derived hepatitis B vaccines do contain trace quantities of yeast protein, but this does not appear to induce clinically significant hypersensitivity to yeast. Prevaccination sera collected from clinical study participants were all positive for antibodies to yeast proteins (50). Following vaccination, some individuals had increases in antiyeast antibody, while in others the level of antibody stayed constant or even declined. Clinical reactions were not more frequent in persons with postvaccination increases in antiyeast antibody (50). Antiyeast IgE was not detected in recipients of yeast-derived hepatitis B vaccine (51).

B. Immunogenicity

A number of dose-response studies have been done using either a 0-, 1-, and 6-month or a 0-, 1-, 2-, and 12-month schedule. Most of the studies were of open design. Some compared antibody responses to yeast-derived and plasma-derived vaccines (either simultaneous comparison with randomization to type of vaccine or sequential use of each vaccine in similar convenience samples). The fact and timing of seroconversion for anti-HBs in initially seronegative individuals were again the outcomes of key interest, but clinical studies of the yeast-derived hepatitis B vaccines also emphasized the maximal titer of the anti-HBs response. This focus derived from previous efficacy studies of plasma-derived vaccine, which showed that persons with a postvaccination titer of at least 10 sample ratio units (10 SRU or S/N) were completely protected against clinically significant hepatitis B infection. A lower positive titer might not afford complete protection. Thus, ≥ 10 S/N (later ≥ 10 mIU/ml) came to be viewed as a "protective" level of anti-HBs (52). Attention was also paid to the "quality" of anti-HBs induced by the yeast-derived vaccines. Studies were undertaken to show that antibody induced by the yeast-derived vaccines was immunologically equivalent to that induced by plasma-derived vaccine.

Clinical studies showed an IgM-to-IgG shift in the anti-HBs formed within 2–4 months of receiving the first dose of either plasma-derived or yeast-derived vaccine (43). Almost all anti-HBs proved to be specific for the *a* determinant of HBsAg regardless of the type of vaccine used to induce it (43,53). The affinity and avidity of antibody for HBsAg were similar whether induced by plasma-derived or yeast-derived vaccine, and both vaccines were able to almost completely absorb the antibody present in the serum from persons vaccinated with either vaccine.

In studies of more than 2000 healthy adults given vaccine at 0, 1, and 6 months, $\geq 96\%$ developed anti-HBs, and the geometric mean antibody titer (GMT) exceeded 1000 mIU/ml (48,49). More than 99% of adults given vaccine at 0, 1, 2, and 12 months developed anti-HBs, with the fourth dose serving as a powerful booster that raised the GMT to more than 10,000 mIU/ml.

Antibody responses to yeast-derived vaccine were diminished in older subjects. In one group of studies, 98% of 20- to 29-year-old adults developed a protective anti-HBs titer (≥ 10 mIU/ml) after three doses of vaccine compared to 89% of vaccinees ≥ 40 years of age (49). Responders in the younger age group had a GMT of nearly 1500 mIU/ml compared to approximately 500 mIU/ml in the older group. Infants, children, and adolescents responded very well to dosages of the yeast-derived hepatitis B vaccine ranging from one-quarter to one-half the adult dosage. The GMTs of anti-HBs in pediatric vaccinees equaled or exceeded that of adult vaccinees, ranging from about 2000 to 4000 mIU/ml (48,49).

Currently available yeast-derived hepatitis B vaccines are similar in consisting of particles of the HBsAg S polypeptide adsorbed to an alum adjuvant. Human immunogenicity is dependent on the tertiary and quaternary structure of these particles, and these properties may differ somewhat between the products. Thus, clinical studies were needed for each vaccine to establish appropriate dosing regimens. For one of the vaccines (RECOMBIVAX HB®, Merck Sharp & Dohme), dosages of 2.5, 5, 10, and 40 μg are recommended for healthy infants and children (5 μg plus HBIG at birth for infants of carrier mothers), adolescents, adults, and dialysis patients, respectively (54,55). For the other yeast-derived hepatitis B vaccine (ENGERIX B®, SmithKline Beecham), the recommended dosages are 10, 20, and 40 μg for infants and children (plus HBIG at birth for infants of carrier mothers), adolescents and adults, and dialysis patients, respectively (55,56).

C. Efficacy

Once the efficacy of plasma-derived hepatitis B vaccines was established, it was not ethical to include a placebo control group in efficacy studies of the yeast-derived vaccines. Other constraints were placed on studies of vaccine efficacy by changes in the epidemiology of hepatitis B. For example, the annual incidence of hepatitis B infection among dialysis patients in the United States had dropped from 3% in 1976 to 0.5% in 1982 following the implementation of various infection control strategies (57). With the emergence of AIDS and efforts to modify the sexual practices of homosexual men, previous estimates of HBV infection rates were considered unreliable bases for new studies of vaccine efficacy in this population. The failure to demonstrate efficacy of plasma-derived hepatitis B vaccine in a study of medical personnel because of an unexpectedly low rate of infection (13) meant that a new study in this population would require many thousands of vaccinees and have to be conducted over a period of several years.

Quasi-efficacy studies were done in cohorts of several high-risk populations, comparing the postvaccination rates of HBV infection to rates that prevailed prior to vaccination. For example, the annual incidence of infection in a group of homosexual men was <1% after vaccination compared to 12% before vaccination (58). This approach is most satisfactory for infants of HBsAg$^+$/HBeAg$^+$ mothers, who have consistently been shown to be at very high risk of infection. Several studies showed that an injection of HBIG at birth followed by a course of yeast-derived hepatitis B vaccine reduced the incidence of chronic HBV infection among these infants by ≥95% (59–61). In one study, vaccine alone was as effective as vaccine plus HBIG (61).

Based on the extensive controlled efficacy studies of plasma-derived hepatitis B vaccines plus the studies of yeast-derived hepatitis B vaccines using historical controls, the induction of anti-HBs is now generally viewed as an acceptable surrogate measure of efficacy for S antigen vaccines.

V. CURRENT AND FUTURE CLINICAL STUDIES

Hepatitis B vaccine remains an active focus for clinical study. This reflects efforts to extend the applications and improve the effectiveness of current vaccines and to develop new investigational vaccine formulations.

A. Duration of Protection

Antibody level does wane after vaccination (62,63). The rate of decline appears to be independent of initial postvaccination titer, but vaccinees with a high starting titer will remain above some benchmark level (e.g., 10 mIU/ml) longer than those with a lower titer.

Long-term follow-up of healthy responders to vaccine in early efficacy studies shows that protection against clinical hepatitis B or antigenemia endures for periods of 5–8 years, even though up to half of the subjects failed to maintain a "protective" level of antibody (64–67). Boosts in the level of anti-HBs ostensibly caused by exposure to HBV, as well as some breakthrough infections manifesting only as seroconversions for anti-HBc, have been observed. Infection with antigenemia was detected in two male homosexual vaccinees, but both had suffered intercurrent HIV infection (65). Among several hundred infants of carrier mothers who responded to vaccine and had antibody at one year of age, only three became carriers of HBV by 5 years of age (67).

The basis for continuing protection in the face of waning antibody is immunological memory. Since hepatitis B infection takes several weeks or months to develop, antibody synthesized by memory cells following exposure to HBV will generally be sufficient to prevent or markedly attenuate infection. The major question for further study is how long will immunological memory last?

Immunological memory is readily monitored through the responses of previous vaccinees to a booster injection of vaccine. A booster dose of vaccine induced a clear anamnestic antibody response in 90–100% of healthy adults and children given a primary vaccine series several years earlier, even though up to half of the subjects had <10 mIU/ml of anti-HBs when the booster was given (68,69). Additional studies of this kind should focus on participants in the earliest vaccine clinical trials, who completed the primary vaccine series at least 10 years ago.

B. Intradermal Administration of Vaccine

Hepatitis B vaccine is recommended for intramuscular injection. However, its cost has stimulated interest in the prospect of intradermal administration using a reduced dosage. A number of studies have been done to evaluate the immunogenicity of hepatitis B vaccine administered intradermally, although most involved small numbers of subjects, and only a few included control groups given vaccine by the intramuscular route. Results have been mixed. Ninety-five percent of young healthy adults given a series of three low-dosage injections of hepatitis B vaccine by the intradermal route developed a protective level of anti-HBs in one study (70). Other investigators, however, found both the seroconversion rate and the GMT for anti-HBs to be significantly lower in adults given a reduced dosage of vaccine by the intradermal route versus a standard dosage by the intramuscular route (71,72). Additional controlled studies are needed. These studies should also assess the quality of antibody induced after intradermal administration of vaccine (e.g., IgM vs. IgG, proportion of anti-HBs specific for the *a* determinant of HBsAg, avidity of anti-HBs for HBsAg).

C. Adjuvants to Increase Vaccine Potency

There are a number of at-risk populations such as patients receiving hemodialysis, alcoholics, persons infected with HIV, organ transplant recipients, persons with cancer, and a small proportion of healthy persons, who respond poorly to existing vaccines and need more potent vaccines or vaccination regimens. One approach to this problem may lie in the use of immune-stimulating lymphokines or other immunomodulators as adjuvants.

Several agents have shown promise in small controlled studies of patients receiving hemodialysis. Thymopentin and interleukin-2 both improved the response to booster doses of hepatitis B vaccine in patients who had failed to develop anti-HBs after a primary course of vaccination (73,74). Patients given vaccine plus recombinant gamma-interferon were also reported to develop antibody sooner and have higher titers than those given vaccine alone (75). Larger controlled studies are needed to confirm the utility of these agents.

D. Flexible Vaccination Schedules

Two schedules are widely recommended for the primary hepatitis B vaccine series. Three doses of vaccine given at intervals of 0, 1, and 6 months typically yields a high seroconversion rate and a relatively high titer of anti-HBs that will persist for an extended period of time. An accelerated schedule, with vaccine given at 0, 1, and 2 months, may increase slightly the proportion of vaccinees with antibody 3–6 months after the first injection. Since the level of antibody after three doses of vaccine is lower the shorter the interval (from 1 to 11 months) between the second and the third dose (76), a fourth dose at 12 months is needed to elicit a high titer of anti-HBs in persons given the first three doses at 0, 1, and 2 months.

A flexible schedule is needed to facilitate broader use of hepatitis B vaccine. The Hepatitis Technical Advisory Group of the World Health Organization recommends that hepatitis B vaccine be integrated into the Expanded Programme on Immunization (77), but local variations in the epidemiology of hepatitis B and the timing of other childhood vaccinations make strict adherence to one or even two schedules for hepatitis B vaccine impractical. The first dose of hepatitis B vaccine should preferably be given at birth, if perinatal infection is common, or else at 6–12 weeks of age when other immunizations (e.g., DTP, OPV) are initiated. The second and third doses of hepatitis B vaccine could be given at various times concurrent with subsequent doses of other childhood vaccines.

Data available from field studies of plasma-derived hepatitis B vaccine in the Gambia and in Venezuela show that vaccine induced a protective level of anti-HBs in 98% of healthy infants and children in spite of large unplanned variations in vaccination schedule (78,79). A small clinical study in the United States showed that 96–100% of healthy infants developed ≥10 mIU/ml of anti-HBs when given plasma-derived hepatitis B vaccine at birth, 2 months, and 4 months of age (80). Additional studies are now being conducted with the yeast-derived hepatitis B vaccines in healthy infants to establish that satisfactory antibody responses can be obtained using a variety of schedules (J. Boscia, SmithKline Beecham, personal communication; G. Calandra, Merck Research Laboratories, personal communication).

E. Multivalent Childhood Vaccines

At present, hepatitis B vaccines are available only in monovalent formulations. Addition of this vaccine to the standard set of pediatric immunizations thus requires the administration of an extra injection to a child on at least three occasions. Acceptance of routine childhood immunization against hepatitis B would be enhanced if HBsAg could be included in polyvalent formulations with other pediatric vaccines. Combinations of HBsAg with the antigens of diphtheria-tetanus-pertussis vaccine and/or *Hemophilus influenzae* type b vaccine should be technically feasible, as all of the existing products are inactivated/purified subunit vaccines incorporating alum as an adjuvant.

The clinical development of polyvalent childhood vaccines containing HBsAg ought to be fairly straightforward. The efficacy of the existing component vaccines has been established. Consequently, controlled, randomized studies of the safety and immunogenicity in infants of an investigational compound vaccine versus the component vaccines should be an adequate basis for licensure. Each of the antigens in the compound vaccine should be at least as immunogenic as they are in the component vaccines, and the compound vaccine should not be more reactogenic than the component vaccines.

F. Vaccines Containing PreS

The surface envelope of HBV contains three proteins. All are translation products of the S gene of HBV, which has three open reading frames (81). The most abundant component, the S protein, is the antigen in currently available yeast-derived hepatitis B vaccines. The M protein, consisting of S plus an additional polypeptide designated PreS2 (M = PreS2+S), is a minor component. A very small fraction of the HBV envelope (ca. 1%) is comprised of the L protein, consisting of M plus a polypeptide segment designated PreS1 (L = PreS1+PreS2+S).

PreS products of the S gene may play a role in inducing immunity to hepatitis B. Anti-PreS develops before anti-HBs during acute hepatitis B infection, and immune elimination of the PreS antigens appears to be predictive of viral clearance and recovery (82,83). Anti-PreS antibodies neutralize the infectivity of HBV in vitro, and chimpanzees immunized with adjuvanted PreS peptides were protected against challenge with HBV (84,85). Thus, a vaccine containing both PreS and S antigens might provide a broader base of protection against hepatitis B infection.

In mice, immune responses to S and to PreS epitopes are regulated independently, and the presence of PreS can augment the immune response to S (86). For example, a strain of mouse that is immunologically nonresponsive to an S antigen vaccine formed both anti-HBs and anti-PreS2 when immunized with a PreS2+S vaccine. The addition of PreS antigens might enhance the immune response of humans to the S antigen in hepatitis B vaccine.

Several recombinant hepatitis B vaccines that include both PreS and S antigens synthesized by genetically engineered yeast or mammalian cell lines have been the subject of human clinical studies (45,47,87,88), and additional development efforts can be expected.

Preclinical and clinical studies of recombinant vaccines made with antigen produced by a transfected mammalian cell line or any cell line containing plasmids that incorporate promoter elements from an oncogenic virus must be monitored closely to ensure that the vaccine does not contain residual DNA with oncogenic potential (89). In addition, since PreS components are involved in binding HBV to hepatocytes, there is at least a theoretical concern that anti-PreS antibodies could interfere with the normal physiological functions of hepatocytes or that anti-idiotypic antibodies to anti-PreS antibodies might precipitate auto-immune disease (90). Consequently, participants in clinical studies of PreS-containing vaccines should be monitored for elevated ALT or other evidence of liver damage.

Given the high protective efficacy of anti-HBs, it is unlikely that improved efficacy can be demonstrated in clinical trials of a vaccine inducing both anti-HBs and anti-PreS antibodies. If vaccines containing both S and PreS antigens are to replace current S antigen vaccines, it will likely be on the basis of superior immunogenicity in randomized, double-blind studies in populations that are hyporesponsive to S antigen vaccine (e.g., patients receiving hemodialysis, older adults, healthy adult nonresponders to a primary vaccine series). A successful candidate vaccine must be as safe and well tolerated as the existing S antigen vaccines. In addition, it should induce earlier seroconversion or development of higher anti-HBs levels than existing S antigen vaccines and/or stimulate formation of anti-PreS antibodies in persons who are deficient in the development of anti-HBs.

REFERENCES

1. H. E. Hopps, B. C. Meyer, and P. D. Parkman, Regulation and testing of vaccines, *Vaccines* (S. A. Plotkin and E. A. Mortimer, eds.), W. B. Saunders Co., Philadelphia, pp. 576–586 (1988).
2. J. C. Petricianni, National and international regulation of new hepatitis B vaccines, *Progress in Hepatitis B Immunization* (P. Coursaget and M. J. Tong, eds.), Colloque INSERM/John Libbey Eurotext Ltd., London, Vol. 194, pp. 11–18 (1990).
3. Code of Federal Regulations, Title 21, parts 600–680, Subchapter F-Biologics. Government Printing Office, Washington, DC, (1985).
4. J. L. Melnick, Historical aspects of hepatitis B vaccine, *Hepatitis B Vaccine* (P. Maupas and P. Guesry, eds.), INSERM Symposium No. 18, Elsevier/North-Holland Biomedical Press, Amsterdam, pp. 23–31 (1981).
5. L. B. Seeff, E. C. Wright, H. J. Zimmerman, et al., Type B hepatitis after needle-stick exposure: Prevention with hepatitis B immune globulin. Final report of the Veterans Administration Cooperative Study, *Ann. Int. Med.*, *88*: 285 (1978).
6. E. E. Reerink-Brongers, H. W. Reesink, H. G. J. Brummelhuis, et al., Preparation and evaluation of heat-inactivated HBsAg as a vaccine against hepatitis B, *Viral Hepatitis: 1981 International Symposium* (W. Szmuness, H. J. Alter, and J. E. Maynard, eds.), Franklin Institute Press, Philadelphia, pp. 437–450 (1982).

7.   P. Adamowicz, G. Gerfaux, A. Platel, et al., Large scale production of an hepatitis B vaccine, *Hepatitis B Vaccine* (P. Maupas and P. Guesry, eds.), INSERM Symposium No. 18, Elsevier/North-Holland Biomedical Press, Amsterdam, pp. 37–49 (1981).

8.   S. Funakoshi, T. Ohmura, T. Fujiwara, et al., Hepatitis B vaccine—the production and testing, *Hepatitis B Vaccine* (P. Maupas and P. Guesry, eds.), INSERM Symposium No. 18, Elsevier/North-Holland Biomedical Press, Amsterdam, pp. 57–66 (1981).

9.   M. R. Hilleman, E. B. Buynak, W. J. McAleer, et al., Hepatitis A and hepatitis B vaccines, *Viral Hepatitis: 1981 International Symposium* (W. Szmuness, H. J. Alter, and J. E. Maynard, eds.), Franklin Institute Press, Philadelphia, pp. 385–397 (1982).

10. J. Pillot, P. Guesry, S. Goueffon, et al., Immunopathological risks of vaccination against hepatitis B virus. An experimental study in chimpanzees, *Hepatitis B Vaccine* (P. Maupas and P. Guesry, eds.), INSERM Symposium No. 18, Elsevier/North-Holland Biomedical Press, Amsterdam, pp. 93–104 (1981).

11. W. Szmuness, C. E. Stevens, H. J. Harley, et al., Hepatitis B vaccine. Demonstration of efficacy in a controlled clinical trial in a high-risk population in the United States, *N. Engl. J. Med.*, *303*: 833 (1980).

12. W. Szmuness, C. E. Stevens, H. J. Harley, et al., Hepatitis B vaccine in medical staff of hemodialysis units. Efficacy and subtype cross-protection, *N. Engl. J. Med.*, *307*: 1481 (1982).

13. J. L. Dienstag, B. G. Werner, B. F. Polk, et al., Hepatitis B vaccine in health care personnel: Safety, immunogenicity, and indicators of efficacy, *Ann. Int. Med.*, *101*: 34 (1984).

14. D. P. Francis, S. C. Hadler, S. E. Thompson, et al., The prevention of hepatitis B with vaccine. Report of the Centers for Disease Control Multi-center Efficacy Trial Among Homosexual Men, *Ann. Int. Med.*, *97*: 362 (1982).

15. D. P. Francis, P. M. Feorino, S. McDougal, et al., The safety of the hepatitis B vaccine. Inactivation of the AIDS virus during routine vaccine manufacture, *JAMA*, *256*: 869 (1986).

16. J. L. Dienstag, B. G. Werner, M. F. McLane, et al., Absence of antibodies to HTLV-III in health workers after hepatitis B vaccination, *JAMA*, *254*: 1064 (1985).

17. G. Papaevangelou, A. Roumeliotou-Karayannis, G. Kallinikos, et al., Lack of antibodies to LAV/HTLV-III in hepatitis B vaccine recipients, *Eur. J. Epidemiol.*, *1*: 323 (1985).

18. C. E. Stevens, No increased incidence of AIDS in recipients of hepatitis B vaccine, *N. Engl. J. Med.*, *308*: 1183 (1983).

19. F. E. Shaw Jr., D. J. Graham, H. A. Guess, et al., Post-marketing surveillance for neurologic adverse events reported after hepatitis B vaccination. Experience of the first three years, *Am. J. Epidemiol.*, *127*: 337 (1988).

20. W. Szmuness, E. E. Stevens, E. J. Harley, et al., The immune response of healthy adults to a reduced dose of hepatitis B vaccine, *J. Med. Virol.*, *8*: 123 (1981).

21. M. R. Hilleman, Immunologic prevention of human hepatitis, *Pers. Biol. Med.*, *27*: 543 (1984).

22. A. McLean, Development of vaccines against hepatitis A and hepatitis B, *Rev. Infect. Dis.*, *8*: 591 (1986).

23. F. Deinhardt, Aspects of vaccination against hepatitis B; passive-active immuniza-

tion schedules and vaccination responses in different age groups, *Scand. J. Infect. Dis.*, *38* (Suppl.): (1983).

24. L-Y. Hwang, R. R. Beasley, C. E. Stevens, et al., Immunogenicity of HBV vaccine in healthy Chinese children, *Vaccine*, *1*: 10 (1983).

25. N. Matsaniotis, C. Kattamis, E. Dionyssopoulou, et al., Immunogenicity of low doses of hepatitis B vaccine in normal children, *Vaccine*, *3*: 297 (1985).

26. G. Papaevangelou, A. Roumeliotou-Karayannis, C. Vissoulis, et al., Immunogenicity of a five-microgram dose of hepatitis B vaccine, *J. Med. Virol.*, *15*: 65 (1985).

27. O. W. Prozesky, C. E. Stevens, W. Szmuness, et al., Immune response to hepatitis B vaccine in newborns, *J. Infect.*, *7* (Suppl. 1): 53 (1983).

28. P. J. Grob, U. Binswanger, K. Zaruba, et al., Immunogenicity of a hepatitis B subunit vaccine in hemodialysis and in renal transplant recipients, *Antiviral Res.*, *3*: 43 (1983).

29. R. W. Steketee, M. E. Ziarnik, and J. P. Davis, Seroresponse to hepatitis B vaccine in patients and staff of renal dialysis centers, Wisconsin, *Am. J. Epidemiol.*, *127*: 772 (1988).

30. C. E. Stevens, H. J. Alter, P. E. Taylor, et al., Hepatitis B vaccine in hemodialysis patients: Immunogenicity and efficacy, *N. Engl. J. Med.*, *311*: 496 (1984).

31. P. R. Guesry, P. Adamowicz, P. Jungers, et al., Vaccination against hepatitis B in high-risk hemodialysis units: a double-blind study, *Viral Hepatitis: 1981 International Symposium* (W. Szmuness, H. J. Alter and J. E. Maynard, eds.), Franklin Institute Press, Philadelphia, pp. 493–507 (1982).

32. R. A. Coutinho, N. Lelie, P. Albrecht-Van Lent, et al., Efficacy of a heat inactivated hepatitis B vaccine in male homosexuals: Outcome of a placebo-controlled double blind trial, *Br. Med. J.*, *286*: 1305 (1983).

33. J. Desmyter, J. Colaert, G. De Groote, et al., Efficacy of heat-activated hepatitis B vaccine in haemodialysis patients and staff: Double-blind placebo-controlled trial, *Lancet*, *2*: 1323 (1983).

34. W. Szmuness, Large-scale efficacy trials of hepatitis B vaccines in the USA: Baseline data and protocols, *J. Med. Virol.*, *4*: 327 (1979).

35. R. P. Beasley, L-Y. Hwang, G. C-Y. Lee, et al., Prevention of perinatally transmitted hepatitis B virus infections with hepatitis B immune globulin and hepatitis B vaccine, *Lancet*, *2*: 1099 (1983).

36. K-J. Lo, Y-T. Tsai, S-D. Lee, et al., Immunoprophylaxis of infection with hepatitis B virus in infants born to hepatitis B surface antigen-positive carrier mothers, *J. Infect. Dis.*, *152*: 817 (1985).

37. D. Pongpipat, V. Suvatte, A. Assateerawatts, Perinatal transmission of hepatitis B virus in Thailand, *Asian Pac. J. Allergy*, *7*: 37 (1985).

38. Z-Y. Xu, C-B. Liu, D. P. Francis, et al., Prevention of perinatal acquisition of hepatitis B virus carriage using vaccine: Preliminary report of a randomized double-blind placebo-controlled and comparative trial, *Pediatrics*, *76*: 713 (1985).

39. R. P. Beasley, L-Y. Hwang, C. E. Stevens, et al., Efficacy of hepatitis B immune globulin for prevention of perinatal transmission of the hepatitis B virus carrier state: Final report of a randomized double-blind placebo controlled trial, *Hepatology*, *3*: 135 (1983).

40. C. E. Stevens, P. T. Toy, M. J. Tong, et al., Perinatal hepatitis B virus transmission in the United States. Prevention by passive-active immunization, *JAMA*, *253*: 1740 (1985).

41. V. C. W. Wong, H. M. H. Ip, H. W. Reesink, et al., Prevention of the HBsAg carrier state in newborn infants of mothers who are chronic carriers of HBsAg and HBeAg by administration of hepatitis-B vaccine and hepatitis-B immunoglobulin. Double-blind randomised placebo-controlled study, *Lancet*, *1*: 921 (1984).

42. W. J. McAleer, E. B. Buynak, R. Z. Maigetter, et al., Human hepatitis B vaccine from recombinant yeast, *Nature*, *307*: 178 (1984).

43. E. A. Emini, R. W. Ellis, W. J. Miller, et al., Production and immunological analysis of recombinant hepatitis B vaccine, *J. Infect.*, *13* (Suppl. A): 3 (1986).

44. J. Petre, F. Van Wijnendaele, B. De Neys, et al., Development of hepatitis B vaccine from transformed yeast cells, *Postgr. Med. J. 63* (Suppl. 2): 73 (1987).

45. F. Tron, F. Degos, C. Brechot, et al., Randomized dose range study of recombinant hepatitis B vaccine produced in mammalian cells and containing the S and preS sequences, *J. Infect. Dis.*, *160*: 199 (1989).

46. M. L. Halliday, J. G. Rankin, N. J. Bristow, et al., A randomized double-blind clinical trial of a mammalian cell-derived recombinant DNA hepatitis B vaccine compared with a plasma-derived vaccine, *Arch. Int. Med.*, *150*: 1195 (1990).

47. H. A. Thoma, A. E. Hemmerling, H. Hotzinger, Evaluation of immune response in a third generation hepatitis B vaccine containing pre-S proteins in comparative trials, *Progress in Hepatitis B Immunization* (P. Coursaget and M. J. Tong, eds.), Colloque INSERM/John Libbey Eurotext Ltd., London, Vol. 194, pp. 11–18 (1990).

48. F. E. Andre, Summary of safety and efficacy data on a yeast-derived hepatitis B vaccine, *Am. J. Med.*, *87* (Suppl. 3A): 14S (1989).

49. D. J. West, Clinical experience with hepatitis B vaccines, *Am. J. Infect. Control*, *17*: 172 (1989).

50. B. A. Zajac, D. J. West, W. J. McAleer, et al., Overview of clinical studies with hepatitis B vaccine made by recombinant DNA, *J. Infect.*, *13* (Suppl. A): 39 (1986).

51. G. Wiedermann, O. Scheiner, F. Ambrosch, et al., Lack of induction of IgE and IgG antibodies to yeast in humans immunized with recombinant hepatitis B vaccines, *Int. Arch. Allergy Appl. Immun.*, *85*: 130 (1988).

52. Centers for Disease Control, Recommendations of the Immunization Practices Advisory Committee: Update on hepatitis B prevention, *MMWR*, *36*: 353 (1987).

53. P. Hauser, P. Voet, E. Simeon, et al., Immunological properties of recombinant HBsAg produced in yeast, *Postgr. Med. J.*, *63* (Suppl. 2): 83 (1987).

54. Recombivax HB (Hepatitis B Vaccine [Recombinant], MSD), Prescribing information, DC7462206, Merck & Co., Inc., West Point, PA, issue date Jan. 1990.

55. Centers for Disease Control, Protection against viral hepatitis. Recommendations of the Immunization Practices Advisory Committee (ACIP), *MMWR*, *39* (RR-2): 1 (1990).

56. Engerix-B (Hepatitis B Vaccine [Recombinant]), Prescribing information, Smith-Kline Beckman Corp., Philadelphia, issue date Sept. 1989.

57. M. J. Alter, M. S. Favero, and J. E. Maynard, Impact of infection control strategies

on the incidence of dialysis-associated hepatitis in the United States, *J. Infect. Dis.*, *153*: 1149 (1986).

58. C. Goilav, H. Prinsen, and P. Piot, Protective efficacy of a recombinant DNA vaccine against hepatitis B in male homosexuals at 36 months, *Vaccine*, *8* (Suppl.): S50 (1990).

59. E. K. Yeoh, W. K. Chang, P. L. S. Ip, et al., A comparative study of recombinant versus plasma vaccine in high risk infants, *J. Med. Virol.*, *21*: 101A (1987).

60. C. E. Stevens, P. E. Taylor, M. J. Tong, et al., Prevention of perinatal hepatitis B virus infection with hepatitis B immune globulin and hepatitis B vaccine, *Viral Hepatitis and Liver Disease* (A. J. Zuckerman, ed.), Alan R. Liss, Inc., New York, pp. 982–988 (1988).

61. Y. Poovorawan, S. Sanpavat, W. Pongpunlert, et al., Comparison of a recombinant DNA hepatitis B vaccine alone or in combination with hepatitis B immune globulin for the prevention of perinatal acquisition of hepatitis B carriage, *Vaccine*, *8* (Suppl.): S56 (1990).

62. D. J. West, K. R. Brown, W. J. Miller, et al., Persistence of anti-HBs in recipients of a yeast recombinant hepatitis B vaccine, *Viral Hepatitis and Liver Disease* (A. J. Zuckerman, ed.), Alan R. Liss, Inc., New York, pp. 1043–1046 (1988).

63. N. Scheiermann, M. Gesemann, C. Maurer, et al., Persistence of antibodies after immunization with a recombinant yeast-derived hepatitis B vaccine following two different schedules, *Vaccine*, *8* (Suppl.): S44 (1990).

64. R. B. Wainwright, B. J. McMahon, L. R. Bulkow, et al., Duration of immunogenicity and efficacy of hepatitis B vaccine in a Yupik Eskimo population, *JAMA*, *261*: 2362 (1989).

65. S. C. Hadler, F. N. Judson, P. M. O'Malley, et al., Studies of hepatitis B vaccine in homosexual men, *Progress in Hepatitis B Immunization* (P. Coursaget and M. J. Tong, eds.), Colloque INSERM/John Libbey Eurotext Ltd., London, Vol. 194, pp. 165–175 (1990).

66. M. J. Tong, C. E. Stevens, P. E. Taylor, et al., Prevention of hepatitis B infection in infants born to HBeAg positive HBsAg positive carrier mothers in the United States. An update, 1989, *Progress in Hepatitis B Immunization* (P. Coursaget and M. J. Tong, eds.), Colloque INSERM/John Libbey Eurotext Ltd., London, Vol. 194, pp. 339–345 (1990).

67. L-Y. Hwang, C-Y. Lee, and R. P. Beasley, Five year follow-up of HBV vaccination with plasma derived vaccine in neonates—evaluation of immunogenicity and efficacy against perinatal transmission, 1990 International Symposium on Viral Hepatitis and Liver Disease, Houston, Abstract No. 247.

68. S. Krugman and M. Davidson, Hepatitis B vaccine: Prospects for duration of immunity, *Yale J. Biol. Med.*, *60*: 333 (1987).

69. C. D. Moyes, A. Milne, and J. Waldon, Very low dose hepatitis B vaccination in the newborn: Anamnestic response to a booster at four years, *J. Med. Virol.*, *30*: 216 (1990).

70. J. A. Clarke, F. B. Hollinger, E. Lewis, et al., Intradermal inoculation with Heptavax-B. Immune response and histologic evaluation of injection sites, *JAMA*, *262*: 2567 (1989).

71. M. L. Gonzalez, M. Usandizaga, P. Alomar, et al., Intradermal and intramuscular route for vaccination against hepatitis B, *Vaccine*, *8*: 402 (1990).

72. P. J. Coleman, F. E. Shaw Jr., J. Serovich, et al., Intradermal hepatitis B vaccination in a large hospital population, *Vaccine*, *9*: 723 (1991).

73. D. Donati and L. Gastaldi, Controlled trial of thymopentin in hemodialysis patients who fail to respond to hepatitis B vaccine, *Nephron*, *50*: 133 (1988).

74. S. C. Meuer, H. Dumann, K-H. Meyer Z. Büschenfelde, et al., Low dose interleukin-2 induces systemic immune responses against HBsAg in immunodeficient non-responders to the hepatitis B vaccination, *Lancet*, *1*: 15 (1989).

75. J. A. Quiroga, I. Castillo, J. C. Porres, et al., Recombinant gamma-interferon as adjuvant to hepatitis B vaccine in hemodialysis patients, *Hepatology*, *12*: 661 (1990).

76. W. Jilg, M. Schmidt, F. Deinhardt, Vaccination against hepatitis B: Comparison of three different vaccination schedules, *J. Infect. Dis.*, *160*: 766 (1989).

77. Y. Ghendon, WHO strategy for the global elimination of new cases of hepatitis B, *Vaccine*, *8* (Suppl.): S129 (1990).

78. S. C. Hadler, M. A. deMonzon, D. R. Lugo, et al., Effect of timing of hepatitis B vaccine doses on response to vaccine in Yucpa Indians, *Vaccine*, *7*: 106 (1989).

79. The Gambia Hepatitis Study Group, Hepatitis B vaccine in the expanded programme of immunizations: The Gambian experience, *Lancet*, *1*: 1057 (1989).

80. J. S. Coberly, N. A. Halsey, T. R. Townsend, et al., Low dose hepatitis B vaccination at birth, 2, and 4 months of age, *Pediat. Res.*, *25*: A176 (1989).

81. P. Tiollais, C. Pourcel, and A. DeJean, The hepatitis B virus, *Nature*, *317*: 489 (1985).

82. A. Budkowska, P. Dubreuil, F. Capel, et al., Hepatitis B virus preS gene-encoded antigenic specificity and anti-preS antibody: Relationship between anti-preS response and recovery, *Hepatology*, *6*: 360 (1986).

83. M. A. Petit, P. Maillard, F. Capel, et al., Immunochemical structure of the hepatitis B surface antigen vaccine II. Analysis of antibody responses in human sera against the envelope proteins, *Molecular Immunology*, *23*: 511 (1986).

84. A. R. Neurath, S. B. H. Kent, K. Parker, et al., Antibodies to a synthetic peptide from the preS 120–145 region of the hepatitis B virus envelope are virus neutralizing, *Vaccine*, *4*: 35 (1986).

85. E. A. Emini, V. Larsen, J. Eichborg, et al., Protective effect of a synthetic peptide comprising the complete preS2 region of the hepatitis B virus surface protein, *J. Med. Virol.*, *28*: 7 (1989).

86. D. R. Milich, A. R. Neurath, S. B. Kent, et al., Enhanced immunogenicity of the preS region of hepatitis B surface antigen, *Science*, *228*: 1195 (1985).

87. S. Iino, H. Suzuki, Y. Akahane, et al., Phase II study of recombinant HB vaccine containing the S and PreS2 antigens, 1990 International Symposium on Viral Hepatitis and Liver Disease, Houston, Abstract No. 292.

88. E. Miskovsky, K. Gershman, M. L. Clements, et al., Comparative safety and immunogenicity of yeast recombinant hepatitis B vaccines containing S or preS2 + S antigens, *Vaccine 9*: 346 (1991).

89. M. R. Hilleman, History, precedent, and progress in the development of mammalian cell culture systems for preparing vaccines: Safety considerations revisited, *J. Med. Virol.*, *31*: 5 (1990).

90. U. Hellstrom, S. Sylvan, M. Kuhns, et al., Absence of preS2 antibodies in natural hepatitis B infection, *Lancet*, *2*: 889 (1986).

9

Overview of Clinical Trials in Low-Endemic Areas

Catherine L. Troisi and F. Blaine Hollinger

Baylor College of Medicine, Houston, Texas

I. FIELD TRIALS WITH PLASMA-DERIVED HEPATITIS B VACCINE

A. Early Studies

The discovery of the Australia antigen, now known as hepatitis B surface antigen (HBsAg) (1), and the subsequent acceptance of its relationship to hepatitis B virus (HBV) (2) allowed researchers for the first time to distinguish between different etiologies of viral hepatitis. As early as 1970, attempts were made to develop vaccines against hepatitis B and the serious sequelae sometimes associated with this infection. The first vaccine for use in humans was prepared by Krugman et al. (3), who heated infectious serum to a temperature of 98°C for one minute. Children who were clients at an institute for the mentally handicapped where hepatitis B was endemic were inoculated intramuscularly with this crude inactivated vaccine. Ten children received one dose, and four children received two doses. Four to eight months later the children were challenged with the unheated infectious serum. Four of the ten children who received one injection of the vaccine were protected from infection, while the clinical disease was of shorter duration in the other six than in the unimmunized controls. All four of the children who received two doses of the vaccine were protected. This early study established the concept that inactivated virus, or its components, could be used as an efficacious vaccine, and research proceeded toward the development of other, more refined, vaccines.

An important step in the eventual development of a vaccine was the early recognition that antibodies directed against the HBsAg envelope of HBV (anti-HBs) were protective. Lander et al. (4) found that patients who developed anti-HBs failed to contract hepatitis after subsequent rechallenge with HBV. Hollinger and other investigators (5–7) reported that no anicteric or icteric hepatitis B developed in 132 transfused recipients whose sera contained anti-HBs prior to blood transfusion. In contrast, 16 of 371 (4.3%) recipients without preexisting anti-HBs experienced clinical hepatitis B. Several other studies have shown that immune globulin containing measurable levels of anti-HBs can prevent hepatitis B when given prior to exposure (8–11).

The first purified subunit vaccines to be evaluated were derived from the plasma of HBsAg-positive carriers (12–14) (see also Chapter 1). These vaccines consisted of HBsAg particles treated with formalin. They were evaluated initially in chimpanzees and were determined to be both safe and efficacious. However, theoretical concerns were raised that these vaccines also may contain host antigens, such as serum proteins, and that these alloantigens may elicit an unfavorable allergic response in some recipients. In 1975, Maupas and colleagues (14) decided that the incidence of HBV infection was so high in hemodialysis centers that this theoretical risk of an allergic response was not an overriding concern. Three doses of vaccine were administered monthly to 46 hemodialysis staff members and, except for mild discomfort at the site of injection, no additional local or systemic reactions were observed. Biochemical tests of liver dysfunction remained normal, and no auto-immune reactions were noted. Seventy-six percent of the volunteers developed anti-HBs by the fifth month, while no subjects developed hepatitis B. In a continuation of this trial (15), three (0, 1, 2 months) or four (0, 1, 2, 12 months) subcutaneous injections of HBsAg were given to 162 staff members and 55 hemodialysis patients. Among the 184 persons who developed a primary antibody response, no clinical evidence of hepatitis was observed, although 9 persons (5%) developed a transient antigenemia. In contrast, HBV occurred in 50 and 87% of nonvaccinated staff and patients, respectively. As observed in subsequent trials, anti-HBs responsiveness was greater among staff members (92%) than among the patients (64%). This prototype vaccine was eventually produced by the Pasteur Institute as Hevac-B.

The first large-scale hepatitis B vaccine study in the United States was initiated by Szmuness et al. in 1978 (16). The aim of this placebo-controlled, randomized, double-blind trial was to determine the efficacy of a plasma-derived vaccine in a homosexual population, a cohort that is at high risk of contracting HBV infection. The vaccine, which was manufactured by Merck Sharp & Dohme (MSD), consisted of a highly purified preparation of HBsAg, subtype *ad*, that was treated with formalin and alum-adsorbed. Additional purification steps included pepsin digestion at low pH and denaturation with urea followed by gel filtration to separate the HBsAg from the urea, pepsin, and any extraneous proteins. These procedures also were capable of inactivating HBV and virtually all other known animal viruses including the human immunodeficiency virus (HIV), which causes AIDS (17). A 40-μg dose was administered intramuscularly at 0, 1, and 6 months to 549 homosexual males. Another 534 gay men received a placebo, which contained all elements of the active vaccine except HBsAg. Side reactions were rare. A low-grade fever was observed in only 2.6% of the vaccinees, a frequency similar to that found in the placebo recipients (2.2%). Over half of all the complaints were about discomfort at the site of injection, and this was more common among the vaccinees. One month after the first injection, 31% of the vaccine group had made specific anti-HBs, and this increased to 96% one month after the third inoculation. Thus, only 4% of the men who received twice the currently recommended dose of plasma-derived vaccine failed to develop an anti-HBs response, although another 5% of those who seroconverted developed an inadequate response, i.e., between 2.1 and 9.9 sample ratio units (SRU).

The vaccine, designated HEPTAVAX B, was shown to be highly efficacious. During the first 26 months of the study, 158 HBV events were recorded. One hundred and twenty-seven (80%) of these occurred in the placebo group, and these cases were distributed evenly throughout the study. In contrast, of the 31 events observed among those given the vaccine, 17 (55%) occurred during the first 105 days after randomization, indicating that their infection probably had taken place near the time of initial vaccination. Of the remaining 15 subjects whose HBV infection occurred after day 105, six (40%) seroconverted for anti-HBc only without detectable HBsAg or a display of clinical symptoms.

Overall, the efficacy ratio (the ratio of incidence in placebo recipients to that in vaccinated subjects) reached 14.0 during months 5–18 of the study, and the reduction in HBV infection was as great as 92%. No HBsAg-positive events were recorded in vaccinees who had received three inoculations and had mounted an adequate immune response (>10 SRU). Thus, the acquisition of anti-HBs is synonymous with protection.

Concurrent with the New York trials, the CDC conducted a randomized, double-blind, placebo-controlled efficacy trial in homosexual males which utilized 20 μg of the MSD vaccine (18). Although seroconversion rates were lower after three injections than in the New York study (85% vs. 96%), vaccination substantially reduced HBV infections, yielding a protective efficacy rate of 98% in responders. The lower seroconversion rate may have been due to any number of factors acting either singularly or in unison. This includes any inherent immunodeficiencies present in the study population, the lower dose of vaccine employed in the CDC trial, or the possibility that the vaccine may have been improperly stored, (e.g., frozen) during and after its shipment, thus potentially lowering its immunogenicity (19,20).

Between months 3 and 15, only 11 (2%) HBV events occurred in 540 vaccine recipients versus 56 (11%) events in the 510 placebo controls. Within the vaccine group, all but one of the 11 HBV events occurred in nonresponders or in poor responders (those with peak anti-HBs levels of <10 SRU). This result is similar to that reported in the New York study, indicating that persons who are unable to mount an adequate immune response to the vaccine remain at risk for acquiring HBV after exposure. As in the previous trial, the vaccine also modified the clinical outcome to concurrent HBV infection by resulting in less severe disease even when administered after apparent exposure to the virus.

HEPTAVAX B was approved by the FDA in 1981 and became generally available in July 1982. The approved dosage is 20 μg for healthy adults and is administered at 0, 1, and 6 months. Twice that amount (40 μg) is recommended for immunosuppressed individuals, e.g., hemodialysis patients, while 10 μg is licensed for use in infants and children 10 years of age and below.

Another randomized, placebo-controlled trial evaluated a relatively impure heat-inactivated (90 seconds at 101–104.5°C and 10 hours at 65°C) plasma-derived HBsAg vaccine prepared by the Central Laboratory of the Netherlands Red Cross Blood Transfusion Service (21). A group of 800 homosexual males received either a placebo or three doses of this vaccine (3 μg each). Hepatitis B attack rates were 24% in the placebo group versus 5% in the vaccine subjects, yielding a protective efficacy ratio of 80%. No HBV infections occurred among the vaccine responders, and side effects were unremarkable.

A number of other large clinical trials (>150 subjects) have been conducted in low-endemic areas using plasma-derived vaccines. Guesry et al. (22), Szmuness et al. (23), and Stevens et al. (24) immunized hemodialysis staff and patients and achieved comparable seroconversion rates (92–96% for staff and 50–64% for patients). Protective efficacy rates ranged from 71–85% for the staff but only 53% for the patients. Clinical trials in neonates in the United States employed both HBIG and 10 or 20 μg plasma-derived vaccine (25). An estimated protective efficacy ratio of 80–86% in infants born to HBeAg-positive mothers was achieved with this regimen.

B. Effect of Vaccine on HBsAg-Positive Subjects

In tandem with these initial field trials, a study was initiated to determine whether this vaccine could ameliorate infection in HBV carriers (26). Sixteen male carriers received 2–6 monthly injections of a 40-μg dose of vaccine (mean number of doses was 4.1 $\pm$ 1.8). Some of the carriers received HBsAg having the same subtype as their chronic infection; others received a heterologous subtype vaccine. Circulating immune complexes were detected in 6 of the 16 vaccinees before immunization, but these levels did not increase subsequently. The 10 subjects who did not have prior evidence of immune complexes did not develop any complexes postinoculation. Elevations in aminotransferase levels

(ALT and AST) were sporadic and did not show a temporal relationship to vaccination. In another study, Barin et al. (27) evaluated the effects of vaccination in children who were HBsAg carriers and compared them with controls. Both studies confirmed that vaccination of carriers was safe but ineffective in eliminating HBsAg from chronically infected individuals.

C. Effect of Hepatitis B Immune Globulin (HBIG) on Vaccine Response

Another question raised initially was whether the simultaneous administration of high concentrations of anti-HBs, in the form of HBIG, might suppress the active immune response to HBsAg vaccine. This was an important consideration since the effectiveness of postexposure prophylaxis generally dictates that HBIG and HBsAg vaccine be given concurrently to achieve rapid protection followed by durable immunity, i.e., passive-active immunity. Szmuness et al. (11) administered HBIG to 20 volunteers one month before beginning a three-dose vaccine schedule (0, 1, and 6 months). Another 26 volunteers received HBIG concurrently with the vaccine, while 44 subjects received only vaccine. One month following the first dose of vaccine, all of the subjects in the first two groups were anti-HBs positive; only one of these became anti-HBs negative during the 8 months of follow-up. No significant differences were observed in the levels of anti-HBs subsequently achieved by the two vaccine groups that received HBIG and the group that did not. Thus, this study implied that simultaneous administration of up to 3.0 ml of HBIG with the first dose of vaccine would not diminish active immunity.

II. FIELD TRIALS WITH RECOMBINANT-DERIVED VACCINES

The next phase of vaccine development utilized genetic engineering in eukaryotic systems (see also Chapter 4). The initial impetus for the development of a genetically engineered vaccine was the appearance in 1982 of the acquired immunodeficiency syndrome (AIDS) in many of the same groups from which the plasma for the plasma-derived vaccine was collected. Even though fear that the human immunodeficiency virus (HIV) might be transmitted by vaccination proved to be groundless, it was felt that a vaccine that did not rely on any human product for its production would enjoy wider acceptance. In addition, it was hoped that a recombinant-derived vaccine might be less expensive to produce and also would lead to more uniformity between lots.

A vaccine produced by MSD was initially administered to 37 subjects with no serious side effects. Anti-*a* antibodies predominated, and there was no appearance of new yeast antibodies or a significant increase in the intensity of existing yeast antibody patterns (28). More reports on this vaccine quickly followed. Jilg et al. (29) studied the response to 10 μg of the vaccine in 30 medical students who were matched by age and sex with 41 subjects who received the plasma-derived vaccine. The geometric mean anti-HBs concentration in the yeast-derived group was less than that of the plasma-derived group for the entire 7-month follow-up interval. No important side effects were observed. Davidson and Krugman (30,31) reported on the results of 5 or 10 μg of the yeast-derived vaccine administered to health-care professionals. They found no differences in immune responses between these recombinant vaccine groups and subjects that received 10 or 20 μg of plasma-derived vaccine a few years earlier. However, historical controls were used, and it should be noted that the group receiving 20 μg of HEPTAVAX B had an exceptionally poor response with a geometric mean anti-HBs level of only 141 mIU/ml at 7 or 8 months. In addition, four different lots of the recombinant vaccine were used, making comparisons between groups difficult. Dandalos et al. (32,33) studied the recombinant vaccine in 110 army recruits and found no serological differences between 5 and 10 μg of this vaccine and 5 μg of the plasma-derived vaccine, but observed that 10 μg of HEPTAVAX B—only half the recommended dose—gave significantly higher immune responses. A reduced dose of recombinant-derived vaccine (2.5 μg) was not found to be as immunogenic as the 5- or 10-μg doses (34). Nonetheless, their study confirmed the safety and immunogenicity of the recombinant-derived vaccine. Heijtink et al. (35) also found reduced geometric mean anti-HBs levels in subjects given the MSD recombinant-derived vaccine when compared to the plasma-derived vaccine. In contrast to the Davidson and Krugman study, both comparison groups received their inoculations concurrently.

Based on these and other studies (36,37), some of which used pooled data (38), a dosage of 10 μg was approved by the FDA in July 1986 for nonimmunosuppressed adults receiving RECOMBIVAX HB, the trade name given the genetically engineered vaccine from MSD However, a number of studies questioned the soundness of this dosage decision (29,39–41). Using a single lot of RECOMBIVAX HB, Hollinger et al. (39) evaluated dosages of 5, 10, and 20 μg in weight-matched, young adult males and found a direct correlation between increased dosage and the immune response. In comparison with adults who had received HEPTAVAX B, immune responses were significantly lower in the 5- and 10-μg RECOMBIVAX HB groups, prompting an editorial that examined the selection of a 10-μg dose for the original RECOMBIVAX HB product (40). Subsequent to this editorial, representatives from MSD (42) presented evidence that a "new and improved" RECOMBIVAX HB vaccine had been formulated that involved both a new purification process and new master seed strain of the yeast. These steps have led to a vaccine that is more immunogenic than the original lots.

Issues have been raised concerning the potency of HBsAg vaccine preparations based on the concentrations recommended by the various manufacturers. The lack of a reference standard for HBsAg makes comparisons of antigen concentrations less meaningful. More important, it is well recognized that quantitation of HBsAg in vaccine, in μg/ml, does not always signify equivalent immunogenicity. Comparability of antigen dose is less important than comparability of immunogenicity per dose. In this regard, the strain of virus or viral gene products employed, the choice of a particular expression vector or expression system, the purification process and method of inactivation, and the type of adjuvant or stabilizers used may have a profound effect on the immunogenicity of a product. Each of these factors are taken into account by the manufacturers when determining the proper dose of vaccine to be used.

Recently, a second yeast-derived vaccine was licensed in the United States. ENGERIX B, a product of SmithKline Biologicals (SB), also uses *S. cerevisiae* as its production system. Initial studies in humans using 2.5, 5, 10, or 20 μg of this vaccine inoculated intramuscularly at 0, 1, and 2 months did not compare favorably with HEPTAVAX B, the plasma-derived vaccine (43). Seroconversion rates reached 100% in both groups, but geometric mean anti-HBs levels were lower in subjects who received the recombinant-derived vaccine (229 vs. 1024 mIU/ml in males; 707 vs. 2328 mIU/ml in females). Wiedermann et al. (44) also found that ENGERIX B did not perform as well as the plasma-derived vaccine when geometric mean anti-HBs levels were measured 3 months after the initial inoculation.

Dahl-Hansen et al. (45) compared the immunogenicity of 20 μg of the SB yeast-derived vaccine with 10 μg of the MSD yeast-derived vaccine, the manufacturers' recommended dosages for each product. Seroconversion rates were equal between the two groups (where seroconversion was defined as >1 mIU/ml), and all vaccinees had anti-HBs levels of $\geq$10 mIU/ml 9 months after the first vaccination. Geometric mean anti-HBs levels were significantly higher at 3, 6, and 9 months in subjects who received the SB vaccine. Although the two groups were not matched for age or weight, the MSD group had younger subjects, which should have afforded an advantage to the MSD vaccine. However, the MSD lot of vaccine which was used in this study was subsequently shown to be less immunogenic than the currently available vaccine and the vaccine tested may have been at a time beyond its verified stability testing. This revelation of a less immunogenic lot (45b) may be of importance to the many individuals who were vaccinated with the earlier lots of MSD yeast-derived vaccine, since a proportion of these vaccinees may not have developed protective levels of anti-HBs. Thus a booster dose with a current batch of vaccine may be needed to establish adequate levels of protection. In another study, Trepo et al. (46) found little difference between the MSD and SB vaccines but reported a significantly better response with a genetically engineered vaccine, also containing PreS2 antigen, that was produced in mammalian (Chinese hamster ovary; CHO) cells.

Clinical trials with the recombinant vaccines have largely been conducted in areas where high endemicity for HBV occurs. Bruguera et al. (47) reported that a four-dose schedule of ENGERIX B (40 μg) given to 43 presumably immunocompromised hemodialysis patients at 0,1,2, and 6 months resulted in an 86% seroconversion rate. Similarly, Van Damme et al. (48) found the SB product to be effective in preventing hepatitis B in institutionalized Down syndrome clients. Finally, Stevens and coworkers (49) immunized 130 neonates of HBeAg-positive mothers in the United States with RECOMBIVAX HB (three doses of 5 μg each given at 0,1,6 months) and a single dose of HBIG at delivery. An estimated protective efficacy ratio of 95% was achieved in this group using this regimen.

III. REACTOGENICITY OF THE VACCINE

Early studies with both the plasma-derived and recombinant-derived vaccines indicated that reactions occurred in only a few individuals and were limited to pain at the injection site and mild elevations in temperatures. In 1981, Hollinger et al. (50,51) reported results from a trial conducted in 198 young adults at low risk of contracting hepatitis B. Eight separate groups of approximately 25 each were selected to receive a plasma-derived, alum-adsorbed HBsAg vaccine produced by the National Institute for Allergy and Infectious Diseases (52). Varying dosages of vaccine and different time intervals were utilized (Table 1). In this randomized, double-blind trial, 70 of the volunteers who initially served as placebo recipients were later crossed over to the vaccine group without their knowledge. Mild pain or discomfort, described as tenderness over the injection site during the first 12 hours that did not require medication for relief, was observed more frequently in those receiving 40 μg of HBsAg (57%) than in those given 20 μg (48%), 10 μg (28%), or a placebo (19%) ($p < 0.001$). In both placebo and vaccine groups, females were more likely to report discomfort than males, and this complaint was also dose-dependent. The frequency of mild pain or discomfort that occurred in the placebo group following their initial inoculation with 40 μg of HBsAg (56%) was virtually identical to that seen in the subjects originally receiving 40 μg of HBsAg vaccine. Systemic reactions were approximately the same in the vaccine and placebo groups, with the exception of slightly increased oral temperatures observed 30 minutes postvaccination. Specifically, an elevated temperature ($>0.5°F$ from an individual's baseline value) was seen in 24% of those receiving 40 μg of vaccine versus 17% of the 20-μg group, 12% of the 10-μg group, and 13% of the placebo group. Although the frequency seen in the 40-μg group was significantly different from that observed in the placebo group ($p < 0.05$), the highest elevation in temperature was only 1.5°F in one case. Females were more likely to have an elevated temperature than were males ($p < 0.05$). These temperature elevations were considered biologically insignificant.

Table 1 Vaccine Schedule and Dose, Maximum Geometric Mean, and Median Anti-HBs Levels (mIU/ml) in Groups Receiving the NIAID Vaccine

Group	Vaccine schedule (month)	Dose (μg)	No. subjects	% Responding	Anti-HBs Response[a] Peak level (geometric) Month	Mean	Median	At final bleeding (geometric) Month	Mean	Median	% Positive
A	0,6	40	24	100	8	781	1367	30	26	41	92
B	0,3,6	40	25	100	8	643	542	30	28	37	88
C	0,1,4	40	25	96	5	771	1225	28	61	60	100
D	0,1,6	40	25	100	7	3338	2902	30	131	161	100
E	0,2,6	40	25	100	7	1303	1674	30	67	85	100
F	0,2,4	40	24	96	6	1848	2869	28	155	148	96
G	0,2,4	20	25	100	5	583	693	28	54	63	96
H	0,2,4	10	25	96	5	277	386	28	30	41	88

[a]Responders only
Source: Ref. 51.

Likewise, the recombinant-derived vaccine has shown few side reactions. Andre (53), in a review of 122 clinical trials involving 40,140 vaccine doses administered, concluded that "no clinically important adverse effect which could be considered as directly related to vaccination has been recorded." Most frequent local complaints were soreness at the injection site (23% of vaccinees) and induration (8%). Fewer symptoms were reported in children than in adults.

The question of vaccination of thimerosal-sensitive persons has been raised. Reactions, though rare, have been cited in the literature (54). Whether allergic reactions are more likely to occur in individuals with an ocular sensitivity to thimerosal, usually associated with the use of contact lenses, has not been evaluated systematically, but nine subjects with a history of ocular sensitivity were vaccinated without adverse effects (55).

Guillain-Barré syndrome, a rare complication of viral vaccination, has been reported after inoculation with the plasma-derived (56) and genetically engineered vaccines (57). However, it is felt that the incidence of this neurological disorder is not any greater among vaccinees than in the general population. Case reports of erythema nodosum following vaccination have been published (58–60). Although de novo development of yeast antibodies have not been reported in vaccine recipients, a case report of a reaction that occurred following vaccination in a yeast-sensitive individual has been cited (61).

IV. FACTORS INFLUENCING IMMUNOGENICITY

A. Vaccine Factors

Characteristics of the vaccine that influence immunogenicity include dosage, number and timing of inoculations, storage of the vaccine, and the use of adjuvants. The incorporation of other epitopes from the S-gene region to enhance antibody response will be discussed in a separate chapter.

1. Dosage and Immunization Schedules

Many field trials evaluating optimal dosage and immunization schedules in humans have been conducted. In the NIAID plasma-derived vaccine study of Hollinger et al. (51) using weight-matched subjects, HBsAg dosage, number of inoculations, and schedules were evaluated (Table 1). The seven schedules included 0,6; 0,1,6; 0,2,6; 0,3,6; 0,1,4; 0,2,4; and 0,2,9 months, with dosages of 10, 20, or 40 μg of HBsAg employed. One month after the first inoculation, the 40-μg group had a significantly higher seroconversion rate than did the other two dosage groups. However, by 6 months this difference had disappeared, and no differences were seen between dosage groups utilizing the same schedule. A total of 98.5% of the recipients made specific anti-HBs after three injections. These data suggest that seroconversion rates have limited usefulness when the immunogenicities of products are compared, except during the initial 1–3 months of a vaccine trial. Geometric mean and median anti-HBs levels were calculated for each vaccine group. The highest peak concentrations were seen in the groups receiving vaccine at 0,1,6 and 0,2,4 months. Slightly lower responses were observed in subjects given vaccine at 0,2,6 and 0,2,9 months. The peak anti-HBs level was directly related to the dosage administered (Table 1; groups F, G, and H). The worst response occurred in subjects who received their 40-μg immunizations at 0,6; 0,3,6; and 0,1,4 months. As expected, based on initial peak geometric concentrations of anti-HBs, persistence of antibody was greatest in the 0,1,6; 0,2,4, and 0,2,6 groups. A good response to the 0,2,4; or 0,2,6 schedule is encouraging since this regimen is similar to that proposed for the universal immunization of infants.

The schedule for administering the vaccine and the number of injections have been the subject of other studies. Currently, two primary immunization series are being employed using three injections at 0,1, and 6 months, or four injections at 0, 1, 2, and 12 months. In general, the 0,1,6 schedule is preferred for pre-exposure prophylaxis of the immunocompetent host, whereas the 0,1,2,(6–12) schedule may be preferable for the immunocompromised patient or for postexposure prophylaxis where a more rapid immune response is preferred. While a 0,1,12 schedule eventually may lead to higher peak anti-HBs responses, (62–64), a potentially undesirable "window of vulnerability" occurring during the interval between months 1 and 12 may restrict its use to groups that have a low risk of hepatitis B infection. In a vaccination study involving more than 1000 Yucpa Indians, Hadler et al. (65) concluded that the response to hepatitis B vaccination is not stringently time dependent and that slight changes in the 0,1,6 schedule did not affect the overall response to the vaccine.

The dosages of hepatitis B vaccines have been studied extensively. As previously cited, initial results with the MSD plasma-derived vaccine indicated that 20 μg of Heptavax-B was equivalent to 40 μg (66). However, this was before the importance of weight-matching, single-lot evaluation, or determination of the peak antibody response levels were appreciated. In addition, comparisons between peak antibody levels at sample ratio units greater than 100 are often suspect because a nonlinear relationship exists between antibody concentration and SRU above that level. Therefore, to compare mean antibody levels, results should be converted to mIU/ml, as described later in this chapter. Studies with the NIAID HBsAg vaccine in weight-matched groups have shown unequivocally that the dose of vaccine administered to a subject is of considerable importance in determining the peak immune response achieved by that individual (39,62,67,68) (Fig. 1). In achieving these results, the importance of using weight-matched groups and the same lot of vaccine cannot be overemphasized (Fig. 2).

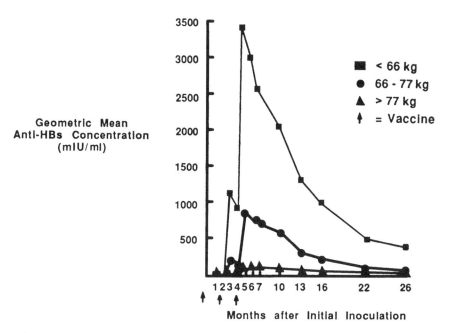

Figure 1   Geometric mean anti-HBs concentration (mIU/ml) as a function of body weight. (From Ref. 62.)

2.   Storage of Vaccine

Another characteristic of the vaccine that can influence the strength of the immune response is the "cold chain." Freezing of the plasma-derived vaccine presumably decreases immunogenicity (19, 69). For this reason, freeze detectors should be included in all vaccine shipments to ensure that this does not occur during any step in the transportation or storage process. In contrast, storage of a recombinant-derived vaccine at temperatures of 37°C for up to 4 weeks did not reduce the immunogenicity of the product in a significant manner (70). This information bodes well for developing nations where refrigeration of vaccine in the field is difficult.

3.   Use of Adjuvants and Biological Response Modifiers

The use of adjuvanted vaccines can favorably influence the immune response. Alum (aluminum phosphate or hydroxide), the most common adjuvant, is clearly superior to aqueous or saline suspensions of vaccine (52,71). Other adjuvants and biological response modifiers have been explored, including taurine, parotin, and lithium as oral adjuvants (72), and murabutide (73), thymopentin

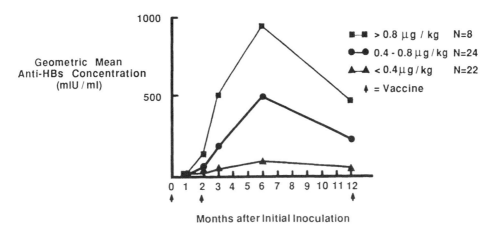

Figure 2 Geometric mean anti-HBs concentration (mIU/ml) as a function of vaccine dose/kg body weight. (From Ref. 51.)

(74–77), gamma inulin (in mice only) (78), and alpha-interferon (79). Results have been varied, with positive effects cited for taurine, parotin, lithium, and gamma inulin, some of which were used to circumvent genetic nonresponsiveness in mice. Murabutide increased the level of antibodies produced in mice and increased the specificity of the response to a synthetic HBsAg polypeptide containing preS antigenic determinants over the response to the tetanus toxoid carrier. Thymopentin, a synthetic pentapeptide that mimics the action of thymopoietin, induces differentiation of thymocytes. The effect appears to depend upon the time of administration of the adjuvant. For example, an enhanced immune response (geometric mean concentration = 77 mIU/ml) was observed in 12 of 13 volunteers administered 50 mg thymopentin subcutaneously three times per week, one week before and 2 weeks after an HBsAg booster inoculation. These subjects had previously either failed to respond to HBsAg or had developed a suboptimal response (75). Donati and Gastaldi (76) also reported success using thymopentin in 40 hemodialysis patients who had previously not responded to the vaccine. Three different schedules were used, but the best results were found when three booster inoculations (5 μg of HEVAC B) were administered one month apart with 50 mg thymopentin given on alternate days between the first and second vaccination (total of 12 doses). In this group, seroconversion rates reached 86% and remained at this level for at least 6 months. Five of the responders developed anti-HBs levels between 16 and 100 mIU/ml, while seven subjects responded with antibody levels higher than 100 mIU/ml. In contrast to these positive results, Grob et al. (74) observed no effect 2 months later when 50 mg thymopentin was given subcutaneously, three times before and after a booster injection of HBsAg, to 14 previously immunized hemodialysis patients. Likewise, three additional doses of HEPTAVAX B in conjunction with 50 mg thymopentin at the time of vaccination, and with or without additional thymopentin injections 3 and 5 days after each vaccine inoculation, had no effect on the response rate one month after the last inoculation in 29 hemodialysis patients.

Interferon, low doses of which have a "primer" effect on the immune system, has been used to reverse human nonresponsivenes to HEPTAVAX B. While no effect was seen in healthy volunteers or in hemodialysis patients, an increase in the immune response to the vaccine was observed in renal transplant patients who were receiving immunosuppressive agents (79). Interleukin-2, a lymphokine that amplifies immune function, also has been shown to enhance the immune response to HBsAg in vitro (80).

B. Host Factors Affecting Immunogenicity

Studies with both plasma-derived and genetically engineered hepatitis B vaccines have shown that many host factors may influence the immune response to the vaccine. These characteristics include age of the subject, weight, genetics, competency of the immune system, smoking status, and the site and route of injection.

1. Age and Weight of Subject

One important factor influencing the immune response is the age of an individual. Increasing age, especially above 30 years, has been shown to independently correlate with a decreasing response to the vaccine (67, 68, 81–83) (Tables 2,3). This probably relates to decreasing immune responses in older individuals.

Suboptimal responses occur in obese persons (51,84,85). Correspondingly, the immune response is inversely related to weight, especially in those subjects who are under 30 years of age (67) (see Figs. 1,2, Table 3). In this regard, it is

Table 2 Anti-HBs Seroconversion Rates in Various Age Groups After Three Injections of HEVAC B® Vaccine

Age (years)	No.	% Anti-HBs positive
61–70	13	69
71–80	16	44
81–90	38	39
91–96	3	33
Total	70	46

Source: Adapted from Ref. 81.

Table 3 Multiple Linear Regression of Age, Weight, Sex, and Dose on Anti-HBs Response to Three Doses of HEPTAVAX B® at 8 Months

	p-Value of F statistic		
Factor	Total ($n = 62$)	Age 10–30 yr ($n = 32$)	Age ≥31 yr ($n = 30$)
Age	<0.05	NS	<0.0005
Weight	<0.001	<0.025	NS
Sex	NS	NS	NS
Dose	<0.01	<0.0005	NS

Source: Ref. 67.

noteworthy that one of the most important criteria for determining the intensity of the immune response in young adults and children is the dosage administered per kilogram of body weight (Fig. 2). Thus, a higher dose/kg of vaccine administered to any given individual will, as might be expected, lead to higher levels of anti-HBs (44,50,62,67,82). Responses in weight-matched males and females revealed that weight, and not gender per se, accounted for the higher response rates seen among females versus males (51,67).

2. Genetics, Host Immune Responses, and Gender

Genetics also may play a role in determining the strength of the immune response in individuals vaccinated under identical circumstances. In one study, white children seemed to respond better to the vaccine than did nonwhite children (Orientals and blacks) (62). When compared to other ethnic groups, anti-HBs levels in the Oriental children were considerably lower throughout the study, but the number of subjects was relatively small. Some studies (86,87) have demonstrated a link between certain HLA antigens such as HLA-DR3 or DR4 and nonresponsiveness to the vaccine. Interestingly, DR3 also has been associated with the HBsAg carrier state and chronic active hepatitis, suggesting that these histocompatibility antigens may predispose individuals to detrimental cell-mediated immune reactions during an HBV infection in addition to modulating the immune response to HBsAg during vaccination.

Immunosuppressed groups, such as hemodialysis patients and those infected with HIV (88–90), respond poorly to vaccination when compared with healthy individuals. Smoking also appears to adversely affect the immunological response to HBsAg, presumably due to elevated levels of T-suppressor cells that occur in smokers (82,83,91).

Gender does not seem to play a role in the immune response to hepatitis B vaccination. While initial studies found that females often responded to the vaccine with higher peak antibody levels than did males (23,35), the key factor in this response may be the weight of the vaccinee and not the gender, e.g., no difference in immune response was observed when males and females were weight-matched (51,92)

3. Site of Inoculation

The site of inoculation is known to influence the outcome of hepatitis B vaccination. Shortly after large-scale vaccination programs were launched in the United States, it became apparent that some individuals were responding poorly to the vaccine. Merck Sharp & Dohme, assisted by the CDC, discovered that subjects inoculated in the buttocks failed to achieve an optimal response when compared to those who received all of their injections intramuscularly in the deltoid region (93–96) (Table 4). Mean seroconversion rates were 92% for those injected in the arm versus 73% for those inoculated only in the buttock, controlling for age and weight. Geometric mean anti-HBs levels also were higher in the former group. The apparent reason for this disparity is that most gluteal injections deliver the vaccine into adipose tissue, which is known to be a poor repository for vaccine (96, 97). A prospective study by Shaw et al. (83) recently confirmed the impropriety of administering hepatitis B vaccine in the buttock versus the arm, even when a 2-inch needle is used for the gluteal injections. Therefore, the current recommendation is to administer all hepatitis B vaccines intramuscularly (or subcutaneously) in the deltoid region (98).

Other routes of inoculation, including both subcutaneous and intradermal, have been extensively evaluated. The potential promise of the intradermal route is that one-tenth of the intramuscular dose can be used, leading to significant cost reduction. This is particularly important in developing countries where hepatitis B infection is endemic. Miller et al. (99) intradermally injected 12 seronegative volunteers with 2 μg of plasma-derived HBsAg vaccine at 0, 1, and 6 months. Specimens obtained one month following the last inoculation revealed that 10 subjects (85%) had seroconverted, yielding a relatively low geometric mean level of 96 mIU/ml. In another study (100,101), nine volunteers were injected

Table 4 Response to Hepatitis B Vaccine by Injection Site Among Hospital Personnel

Injection site	No. tested	% with Anti-HBs
Arm	3838	92
Mixed	1071	86
Buttock	4867	73

Source: Adapted from Ref. 93.

intradermally with HEPTAVAX B: four injections of 2 μg HBsAg at different sites on day one of the trial, then 5 μg of vaccine at months 1 and 6. Their response was compared with a group of 10 subjects who received 20 μg of vaccine by the intramuscular route at months 0 and 1, followed by 5 μg of HBsAg given intradermally and 15 μg given intramuscularly at month 6. Results showed that while 100% of both groups seroconverted after the final injection, the group receiving HBsAg by the intramuscular route achieved a much higher peak geometric mean antibody level (4916 vs. 500 mIU/ml). Although rates of antibody decline were similar in the two groups, the intramuscular group had higher antibody levels 19–21 months after the initial injection. The percentage of skin reactions were similar in both groups, and the investigators concluded that the intradermal route was safe but inferior to intramuscular immunization. Wahl and Hermodsson (102) compared serological responses to 20 μg of HEPTA-VAX-B injected intramuscularly ($N = 16$) with 2 μg injected intradermally ($N = 21$) or subcutaneously ($N = 21$) in a three-dose regimen. While the low-dose subcutaneous route yielded suboptimal results at 7 months (seroconversion rate = 63%; geometric mean anti-HBs concentration = 30 mIU/ml), the 2-μg intradermal and 20-μg intramuscular routes of administration produced comparable geometric mean antibody levels (1000 vs. 3000 mIU/ml) and seroconversion rates (100% versus 94%).

Other researchers have confirmed the lower immunogenicity of the intradermal route for administering the hepatitis B vaccine, in addition to its safety (103–108). Clarke et al. (106) inoculated 92 volunteers intradermally at 0, 1, and 6 months with 2 μg of HEPTAVAX B. Anti-HBs levels greater than 10 mIU/ml were detected in 95% of the subjects at one year, while 78% had levels >100 mIU/ml. Induration at the site of inoculation was present in 18% of the participants at month 6 but had resolved in all subjects by one year. Macules were observed at the inoculation site in 63% of the volunteers at one year, but these continued to fade with time. Over 99% of the participants queried stated that they would recommend this route to their colleagues. Skin biopsies of seven volunteers 2 months after vaccination showed an essentially normal upper dermis in two subjects with absent or low antibody response, while subjects who had responded well to the vaccine showed a prominent chronic lymphoid reaction with lympho-plasma histocytic infiltrates. However, no correlation could be made between the external skin reaction and antibody concentration at either month 6 or one year. Finally, Horowitz et al. (82) looked at the potential advantages of the intradermal route as a mechanism for boostering recipients who had completed their basic intramuscular immunization series. They concluded that an intradermal booster works well in those individuals who had initially responded to the vaccine by the intramuscular route. However, intradermal inoculation does not improve response rates in non- or hyporesponders previously vaccinated intramuscularly (109).

One of the major problems with intradermal inoculation, especially in mass immunization campaigns, is the relative difficulty of assuring intradermal versus subcutaneous placement of the vaccine. In addition, it is physically more dificult to vaccinate neonates by this route. Intradermal administration can be performed by jet injectors, but this also is less reliable than by needle. Lemon et al. (110) assessed the feasibility of mass inoculation against HBV with HEPTAVAX B by automatic jet injection, which delivers vaccine subcutaneously. Administration was safe and effective and resulted in 79% of the participants reaching a level of 10 SRU of anti-HBs or higher. Although this rate is lower than one might expect from intramuscular administration, it should be noted that less than 20 μg was received by some recipients in the second dose due to injector malfunction.

In summary, intradermal inoculation with either the plasma-derived or yeast-derived vaccine, although safe, has not led to equivalent levels of anti-HBs in most studies (106,108,111-114). As anticipated, among those who were given intradermal inoculations, peak antibody levels remained age and weight (or gender) dependent. None of these results should be surprising given the fact that the intramuscular route employs ten times the amount of antigen. To compensate for this disparity in the quantity of HBsAg and to guarantee adequate immunogenicity, the number of injections could be increased. To investigate this issue, Heijtink et al. (115) immunized 165 medical students either by the intramuscular or intradermal route with 2 μg plasma-derived HBsAg given four times at 0, 1, 2, and 6 months. They found that protective immunity (>10 mIU/ml) and the geometric mean concentrations of anti-HBs at month 7 were comparable in the two groups (90% and 533 mIU/ml in the intramuscular group vs. 94% and 541 mIU/ml in the intradermal group). These data suggest that low-dose intramuscular vaccine, given at least four times, may be acceptable for mass immunization of young adults if cost is a factor. A booster dose at 12 months for those with anti-HBs responses <1000 mIU/ml at month 7 should enhance long-term immunity in these subjects.

V. DURATION OF ANTIBODY

Reporting of results from clinical trials in terms that allow comparison between studies is necessary if antibody responses are to be analyzed in a meaningful way. Hollinger and coworkers (50,51,106) have provided a calculation for determining mIU/ml (IU/L) using a World Health Organization anti-HBs reference standard diluted to contain 125 mIU/ml. By employing a sample to reference standard ratio (S-N/R-N) in counts per minute (where N is the mean negative control value), in the following regression sample, a concentration of anti-HBs in mIU/ml can be obtained:

mIU/ml $= 130.75 \ (e^{0.66765 \ (S/R)} - 1)$ (reciprocal of dilution)

Dilutions are usually required when anti-HBs levels exceed 200 mIU/ml.

Initial studies (18,116) suggested that an antibody response of 10 mIU/ml or greater might be necessary for complete protection from HBV infection. Peak anti-HBs should be determined 1–3 months after the last inoculation. The reason for this is twofold. First, it is important to know if the subject has failed to respond to the vaccine and thus remains susceptible to HBV should exposure occur. Second, the anti-HBs concentration can be used to estimate when anti-HBs levels may decline to 10 mIU/ml or less. When the peak antibody level is assessed, vaccinees can be segregated into four groups—nonresponders (no anti-HBs produced), inadequate responders (anti-HBs levels between 1 and 10 mIU/ml), low responders (10–100 mIU/ml), and adequate responders (>100 mIU/ml). In general, a direct relationship exists between the peak antibody level achieved by an individual and the time required until the anti-HBs level drops to 10 mIU/ml, i.e., the regression slope is similar regardless of the peak anti-HBs concentration (51,117). A regression formula can be used to predict when a specified antibody level (e.g., 10 mIU/ml) will be reached. Because the slope is not linear, and also varies from person to person, the actual interval required to reach this low level may be longer or shorter. Nevertheless, the following mathematical expression has been used to obtain this information:

$$x \ (months) = \frac{\ln y}{0.132}$$

where ln y is the difference between the natural logarithm of the observed anti-HBs level and the designated endpoint. A level of 10 mIU/ml is usually chosen since immunity may be compromised below this concentration. In general, the $T_{1/2}$ for vaccine-induced anti-HBs is about 6 months for most individuals.

Duration of antibody in the general population following vaccination has been a subject of great interest. Hadler et al. (118) reevaluated serological responses in 773 homosexual male participants 7 years after their initial inoculation in the CDC vaccine trial. While 82% of the subjects initially had peak levels of antibody greater than 9.9 SRU, 22% of these had undetectable anti-HBs values within this interval, and only 48% had antibody concentrations greater than 10 SRU. The persistence of antibody was directly related to the maximum antibody peak attained after the primary immunization series, and a stepwise regression showed that no other variable was involved.

In another study of gay men in which 40 μg of plasma-derived HBsAg (twice the currently licensed dose) was administered, follow-up at 4.5 years revealed that 9% of vaccine responders had become anti-HBs negative, while another

20% had levels less than 10 S/N (119). Thus, 71% retained anti-HBs levels considered protective. Gibas et al. (120) also found that anti-HBs persisted above 10 mIU/ml for 5 years in 76% of health-care workers.

In interpreting these data on persistence of anti-HBs, it should be recognized that only 14–23% of the original vaccine subjects were evaluated at the longest follow-up interval. Thus, any statements about persistence of antibody applies only to the small subset of the entire population that was sampled. In addition, the role of natural anamnestic responses in maintaining antibody levels in these high-risk groups cannot be easily dismissed, especially when the annual incidence of infection approaches 13–17% (121). Durability of immunity obtained with the plasma-derived vaccine may not be observed with the yeast-derived product whose immunogenicity is lower (see below).

Other studies of long-term persistence of anti-HBs following vaccination with the plasma-derived vaccine have indicated that anti-HBs levels remain above 10 mIU/ml in 68% of responders after 3 years and 52–55% after 4 years (122,123). Wainwright et al. (123,124), in a study of 1630 susceptible Yupik Eskimos, found that 74% of those who initially had an anti-HBs response of 10 mIU/ml or greater following their basic immunization series retained antibody at that level for at least 7 years. Only 5% of the original group failed to achieve this level of immunity. Initial antibody level was a strong predictor of antibody persistence.

Because the yeast-derived vaccine has not been in existence as long as the plasma-derived vaccine, there are few long-term studies that evaluate antibody persistence. Hollinger et al. reevaluated 105 paramedics 24 months after their initial immunization with 5, 10, or 20 μg of the early lots of RECOMBIVAX HB (39). The rate of decline of the geometric mean anti-HBs levels was similar to that observed with the plasma-derived vaccine and, from months 18 to 24, these levels had declined from 10 to 1.8 mIU/ml, from 89 to 14 mIU/ml, and from 189 to 26 mIU/ml in the groups receiving 5, 10, or 20 μg of RECOM-BIVAX HB, respectively (unpublished data).

VI. BOOSTER INOCULATIONS

There are at least two situations where hepatitis B booster inoculations might be warranted (see also Chapter 17). The first is to augment an inadequate or nonresponse to the basic immunization series. Although it is generally accepted that hyporesponders are more likely to improve their level of immunity following a booster inoculation than are nonresponders (69, 82), most people would agree that both groups should be reimmunized with one or two injections of vaccine. In one study, 20 nonresponders to three doses of HEPTAVAX B were given additional inoculations (125). Five subjects (25%) reacted after one booster, three more after two boosters (total of 40%), and only one more after a third booster. In general, the peak geometric mean anti-HBs concentration is lower in hyporesponders after a booster injection than in those who initially developed an adequate response to the vaccine. An increased dosage, e.g., twice the recommended amount, could be considered for the booster inoculation(s) in nonresponders as could a switch from plasma-derived to yeast-derived vaccine or vice versa, depending on which was used for the initial series. However, recent studies indicate that recombinant-derived revaccination may not be effective in eliciting a response in nonresponders to the plasma-derived vaccine (126). Even low responders (10–100 mIU/ml) should be encouraged to receive a single booster inoculation in 1–2 years.

The second reason for booster inoculations is to raise declining anti-HBs levels after an adequate response to the vaccine has been achieved. Because live, attenuated hepatitis B vaccines are not available, it has been assumed that booster injections would be necessary for normal responders as they are for most inactivated or subunit vaccines. The question of when to administer booster inoculations has been given much consideration (122,127–129). To some extent, it may depend on the particular risk group being studied. Jilg et al. (127) proposed that if the antibody level in adults was less than 100 mIU/ml after completing the basic immunization series, then a booster should be given within 6 months; if 101–1000 mIU/ml, the antibody levels should be reevaluated in 1–2 years. However, if anti-HBs levels were >10,000 mIU/ml, reevaluation could be extended for 4–6 years. Those individuals who had levels <10 mIU/ml should be revaccinated immediately. Coursaget et al. (130) stated that the optimal time for a booster inoculation in children 5–6 years after the initial vaccination.

While it may ultimately be established that at-risk populations will be protected against clinical infection by a natural anamnestic response even if their antibody levels decline to less than 10 mIU/ml (31,120,123,131), the data for this conclusion are fragmentary. However, it is comforting to know that few, if any, relevant clinical infections have been recorded among vaccine responders who have been followed for 7–9 years. For example, during the initial large-scale field trials conducted in homosexual populations or the Eskimos, exposure to HBV either did not produce infection or caused only low levels of viral replication (123, 124, 128). In the CDC study of homosexual males, reviewed by Hadler et al. (118), 24% of 134 non- or hyporesponders had serological and/or clinical evidence of HBV infection (anti-HBc seroconversion), with half displaying HBsAg in the sampled specimen. Six (4.5%) of these subjects became persistently infected. Conversely, only 8% of the 634 responders acquired HBV during follow-up, and none of these had clinical symptoms or became persistently infected. Only 2 (0.3%) had detectable HBsAg at the time they were sampled, and both of these individuals were positive for HIV. Most of the HBV events observed in the vaccine responders were delayed for 4–9 years, and 72% occurred in those whose anti-HBs levels had declined to <10 SRU. At issue in this study is the incomplete follow-up of vaccinees and their contacts so that risk cannot be comprehensively assessed. Regardless, similar results were found in the Yupik Eskimo trial in Alaska (124) in which only five responders (0.3%) out of 1548 developed anti-HBc during a 7-year follow-up period and none displayed HBsAg or clinical hepatitis.

The controversy over whether to recommend booster doses centers on the majority of vaccinees who are considered to have made an adequate response (>100 mIU/ml). One group of experts has gone on record as favoring at least one booster inoculation approximately 5–7 years following the basic series of immunizations (129). Another group of experts recommends that no booster doses are necessary at this time (98). Whether these recommendations can be applied implicitly to persons who have received the less immunogenic recombinant products cannot be determined at this time.

In summary, control of hepatitis B infection by vaccination is within our grasp. Questions to be resolved include how nonresponders and immunosuppressed groups will be managed, what type of vaccine will provide the most complete protection, whether routes of injections, other than intramuscular, can be used with the same excellent results, and the necessity and timing of booster inoculations. However, as long as carriers exist, eradication of hepatitis B will not be feasible due to the existence of vaccine nonresponders and intrauterine infection.

REFERENCES

1. B. Blumberg, H. Alter, S. Visnich, A "new" antigen in leukemia sera, *JAMA*, *191*: 541 (1965).
2. A. Prince, An antigen detected in the blood during the incubation period of serum hepatitis, *Proc. Natl. Acad. Sci. USA*, *60*: 814 (1968).
3. S. Krugman, J. P. Giles, J. Hammond, Viral hepatitis type B (MS-2 strain): Studies on active immunization, *JAMA*, *217*: 41 (1971).
4. J. J. Lander, J. P. Giles, R. H. Purcell, S. Krugman, Viral hepatitis type B (MS-2 strain): Detection of antibody after primary infection, *N. Engl. J. Med.*, *285*: 303 (1971).
5. H. J. Alter, P. V. Holland, R. Purcell, J. Lander, S. Feinstone, A. Morrow, P. Schmidt, Posttransfusion hepatitis after exclusion of commercial and hepatitis-B antigen-positive donors, *Ann. Intern. Med.*, *77*: 691 (1972).
6. F. B. Hollinger, J. Werch, J. L. Melnick, A prospective study indicating that double-antibody radioimmunoassay reduces the incidence of post-transfusion hepatitis B, *N. Engl. J. Med.*, *290*: 1104 (1974).
7. F. B. Hollinger, R. D. Aach, G. L. Gitnick, J. Roche, J. Melnick, Limitations of solid-phase radioimmunoassay for HBsAg in reducing frequency of post-transfusion hepatitis, *N. Engl. J. Med.*, *289*: 385 (1973).
8. A. M. Courouce-Pauty, S. Delons, J. P. Soulier, Attempt to prevent hepatitis B by using specific anti-HBs immunoglobulin, *Am. J. Med. Sci.*, *270*: 375 (1975).
9. S. Iwarson, A. Erikosen, S. Hermodsson, H. Kjellman, C. Ljunqren, D. Selander,

Hepatitis B immune globulin in prevention of hepatitis B among hospital staff members, *J. Inf. Dis., 135*: 473 (1977).

10. W. Szmuness, A. M. Prince, M. Goodman, C. Ehrich, R. Pick, M. Ansari, Hepatitis B immune serum globulin in prevention of nonparenterally transmitted hepatitis B, *N. Engl. J. Med., 290*: 701 (1980).

11. W. Szmuness, C. E. Stevens, W. R. Oleszko, A. Goodman, Passive-active immunisation against hepatitis B: immunogenicity studies in adult Americans, *Lancet, 1*: 575 (1981).

12. R. H. Purcell, J. L. Gerin, Hepatitis B subunit vaccine: A preliminary report of safety and efficacy tests in chimpanzees, *Am. J. Med. Sci., 270*: 395 (1975).

13. M. R. Hilleman, E. B. Buynak, R. R. Roehm, A. Tytell, A. Bertland, G. Lampson, Purified and inactivated human hepatitis B vaccine. Progress report, *Am. J. Med. Sci., 270*: 401 (1975).

14. P. Maupas, A. Goudeau, P. Coursaget, J. Drucker, Immunization against hepatitis B in man, *Lancet, 1*: 1367 (1976).

15. P. Maupas, A. Goudeau, P. Coursaget, J. Drucker, F. Barin, M. Andre, Immunization against hepatitis B in man: A pilot study of two years duration, *Viral Hepatitis* (G. Vyas, S. Cohen, R. Schmid, eds.), Franklin Institute Press, Philadelphia, p. 539 (1978).

16. W. Szmuness, C. E. Stevens, E. J. Harley, E. Zang, W. Oleszko, D. William, R. Sadovsky, J. Morrison, A. Kellner, Hepatitis B vaccine. Demonstration of efficacy in a controlled clinical trial in a high-risk population in the United States, *N. Engl. J. Med., 303*: 833 (1980).

17. Report of an Inter-Agency Group, Hepatitis B virus vaccine safety, *MMWR, 31*: 465 (1982).

18. D. P. Francis, S. C. Hadler, S. E. Thompson, J. Maynard, D. Ostrow, N. Altman, E. Braff, P. O'Malley, D. Hawkins, F. Judson, K. Penley, T. Nylund, G. Christie, F. Meyers, J. Moore, A. Gardner, I. Doto, J. Miller, G. Reynolds, B. Murphy, C. Schable, B. Clark, J. Curran, A. Redeker, The prevention of hepatitis B with vaccine. Report of the Centers for Disease Control multicenter efficacy trial among homosexual men, *Ann. Intern. Med., 97*: 362 (1982).

19. A. A. McLean, R. Shaw, Hepatitis B virus vaccine, *Ann. Intern. Med., 97*: 451 (1982).

20. S. Klotz, R. Normand, R. Silberman, Hepatitis B vaccine in healthy hospital employees, *Infect. Control, 7*: 365 (1986).

21. R. Coutinho, N. Lelie, P. Albrecht van Lent, E. Reerink-Brongers, L. Stoutjesdijk, P. Dees, J. Nivand, J. Huisman, H. Reesink, Efficacy of a heat-inactivated hepatitis B vaccine in male homosexuals: outcome of a placebo-controlled double blind trial, *Br. Med. J., 286*: 1305 (1983).

22. P. Guesry, P. Adamowitz, P. Jungers, A. M. Courouce, A. LaPlanch, B. LaCour, E. Benhamou, Vaccination against hepatitis B in high risk hemodialysis units: A double-blind study, *Viral Hepatitis—1981 International Symposium* (W. Szmuness, H. Alter, J. Maynard, eds.), Franklin Institute Press, Philadelphia, p. 493 (1982).

23. W. Szmuness, C. E. Stevens, E. J. Harley, E. Zang, H. Alter, P. Taylor, A. DeVera, G. Chen, A. Kellner, Hepatitis B vaccine in medical staff of hemodialysis units. Efficacy and subtype cross-protection, *N. Engl. J. Med., 307*: 1481 (1982).

24. C. Stevens, H. Alter, P. Taylor, E. Zang, E. Harley, W. Szmuness, and the Dialysis Vaccine Study Group, Hepatitis B vaccine in patients receiving hemodialysis, *N. Engl. J. Med.*, *311*: 496 (1984).

25. C. Stevens, P. Taylor, M. Tong, P. Toy, G. Vyas, E. Zang, S. Krugman, Prevention of perinatal hepatitis B virus infection with hepatitis B immune globulin and hepatitis B vaccine, *Viral Hepatitis and Liver Disease* (A. Zuckerman, ed.), Alan R. Liss, New York, p. 982 (1988).

26. J. L. Dienstag, C. E. Stevens, A. K. Bhan, W. Szmuness, Hepatitis B vaccine administered to chronic carriers of hepatitis B surface antigen, *Ann. Intern. Med.*, *96*: 575 (1982).

27. F. Barin, B. Yvonnet, A. Goudeau, P. Coursaget, J. P. Chiron, F. Denis, I. Diop Mar, Hepatitis B vaccine: Further studies in children with previously acquired hepatitis B surface antigenemia, *Infect. Immun.*, *41*: 83 (1983).

28. E. M. Scolnick, A. A. McLean, D. J. West, W. McAleer, W. Miller, E. Buynak, Clinical evaluation in healthy adults of a hepatitis B vaccine made by recombinant DNA, *JAMA*, *251*: 2812 (1984).

29. W. Jilg, B. Lorbeer, M. Schmidt, B. Wilskee, G. Zoulek, F. Dienhardt, Clinical evaluation of a recombinant hepatitis B vaccine, *Lancet*, *2*: 1174 (1984).

30. M. Davidson, S. Krugman, Immunogenicity of recombinant yeast hepatitis B vaccine, *Lancet*, *1*: 108 (1985).

31. M. Davidson, S. Krugman, Recombinant yeast hepatitis B vaccine compared with plasma-derived vaccine: Immunogenicity and effect of a booster dose, *J. Infect.* (Suppl. A), *13*: 31 (1986).

32. E. Dandalos, A. Roumeliotou-Karayannis, S. C. Richardson, G. Papaevangelou, Safety and immunogenicity of a recombinant hepatitis B vaccine, *J. Med. Virol.*, *17*: 57 (1985).

33. G. Papaevangelou, E. Dandolos, A. Roumeliotou-Karayannis, S. Richardson, Immunogenicity of recombinant hepatitis B vaccine, *Lancet*, *1*: 455 (1985).

34. A. Roumeliotou-Karayannis, E. Dandalos, S. C. Richardson, G. Papaevangelou, Immunogenicity of a reduced dose of recombinant hepatitis B vaccine, *Vaccine*, *4*: 93 (1986).

35. R. A. Heijtink, J. Kruining, M. Bakker, S. Schalm, Immune response after vaccination with recombinant hepatitis B vaccine as compared to that after plasma-derived vaccine, *Antiviral Res.* (Suppl. 1), *1*: 273 (1985).

36. M. R. Hilleman, Yeast recombinant hepatitis B vaccine, *Infection*, *15*: 3 (1987).

37. C. Tsakalakis, S. C. Richardson, A. Roumeliotou-Karayannis, G. Papaevangelou, Immunogenicity of low doses of recombinant hepatitis B vaccine in young males, *Vaccine*, *6*: 328 (1988).

38. B. A. Zajac, D. J. West, W. J. McAleer, E. Scolnick, Overview of clinical studies with hepatitis B vaccine made by recombinant DNA, *J. Infect.* (Suppl. A), *13*: 39 (1986).

39. F. B. Hollinger, C. Troisi, P. Pepe, Anti-HBs response to vaccination with a human hepatitis B vaccine made by recombinant DNA technology in yeast, *J. Infect. Dis.*, *153*: 156 (1986).

40. F. B. Hollinger, Hepatitis B vaccines—to switch or not to switch, *JAMA*, *257*: 2634 (1987).

41. L. Butterly, E. Watkins, J. Dienstag, Recombinant-yeast-derived hepatitis B vaccine in healthy adults, *J. Med. Virol.*, *27*: 155 (1989).

42. R. J. Gerety, R. W. Ellis, B. A. Zajac, D. West, Two superb vaccines against hepatitis B in Mexican standoff, *JAMA*, *259*: 2403 (1988).

43. E. Kuwert, N. Scheiermann, M. Gesemann, D. Paar, A Safary, E. Simoen, P. Hauser, F. Andre, Dose range study in healthy volunteers of a hepatitis B vaccine produced in yeast, *Antiviral Res.* (Suppl. 1): 281 (1985).

44. G. Wiedermann, N. Scheiermann, P. Goubau, F. Ambrosch, M. Gesemann, C. De Bel, P. Kremsner, D. Paar, C. Kunz, P. Hauser, E. Simoen, A. Safary, F. Andre, J. Desmyter, Multicentre dose range study of a yeast-derived hepatitis B vaccine, *Vaccine*, *5*: 179 (1987).

45. E. Dahl-Hansen, J. Siebke, S. Froland, M. Degre, Immunogenicity of yeast-derived hepatitis B vaccine from two different producers, *Epidemiol. Infect.*, *104*: 143 (1990).

45b. D. J. West, B. A. Zajac, R. W. Ellis, R. J. Gerety, Improved immunogenicity of a yeast derived recombinant hepatitis B vaccine. *Infektionsklinik 1*: 3 (1988).

46. C. Trepo, P. Rougier, M. Gassin, F. Derby, F. Zoulim, P. Lery, A. Saury, Preliminary results of a randomized comparative immunogenicity study of three recombinant HBV vaccines in healthy medical personnel, *Progress in Hepatitis B Immunization* (P. Coursaget, M. Tong, eds.), Colloque INSERM, Vol. 194, p. 239 (1990).

47. M. Bruguera, M. Cremades, J. Rodicio, J. Alcazar, A. Olliver, G. Del Rio, M. Estebanmur, Immunogenicity of a yeast-derived hepatitis B vaccine in hemodialysis patients, *Am. J. Med.* 87 (Suppl. 3A): 30 (1989).

48. P. Van Damme, R. Vranckx, A. Meheus, Immunogenicity of a recombinant DNA hepatitis B vaccine in institutionalized patients with Down's syndrome, *Vaccine 8* (Suppl.): S53. (1990).

49. C. Stevens, P. Taylor, M. Tong, P. Toy, G. Vyas, P. Nair, J. Weissman, S. Krugman, Yeast recombinant hepatitis B vaccine. Efficacy with hepatitis B immune globulin in prevention of perinatal hepatitis B virus transmission, *JAMA*, *257*: 2612 (1987).

50. F. B. Hollinger, E. Adam, D. Heiberg, J. Melnick, Response to hepatitis B vaccine in a young adult population, *Viral Hepatitis* (W. Szmuness, H. J. Alter, J. E. Maynard, eds.), Franklin Institute Press, Philadelphia, p. 451 (1981).

51. F. B. Hollinger, E. Adam, J. Zahradnik, D. Heiberg, C. Troisi, J. Melnick, Hepatitis B vaccine. Final progress report, covering July 1979–Dec 1982. NIAID, March 1983.

52. V. J. McAuliffe, R. H. Purcell, J. L. Gerin, F. Taylor, Current status of the NIAID hepatitis B vaccines. *Viral Hepatitis* (W. Szmuness, H. J. Alter, and J. E. Maynard, eds.), Franklin Institute Press, Philadelphia, p. 425 (1981).

53. F. E. Andre, Overview of a 5-year clinical experience with a yeast-derived hepatitis B vaccine, *Vaccine*, *8* (Suppl.): 74

54. R. Rietschel, R. Adams, Reactions to thimerosal in hepatitis B vaccines, *Dermatol. Clin.*, *8*: 161 (1990).

55. L. Kirkland, Ocular sensitivity to thimerosal: A problem with hepatitis B vaccine?, *So. Med., J.*, *83*: 497 (1990).

56. F. Shaw, D. Graham, H. Guess, J. Milstien, J. Johnson, G. Schatz, S. Hadler, J. Kuritsky, E. Hiner, D. Bregmon, J. Maynard, Postmarketing surveillance for neurologic adverse reactions reported after hepatitis B vaccination: Experience of the first three years, *Am. J. Epidemiol.*, *127*: 337 (1988).

57. P. G. Tuohy, Guillain-Barre syndrome following immunisation with synthetic hepatitis B vaccine, *N. Z. Med. J.*, *102*: 672 (1989).

58. M. Nutini, F. Marie, C. Loucq, F. Tron, Hepatitis B vaccine: Clinical experience and safety, *Lancet*, *2*: 1301 (1983).

59. C. DiGusto, J. Bernhard, Erythema nodosum provoked by hepatitis B vaccine, *Lancet*, *2*: 1042 (1986).

60. P. L. Goolsby, Erythema nodosum after RECOMBIVAX-HB hepatitis B vaccine, *N. Engl. J. Med.*, *321*: 1198 (1989).

61. C. Brightman, G. Scadding, L. Dumbreck, Y. Latchman, J. Brostoff, Yeast-derived hepatitis B vaccine and yeast sensitivity, *Lancet*, *1*: 903 (1989).

62. J. M. Zahradnik, D. Heiberg, F. B. Hollinger, Hepatitis B vaccine: Immune responses in children from families with an HBsAg carrier, *Vaccine*, *3*: 407 (1985).

63. W. Jilg, M. Schmidt, F. Deinhardt, Prolonged immunity after booster doses of hepatitis B vaccine, *J. Infect. Dis.*, *157*: 1267 (1988).

64. W. Jilg, M. Schmidt, F. Deinhardt, Vaccination against hepatitis B: Comparison of three different vaccination schedules, *J. Infect. Dis.*, *160*: 766 (1989).

65. S. Hadler, M. Alcala de Manzon, D. Lugo, M. Perez, Effect of timing of hepatitis B vaccine on response to vaccine in Yucpa Indians, *Vaccine*, *7*: 106 (1989).

66. W. Szmuness, C. E. Stevens, E. J. Harley, E. Zang, P. Taylor, H. Alter, and the Dialysis Vaccine Trial Group, The immune response of healthy adults to a reduced dose of hepatitis B vaccine, *J. Med. Virol.* *8*: 123 (1981).

67. C. L. Troisi, D. A. Heiberg, F. B. Hollinger, Normal immune response to hepatitis B vaccine in patients with Down's syndrome, *JAMA*, *254*: 3196 (1985).

68. E. K. Yeoh, C. Lai, W. Chang, H. Yo, Comparison of the immunogenicity, efficacy and safety of 10 μg and 20 μg of a hepatitis B vaccine: A prospective randomized trial, *J. Hyg. Camb.*, *96*: 491 (1986).

69. D. Ostrow, J. Goldsmith, S. Kalish, J. Chmiel, S. Hadler, J. Phair, Nonresponse to hepatitis B vaccine in homosexual men, *Sex. Transm. Dis.*, *14*: 92 (1987).

70. M. Just and R. Berger, Immunogenicity of a heat-treated recombinant DNA hepatitis B vaccine, *Vaccine*, *6*: 399 (1988).

71. Y. Sanchez, I. Ionescu-Matiu, J. L. Melnick, G. Dreesman, Comparative studies of the immunogenic activity of hepatitis B surface antigen (HBsAg) and HBsAg polypeptides, *J. Med. Virol.*, *11*: 115 (1983).

72. S. Kuriyama, T. Tsujii, S. Ishizaka, E. Kikuchi, K. Kinoshita, K. Nishimura, K. Kitagami, Enhancing effects of oral adjuvants on anti-HBs responses induced by hepatitis B vaccine, *Clin. Exp. Immunol.*, *72*: 383 (1988).

73. G. Przewlocki, F. Audibert, M. Jolivet, L. Chedid, S. Kent, A. R. Neurath, Production of antibodies recognizing a hepatitis B virus (HBV) surface antigen by administration of murabutide associated to a synthetic pre-S HBV peptide conjugated to a toxoid carrier, *Biochem. Biophys. Res. Comm.*, *140*: 557 (1986).

74. P. J. Grob, U. Binswanger, A. Blumberg, H. Gloor, A. Hany, W. Herwig, H.

Iselin, K. Zaruba, K. Bolla, Thymopentin as adjuvant to hepatitis B vaccination. Results from three double-blind studies, *Surv. Immunol. Res.*, *4* (Suppl. 1): 107. (1985).

75. K. Zaruba, P. J. Grob, K. Bolla, Thymopentin as adjuvant therapy to hepatitis B vaccination in formerly non- or hyporesponding hemodialysis patients, *Surv. Immunol. Res.*, *4* (Suppl. 1) 102 (1985).

76. D. Donati, L. Gastaldi, Controlled trial of thymopentin in hemodialysis patients who fail to respond to hepatitis B vaccination, *Nephron*, *50*: 133 (1988).

77. S. Pagani, L. Cruciani, M. Chianelli, E. Procaccini, P. Pozzilli, Thymopentin administration and increase of seroconversion after B-hepatitis vaccine in diabetic patients, *Diabetes Res.*, *12*: 199 (1989).

78. D. E. Leslie, S. Nicholson, M. Dimitrakakis, N. Johnston, I. D. Gust, Humoral immune responses in mice using gamma inulin preparations as adjuvants for hepatitis B vaccines, *Immunol. Cell Biol.*, *68*: 107 (1990).

79. P. J. Grob, H. I. Joller-Jemelka, U. Binswanger, K. Zarub, C. Descoeudres, M. Fernex, Interferon as an adjuvant for hepatitis B vaccination in non- and low-responder populations, *Eur. J. Clin. Microbiol.*, *3*: 195 (1984).

80. S. Kakumu, A. Fuji, H. Tahara, K. Yoshioka, N. Sakamot, Enhancement of antibody production to hepatitis B surface antigen by interleukin 2, *J. Clin. Lab. Immunol.*, *26*: 25 (1988).

81. F. Denis, M. Mounier, L. Hessel, J. Michel, N. Gualde, F. Dubois, F. Barin, A. Goudeau, Hepatitis B vaccination in the elderly, *J. Infect. Dis.*, *149*: 1019 (1984).

82. M. M. Horowitz, W. B. Ershler, W. P. McKinney, R. Battiola, Duration of immunity after hepatitis B vaccination: Efficacy of low-dose booster vaccine, *Ann. Intern. Med.*, *108*: 185 (1988).

83. F. E. Shaw, Jr., H. A. Guess, J. M. Roets, F. Mohr, P. Coleman, E. Mandel, R. Roehm, W. Talley, S. Hadler, The effect of anatomic injection site, age, and smoking on the immune response to hepatitis B vaccination, *Vaccine*, *7*: 425 (1989).

84. D. J. Weber, W. A. Rutala, G. P. Samsa, J. Santimaw, S. Lemon, Obesity as a predictor of poor antibody response to hepatitis B plasma vaccine, *JAMA*, *254*: 3187 (1985).

85. D. Weber, W. Rutala, G. Samsa, S. Bradshaw, S. Lemon, Impaired immunogenicity of hepatitis B vaccine in obese persons, *N. Engl. J. Med.*, *314*: 1393 (1986).

86. M. Varla-Leftherioti, M. Papanivolaou, M. Spyropoubu, H. Vallindra, P. Tsiroyianni, N. Tassopoulos, H. Kapasouri, C. Stavropoulos-Giokas, HLA-associated non-responsiveness to hepatitis B vaccine, *Tissue Antigens*, *35*: 60 (1990).

87. H. Watanabe, M. Okumura, K. Hirayama, T., Sasazuki, HLA-Bw54-DR4-DRw53-DQw4 haplotype controls non-responsiveness to hepatitis B surface antigen via CD8-positive suppressor T cells, *Tissue Antigens*, *36*: 69 (1990).

88. C. A. Carne, I. V. Weller, J. Waite, M. Briggs, F. Pearce, M. Adler, R. Tedder, Impaired responsiveness of homosexual men with HIV antibodies to plasma derived hepatitis B vaccine, *Br. Med. J.*, *294*: 866 (1987).

89. A. C. Collier, L. Corey, V. L. Murphy, H. H. Handsfield, Antibody to human

immunodeficiency virus (HIV) and suboptimal response to hepatitis B vaccination, *Ann. Intern. Med.*, *109*: 101 (1988).

90. R. Loke, I. Murray-Lyon, J. Coleman, B. Evans, A. Zuckerman, Diminished response to recombinant vaccine in homosexual men with HIV antibody, *J. Med. Virol.*, *31*: 109 (1990).

91. M. J. Nowicki, M. J. Tong, R. E. Bohman, Alterations in the immune response of nonresponders to the hepatitis B vaccine, *J. Infect. Dis.*, *152*: 1245 (1985).

92. F. B. Hollinger, C. Troisi, D. Heilberg, Y. Sanchez, G. Dreesman, J. Melnick, Response to a hepatitis B polypeptide vaccine in micelle form in a young adult population. *J. Med. Virol.*, *19*: 229 (1986).

93. A. A. McLean, H. A. Guess, E. M. Scolnick, Suboptimal response to hepatitis B vaccine given by injection into the buttock, *MMWR*, *34*: 105, (1985).

94. T. Ukena, H. Esber, R. Bessette, T. Parks, B. Crocker, F. Shaw, Site of injection and response to hepatitis B vaccine, *N. Engl. J. Med.*, *313*: 579 (1985).

95. F. de Lalla, E. Rinaldi, D. Santoro, G. Pravettoni, Immune response to hepatitis B vaccine given at different injection sites and by different routes: A controlled randomized study, *J. Epidemiol.*, *4*: 256 (1988).

96. A. Cockcroft, P. Soper, C. Insall, Y. Kennard, S. Chapman, C. Gooch, P. Griffiths, Antibody response after hepatitis B immunisation in a group of health care workers, *Br. J. Ind. Med.*, *47*: 199 (1990).

97. S. M. Lemon, D. J. Weber, Immunogenicity of plasma-derived hepatitis B vaccine: Relationship to site of injection and obesity, *J. Gen. Intern. Med.*, *1*: 199 (1986).

98. Advisory Committee on Immunization Practices: Protection against viral hepatitis. *MMWR*, *39* (Suppl. 2): 1 (1990).

99. K. Miller, R. Gibbs, M. Mulligan, T. Nutman, D. Francis, Intradermal hepatitis B virus vaccine: Immunogenicity and side-effects in adults, *Lancet*, *22*: 1454 (1983).

100. G. Zoulek, B. Lorbeer, W. Jilg, F. Deinhardt, Evaluation of a reduced dose of hepatitis B vaccine administered intradermally, *J. Med. Virol.*, *14*: 27 (1984).

101. G. Zoulek, B. Lorbeer, W. Jilg, F. Deinhardt, Antibody responses and skin reactivity after intradermal hepatitis B virus vaccine, *Lancet, 14*: 27 (1984).

102. M. Wahl, S. Hermodsson, Intradermal, subcutaneous or intramuscular administration of hepatitis B vaccine side effects and antibody response, *J. Infect. Dis.*, *19*: 617 (1987).

103. R. R. Redfield, B. L. Innis, R. M. Scott, H. G. Cannon, W. Bancroft, Clinical evaluation of low-dose intradermally administered hepatitis B virus vaccine. A cost reduction strategy. *JAMA*, *254*: 3203 (1985).

104. W. L. Irving, M. Alder, J. B. Kurtz, B. Juel-Jensen, Intradermal vaccination against hepatitis B, *Lancet, 2*: 1340 (1986).

105. I. H. Frazer, B. Jones, M. Dimitrakakis, I. MacKay, Intramuscular versus low-dose intradermal hepatitis B vaccine. Assessment by humoral and cellular immune response to hepatitis B surface antigen, *Med. J. Aust.*, *146*: 242 (1987).

106. J. A. Clarke, F. B. Hollinger, E. Lewis, L. Russell, C. Miller, A. Huntley, N. Flynn, Intradermal inoculation with HEPTAVAX-B: Immune response and histologic evaluation of injection sites, *JAMA*, *262*: 2567 (1989).

107. J. Hayashi, S. Kashiwagi, A. Noguchi, K. Nashima, H. Ikematsu, W. Kajiyama,

Intradermal hepatitis B vaccine for mentally retarded patients, *J. Infect.*, *19*: 119 (1989).

108. J. Bryan, M. Sjogren, M. Iqbal, A. Khattock, S. Nabi, A. Ahmed, B. Cox, A. Morton, J. Shuck, P. MacCarthy, P. Perine, I. Malik, L. Legters, Comparative trial of low-dose intradermal, recombinant- and plasma-derived hepatitis B vaccines, *J. Infect. Dis.*, *162*: 789 (1990).

109. C. Fessard, O. Riche, J. H. M. Cohen, Intramuscular versus subcutaneous injection for hepatitis B vaccine, *Vaccine*, *6*: 469 (1988).

110. S. M. Lemon, R. M. Scott, W. H. Bancroft, Subcutaneous administration of inactivated hepatitis B vaccine by automatic jet injection. *J. Med. Virol.*, *12*: 129 (1983).

111. C. A. Morris, P. R. Oliver, F. Reynolds, J. Selkon, Intradermal hepatitis B immunization with yeast-derived vaccine: Serological response by sex and age, *Epidem. Inf.*, *103*: 387 (1989).

112. T. Wilkins, Y. Cossart, Low-dose intradermal vaccination of medical and dental students, *Med. J. Aust.*, *152*: 140 (1990).

113. M. L. Gonzalez, M. Usandizaga, P. Alomar, F. Salva, F. Martin, M. J. Erroz, R. Lardinois, Intradermal and intramuscular route for vaccination against hepatitis B, *Vaccine*, *8*: 402 (1990).

114. J. Wistrom, B. Settergren, A. Gustafsson, P. Juto, R. Norrby, Intradermal vs. intramuscular hepatitis B vaccinations, *JAMA*, *264*: 181 (1990).

115. R. Heijtink, R. Knol, S. Schalm, Low-dose (2 micrograms) hepatitis B vaccination in medical students: comparable immunogenicity for intramuscular and intradermal routes, *J. Med. Virol.*, *27*: 151 (1989).

116. W. Szmuness, C. E. Stevens, E. A. Zang, E. Harley, A. Kellner, A controlled clinical trial of the efficacy of the hepatitis B vaccine (Heptavax B): A final report, *Hepatology*, *1*: 377 (1981).

117. W. Jilg, F. Deinhardt, Results of immunisation with a recombinant yeast-derived hepatitis B vaccine. *J. Infect.*, *13*: 47 (1986).

118. S. Hadler, P. Coleman, P. O'Malley, F. Judson, N. Altman, Evaluation of long term protection by hepatitis B vaccine for seven to nine years in homosexual men, *Viral Hepatitis and Liver Disease* (F. B. Hollinger, S. M. Lemon, H. S. Margolis, eds.), Williams & Wilkins, Baltimore (1992).

119. C. E. Stevens, P. E. Taylor, M. J. Tong, P. Toy, G. Vyas, Hepatitis B vaccine: An overview, *Viral Hepatitis and Liver Disease* (G. N. Vyas, J. L. Dienstag, and J. H. Hoofnagle, eds.), Grune & Stratton, Orlando, p. 275 (1984).

120. A. Gibas, E. Watkins, C. Hinkle, J. Dienstag, Long-term persistence of protective antibody after hepatitis B vaccination of healthy adults, *Viral Hepatitis and Liver Disease* (A. J. Zuckerman, ed.), Alan R. Liss, Inc., New York, p. 998 (1988).

121. M. Pasko, T. Beam, Persistence of anti-HBs among health care personnel immunized with hepatitis B vaccine, *Am. J. Public Health*, *80*: 590 (1990).

122. G. Barnas, L. Hanacik, Hepatitis B vaccine: Persistence of antibody following immunization, *Infect. Cont. Hosp. Epid.*, *9*: 147 (1988).

123. R. Wainwright, B. McMahon, L. Bulkow, D. Hall, M. Fitzgerald, A. Harpster, S. Hadler, A. Lanier, W. Heyward, Duration of immunogenicity and efficacy of hepatitis B vaccine in a Yupik Eskimo population, *JAMA*, *261*: 2362 (1989).

124. R. Wainwright, B. McMahon, L. Bulkow, A. Parkinson, A. Harpster, S. Hadler, Duration of immunogenicity and efficacy of hepatitis B vaccine in a Yupik Eskimo population, *Viral Hepatitis and Liver Disease* (F. B. Hollinger, S. M. Lemon, and H. S. Margolis, eds.), Williams & Wilkins, Baltimore, (1992).

125. D. E. Craven, A. L. Awdeh, L. M. Kunches, E. Yunis, J. Dienstag, B. Werner, F. Polk, D. Snydman, R. Platt, C. Crumpacker, G. Grady, C. Alper, Nonresponsiveness to hepatitis B vaccine in health care workers. Results of revaccination and genetic typings, *Ann. Intern. Med, 105*: 356 (1986).

126. J. Y. Weissman, M. M. Tsuchiyose, M. J. Tong, R. Co., K. Chin, R. Ettenger, Lack of response to recombinant hepatitis B vaccine in nonresponders to the plasma vaccine, *JAMA, 260*: 1734 (1988).

127. W. Jilg, M. Schmidt, F. Deinhardt, R. Zachoval, Hepatitis B vaccination: How long does protection last? *Lancet, 2*: 458 (1984).

128. S. C. Hadler, D. P. Francis, J. E. Maynard, S. Thompson, F. Judson, D. Echenberg, D. Ostrow, P. O'Malley, K. Penley, N. Altman, E. Braff, G. Shipman, P. Coleman, E. Mandel, Long-term immunogenicity and efficacy of hepatitis B vaccine in homosexual men, *N. Engl. J. Med., 315*: 209 (1986).

129. Hepatitis B expert panel, Immunization against hepatitis B, *Lancet, 2*: 875 (1988).

130. P. Coursaget, B. Yvonnet, J. Chotard, M. Sarr, P. Vincelot, R. N'Doye, I. Diop Mar, J. Chiron, Seven-year study of hepatitis B vaccine efficacy in infants from an endemic area (Senegal), *Lancet, 2*: 1143 (1986).

131. R. Berger, M. Just, F. Andre, A. Safary, Boosting against hepatitis B: Must it be done when titers disappear? *Viral Hepatitis and Liver Disease* (A. J. Zuckerman, ed.), Alan R. Liss, Inc., New York, p. 1006 (1988).

10

Overview of Clinical Studies in Developing Countries

Pierre Coursaget

*Laboratoire de Microbiologie,
Tours, France*

Mark A. Kane

*World Health Organization,
Geneva, Switzerland*

I. CHALLENGES AND GOALS OF CLINICAL STUDIES IN DEVELOPING COUNTRIES

A. Rationale and Necessity for Clinical Studies in Developing Countries

Following vaccine development in the laboratory, phase one and two clinical studies are performed by the vaccine manufacturers to establish the safety, immunogenicity, and efficacy of their vaccine, to determine the optimal dose and schedules for immunization, and to obtain licensure from national control authorities. Such studies are done by specially chosen investigators, who will ensure careful adherence to the protocols. Vaccine is carefully shipped and stored, vaccinators are specially trained, and enormous effort is made to ensure that vaccine recipients receive vaccine on schedule and are not lost to follow-up.

Such studies, many of which are done in areas of low endemicity, establish optimal vaccine immunogenicity and efficacy. There are many instances of vaccines not working as well under "field conditions," and experience has taught investigators and public health officials that evidence of good safety, immunogenicity, and efficacy must be obtained under varying conditions in many parts of the world.

The epidemiology of HBV infection varies greatly in different parts of the world (discussed in Chapter 7), and target populations, the optimal age of immunization, and other aspects of immunization strategy may vary as well.

209

Vaccine performance must be established in different age groups, under various levels of endemicity, and under conditions appropriate for use in developing countries.

For example, in many developed countries infants of carrier mothers are given both hepatitis B immune globulin (HBIG) and hepatitis B (HB) vaccine at the time of birth. This strategy is not appropriate for most developing countries because the serological status of mothers is not investigated and HBIG is not available. Therefore, trials examining vaccine strategies appropriate for developing countries must be undertaken in those areas. Most vaccine used in the world is delivered through the Expanded Programme on Immunization (EPI), which is a network of global, regional, national, and local programs reaching the village level in most developing countries. Any vaccine for infants must be accepted and integrated within the framework of the EPI or there will be little chance of its widespread use in most developing countries.

Integration into the EPI requires operational research into such issues as interference with other antigens, optimal ways to integrate the vaccine into EPI schedules, and the immunogenicity and efficacy of vaccine under conditions of missed doses and varying schedules found in actual vaccination programs. In addition, the cost of HB vaccines has induced many investigators to examine the performance of lower doses of vaccine and alternate routes of administration.

For hepatitis B vaccines, the schedules used in phase one and two clinical trials often did not correspond to EPI scheduled visits, which may vary from country to country. Thus, clinical studies must be done to examine how HB vaccine can be integrated into EPI schedules without requiring additional visits. Other studies have been performed to ascertain the local cost-effectiveness of HBV vaccination in various epidemiological and geographical situations, to investigate logistical problems related to the stability of HB vaccine, and to determine the impact that addition of HB vaccine will have on the cold chain.

This chapter will review and discuss clinical studies on HB vaccine that have been done in developing countries outside of the Far East and the Pacific Basin. Studies in areas of low endemicity and the Far East will be discussed in other chapters.

B. HBV Epidemiology

It is estimated that 2000 million individuals have been infected by HBV, resulting in 300 million chronically infected persons who are at high risk of illness and death from chronic active hepatitis, cirrhosis, and primary hepatocellular carcinoma (PHC). These chronic carriers, and those acutely infected with HBV, also constitute an infectious pool responsible for the continued transmission of the disease.

In most developing countries HBV infection is of moderate to high endemicity, with 5–15% of the population chronically infected carriers of HBV, and 50–90% of the population having serological evidence of past HBV infection.

Most HBV transmission takes place during childhood either from infected mothers to their newborns (perinatal tansmission) or from infected child to a susceptible child. The relative importance of perinatal transmission depends on the frequency of carrier mothers in the population and on the percent of carrier mothers who have high titers of circulating virus, indicated by their being positive to the HB "e" antigen (HBeAg) or having high titers of HBV DNA in the serum.

Approximately 70–90% of infants of HBeAg-positive carrier mothers will become chronic carriers unless they receive HB vaccine and possibly HBIG at birth. In Asia, approximately 40% of HBV carrier mothers are also HBeAg positive, whereas in Africa, Europe, South America, and the Middle East, this proportion is usually around 13%, and almost never exceeds 20% (1–3). Thus, the relative importance of perinatal transmission is much greater for Asia than for most of the rest of the world. In parts of the world where perinatal infection is important it is desirable to give the first dose of HB vaccine at birth. This may or may not be feasible in developing country immunization programs.

Child-to-child transmission is the most common mode of transmission even in Asia. Child-to-child transmission at an early age leads to high levels of the carrier state (4), but most children who escape perinatal transmission are not infected during the first 6 months of life because of passive antibody protection from their mothers, in many cases, and lack of exposure to the virus (1). This allows time to immunize the child before exposure to HBV, a situation in which the vaccine may have an efficacy exceeding 95%.

II. OVERVIEW OF SAFETY AND IMMUNOGENICITY RESULTS IN DEVELOPING COUNTRIES

A. Safety

Since the pioneering work of P. Maupas and colleagues in 1978 (5–7), many controlled immunization studies have been undertaken in developing countries using various immunization protocols and vaccine formulations. The initial clinical trials of the vaccine reported that neither serious local nor systemic reactions were observed after administration of HB vaccine, regardless of the HBV serological status before immunization or the age of the recipients. Only minor adverse events, including soreness and erythema at the site of injection and mild fever, are mentioned. These studies have shown that hepatitis B vaccine can be safely incorporated into EPI programs in the developing world.

B. Immunization of Newborns and Children

Studies in infants and newborns in high-risk area have been reported using two plasma-derived and one recombinant vaccine (8–25). Table 1 and 2 summarize the results on immune response from these studies. Caution must be used in making direct comparisons of the results of these studies because the dosage of vaccine varied from 2 to 20 μg with different vaccines, and the age at vaccination and the schedule of immunization varied widely in these 16 studies.

Clinical trials have been conducted in newborn infants: six in Africa and one in the Middle East. Plasma-derived vaccine contained 5 μg of HBsAg for the Pasteur-Mérieux (PM) vaccine and 10 μg in studies with the Merck Sharp & Dohme (MSD) vaccine.

In five studies, three doses of vaccine were given at 0-, 1-, and 6–12-month intervals, and in two studies four doses were given with a schedule of 0, 1–2, 2–4, 9–12. Anti-HBs was detected in 94–100% of the infants with geometric mean anti-HBs titer ranging from 210 to 2640 mIU/ml.

Ten clinical studies were performed on the potency of HB vaccine in 1- to 24-month-old infants in endemic areas. Plasma-derived vaccines were used, except in one study, which used a mammalian cell–derived recombinant vaccine (51).

Using dosage and schedules recommended by the manufacturers, and with the third or fourth dose being given at least 6 months after the first dose, anti-HBs was detected in 95–100% of the infants with geometric mean titers of 427–3864 mIU/ml. Somewhat lower proportions of protected infants (81–95%) were observed when vaccine was given at a lower dosage (2 μg), with geometric mean titers ranging from 200 to 1650 mIU/ml (10,12,20). It should be noted that

Table 1 Seroconversion After HB Vaccination in Newborns from Developing Countries

Country	Ref.	Type	Dose	Schedule (months)	Seroconversion (%)	GMT (MIU/ml)
Senegal	11	plasma (PM)	5 μg	0,1,2,12	94	2400
Senegal	23	plasma (PM)	5 μg	0,1,2,9	100	2640
Gambia	22	plasma (MSD)	10 μg	0,2,4,9	98	1920
Burundi	13	plasma (PM)	5 μg	0,2,12	96	214
Kenya	14	plasma (PM)	5 μg	0,1,7	94	800
South Africa	9	plasma (MSD)	10 μg	0,1,6	94	—
Gambia	15	plasma (PM)	5 μg	0,1,6	100	—
Saudi Arabia	19	plasma (PM)	5 μg	0,1,6	100	210

Table 2 Seroconversion After HB Vaccination in Children from Developing Countries

Country	Ref.	Vaccine			Seroconversion (%)	GMT (mIU/ml)
		Type	Dose	Schedule (months)		
Senegal	51	recombinant (PM)	20 μg	0,2,6	100	2845
Gambia	24	plasma (MSD)	20 μg	0,2,4	100	926
Gambia	24	plasma (MSD)	10 μg	0,1,3,8	97[a]	5431
South Africa	25	plasma (MSD)	10 μg	0,2,3.5	97	—
Zambia	21	plasma (MSD)	10 μg	0,1,6	100	—
Senegal	14	plasma (PM)	5 μg	0,1,2,12	99	1450
Senegal	10	plasma (PM)	5 μg	0,2,12	96	427
Senegal	10	plasma (PM)	5 μg	0,2,6	95	850
Senegal	51	plasma (PM)	5 μg	0,2,6	100	3864
Senegal	16	plasma (PM)	5 μg	0,3,6	100	1065
Nigeria	12	plasma (PM)	5 μg	0,1,2	88	—
Senegal	17	plasma (PM)	2 μg	0,1,2,6	95	1650
Ethiopia	20	plasma (PM)	2 μg	0,1,2,6	84[a]	940
Senegal	17	plasma (PM)	2 μg	0,2,6	85	200
Nigeria	12	plasma (PM)	2 μg	0,1,2	81	—

[a]$\geq$ 10 mIU/ml.

results comparable to the full dosage were obtained with 2 μg of vaccine given according to a four-dose schedule.

From this point of view, the use of four lower doses of vaccine, which has the advantage of reducing vaccine cost, must be balanced against the increased cost and difficulties of delivering four instead of three doses of HB vaccine. Many public health officials, and the manufacturers themselves, are more comfortable with more rather than less HBsAg in each dose, citing the fact that vaccine shipping and storage conditions, injection techniques, training of vaccinators, and the immune competence of vaccine recipients vary widely under field conditions. From these data it can be concluded that a wide range of schedules may be used to obtain a good immune response in both newborns and older children, allowing the vaccine to be used in a wide range of EPI schedules.

In one controlled study (51) infants were randomly selected to receive either plasma-derived vaccine or a recombinant vaccine produced in mammalian cells. This study found that mammalian recombinant vaccine was as safe as the plasma derived product. Antibodies directed against S and preS2 epitopes appeared more rapidly in infants immunized with the recombinant vaccine. However, after

completion of vaccination all infants in both groups had protective and comparable levels of anti-HBs antibodies.

1. Long-Term Persistence of Anti-HBs Antibodies

Long-term follow-up for anti-HBs antibody persistence has continued among the
vaccine recipients of four different studies (24,26–28). All four studies have
been performed with plasma-derived vaccines: 10 μg of MSD vaccine in Venezuela, 10 and 20 μg MSD vaccine in Gambia, and 5 μg of PM vaccine in
Senegal. One year after the first dose of vaccine, 98–100% of the infants had
evidence of anti-HBs antibodies, with geometric mean titer ranging from 926 to
1920 (Table 3, Fig. 1). Two years after the first dose the proportion of anti-HBs
positive infants was still 95–99%, however, the geometric mean titers had fallen
to values ranging from 214 to 767 mIU/ml. The higher values were observed in
older children (26).

The proportion of anti-HBs positive infants decreased very slowly 3, 4, 5, and
6 years after the first dose of vaccine. In the Senegalese study, approximately
90% of them are still anti-HBs positive up to 6 years after the first dose. At that
time the anti-HBs geometric titer was calculated to be 60 mIU/ml.

In Senegal some infants receiving a three-dose protocol have also been
followed for 6 years (28). A similar anti-HBs response to the vaccine was
observed in this population; however, 6 years later only 70% of them had
anti-HBs levels greater than 10 mIU/ml compared to 85% in those receiving a
four-dose protocol. Anti-HBs geometric mean titers were of 36 and 60 mIU/ml,
respectively.

A booster dose was given to 59 of these infants 6–7 years after the first dose.
The geometric mean titer increased from 62 mIU/ml at the time of revaccination
to 733 mIU/ml 4 months later and then decreased to 427 mIU/ml after 7 months
and to 198 mIU/ml after 12 months. This decrease is similar to the antibody
decay observed after immunization.

2. Efficacy of Hepatitis B Vaccine in Developing Countries

Various possible outcomes may be measured in efficacy studies of vaccines.
Protection against infection, acute disease, the development of the carrier state,
chronic liver disease, and primary liver cancer are possible outcomes of these
studies. The Gambia Hepatitis Intervention Study is the only current study
designed to measure a reduction in liver cancer several decades from now,
although, hopefully, cancer registries in many countries will document this
reduction. Most efficacy studies looked at infants of HBeAg-positive carrier
mothers, because the rate of chronic infection in the untreated groups was so high
that efficacy could be established with relatively small studies in short periods of
time.

Many of the following studies look at the reduction of the carrier state in

Table 3 Long-Term Persistence of Anti-HBs Antibodies in Immunized Infants

Time after immunization (yr)	Country	Ref.	Vaccine			Seroconversion (%)	GMT (mIU/ml)
			Type	Content	Schedule (months)		
1	Gambia	24	plasma (MSD)	20 μg	0,2,4	100	926
	Gambia	27	plasma (MSD)	10 μg	0,2,4,9	98	1920
	Senegal	28	plasma (PM)	5 μg	0,1,2,12	99	1458
2	Venezuela	26	plasma (MSD)	10 μg	0,1,6	99	767
	Gambia	27	plasma (MSD)	10 μg	0,2,4,9	95	524
	Senegal	28	plasma (PM)	5 μg	0,1,2,12	97	214
3	Gambia	27	plasma (MSD)	10 μg	0,2,4,9	95	376
	Senegal	28	plasma (PM)	5 μg	0,1,2,12	96	213
4	Gambia	24	plasma (MSD)	20 μg	0,2,4	95[a]	75
	Senegal	28	plasma (PM)	5 μg	0,1,2,12	100	152
5	Senegal	28	plasma (PM)	5 μg	0,1,2,12	93	82
6	Senegal	28	plasma (PM)	5 μg	0,1,2,12	90	60

[a] ≥10 mIU/ml.

cohorts of children followed for several years. These types of studies are extremely valuable, for they tell us the efficacy of vaccine in preventing the carrier state under actual field conditions in developing countries and will tell us if and when booster doses become necessary. No HBIG was used in these studies.

The efficacy was established by comparison of HBsAg-positive and/or anti-HBc-positive events in immunized infants and controls. Efficacy after one year was reported for five studies (Table 4) including newborns and infants from endemic areas (13,20,28–30). In the vaccine group, HBsAg-positive infection was reported in 0.0–1.5% of the recipients compared to 2.3–9.6% in control groups. Efficacy was calculated to be 70–100%. High levels of protection were observed with low doses of vaccine and with schedules of immunization of three doses at one-month intervals. The lower efficacy rate was observed in older infants, since HBV infections were due to HBV infection before completion of immunization and, in a small proportion, to nonresponders.

Two years after immunization, efficacy of vaccine was reported in four different trials with HBsAg-positive events ranging from 0.0 to 1.0% among

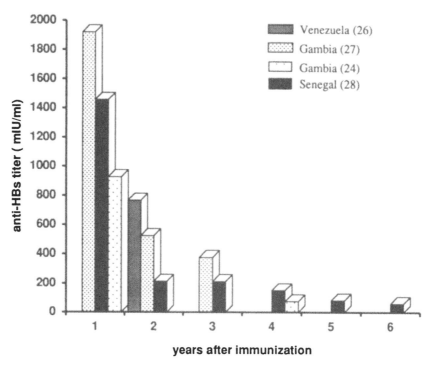

Figure 1   Long-term persistence of anti-HBs antibodies in infants from developing countries immunized with hepatitis B vaccines.

vaccinees compared to 8.4–15.8% in the control population groups. The efficacy after 2-year follow-up was calculated to be 88–100%.

Efficacy after a longer period of follow up was reported in several studies. Efficacy remained high after 3 years in the Gambian study, where only 0.7% of the vaccinees were HBsAg-positive compared to 13.0% of control children. In the Senegalese study, efficacy was very high after 4 years, where up to 90% of HBsAg-positive infections were prevented. However, this study reported a reduction in protection after 6 years of follow-up, where 4.6% of the vaccinated infants tested positive for HBsAg compared to 21.2% of the control group, a protective efficacy rate of 78%. The efficacy was very high after the last dose of vaccine (dose three or four) since no new HBsAg infection was observed during the 4 years period following completion of immunization.

C.   Hepatitis B Immunization of Adults in Countries of High or Intermediate Endemicity

In areas of high incidence of HBV infection, the concept of high-risk groups among the adult population, as they are defined in areas of low endemicity, has

Table 4   Efficacy of Hepatitis B Vaccine in Developing Countries

Time after immunization (yr)	Country	Ref.	Vaccine Type	Dose	Schedule (months)	HBsAg+ infection (%) Vaccine group	Control group	Protective efficacy
1	Senegal	28	plasma (PM)	5 μg	0,1,2,12	1.5	5.0	70
	Burundi	13	plasma (PM)	5 μg	0,2,12	0.0	6.8	100
	Senegal	28	plasma (PM)	5 μg	0,2,12	0.0	5.0	100
	Nigeria	13	plasma (PM)	2 μg	0,1,2	1.1	9.6	89
	Ethiopia	20	plasma (PM)	2 μg	0,1,6	0.0	2.3[a]	100
2	Gambia	30	plasma (MSD)	10 μg	0,2,4,9	0.3		96
	Burundi	13	plasma (PM)	5 μg	0,2,12	0.0	15.8	100
	Senegal	28	plasma (PM)	5 μg	0,1,2,12	1.0	8.4	88
	Senegal	28	plasma (PM)	5 μg	0,2,12	0.0	8.4	100
3	Gambia	30	plasma (MSD)	10 μg	0,2,4,9	0.3		99
4	Senegal	28	plasma (PM)	5 μg	0,1,2,12	1.7	19.3	91
	Senegal	28	plasma (PM)	5 μg	0,2,12	2.0	19.3	90
6	Senegal	28	plasma (PM)	5 μg	0,1,2,12	4.6	21.2	78

[a]7 months after immunization.

less relevance since only a small proportion of the adult population is still at risk of infection. The cost of immunizing these groups and the technical and programmatic difficulties of adult immunization programs in developing countries make this control strategy problematic in many areas. However, immunization was investigated in two groups of adults: medical personnel and pregnant women (Table 5).

Seronegative medical personnel in an intermediate or highly endemic area are at a high risk of infection, and selection of seronegative individuals is easily done if HBV antibody testing is available. Immunization of medical personnel was evaluated in four different studies (31–34). High seroconversion rates were observed with both plasma and recombinant vaccines. Two 20-μg doses were sufficient to obtain a 96% anti-HBs seroconversion in a population from India (32). However, the same vaccine gave a rather low (67%) seroconversion rate at the 10 mIU/ml levels in the general population from an high endemic African country (21).

Immunized pregnant women will passively transfer protective levels of anti-

Table 5 Hepatitis B Immunization of Seronegative Adults in Countries of High or Intermediate Endemicity for HBV Infections

Country	Ref.	Population groups	Vaccine Schedule (months)	Type	Dose	Seroconversion (%)
Senegal	35	pregnant women	0,1	plasma (PM)	5 μg	72
Nigeria	12	pregnant women	0,1	plasma (MSD)	20 μg	85
India	32	medical personnel	0,1	plasma (MSD)	20 μg	96
Senegal	35	pregnant women	0,1,2	plasma (PM)	5 μg	95
Pakistan	33	students	0,1,5	recombinant (MSD)	10 μg	94[a]
Zambia	21	general population	0,1,6	plasma (MSD)	20 μg	67[a]
Brazil	34	medical personnel	0,1,6	plasma (MSD)	20 μg	98
Ivory Coast	31	medical personnel	0,1,2,12	plasma (PM)	5 μg	93

[a]$\geq$10 mIU/ml.

HBs antibodies to their newborns. Such protection usually last about 3–6 months and should persist until the child is taken for immunization.

Two studies (12,35) were developed with the aim to reinforce the protection of infants through immunization of their mother during pregnancy. Only two to three doses of vaccine could be administered before delivery. Anti-HBs seroconversion rates were 72–85% with two doses and 95% with three doses at one-month intervals; however, this schedule produced relatively low anti-HBs titers. This vaccination of pregnant women ensured the transmission of passive anti-HBs antibodies in 60% of the newborn babies as against 32% in children born to nonimmunized mothers. However, such protection was of short duration, was difficult to apply in rural areas in developing countries, and, most importantly, provided no protection for children born to HBsAg-positive mothers, who represent the major risk of infection for their infants during the first months of life.

III. OVERVIEW OF DATA RELATED TO THE SITUATION IN DEVELOPING COUNTRIES

A. Studies Related to the Reduction in Number of Doses, Spacing of Doses, Route of Administration, and Immunization of Particular Groups

1. Number of Doses

In developing countries, there is frequent noncompliance with immunization teams' appointments, and a portion of infants received incomplete immunization protocols. Retrospective study was undertaken to determine the potency and efficacy of hepatitis B vaccine whether infants received only one or two doses or the classical three or four-dose protocols.

Only 24% of infants receiving one dose of vaccine were found to be anti-HBs positive at the 10 mIU/ml level 12–24 months after injection (Table 6). This proportion is 75% in those receiving two doses and reached 94–97% in those receiving three or four doses. Accordingly, high anti-HBs titers (>1000 mIU/ml) were rarely detected in infants receiving one or two doses of vaccine. From these data it could be concluded that infants receiving incomplete immunization protocols will be poorly protected since a large portion of them did not seroconvert or had low anti-HBs titers, and it is expected that many HBsAg-positive infections will occur in this group of infants. However, long-term efficacy data argues against such a conclusion, since only one or two doses of vaccine were found to be 70% effective against HBsAg/anti-HBc–positive events after 5–7 years. These preliminary results were confirmed recently by similar data (24) in which infants receiving nonadjuvated intradermal vaccine responded poorly to the vaccine in terms of both seroconversion rate and anti-HBs titers, but were highly protected against HBsAg carriage in a 5-year follow-up study.

It must be noted that in these two groups of infants many HBsAg-negative, anti-HBc–positive infections were observed. These results are very promising for the implementation of mass immunization since the overall efficacy on the reduction of the chronic carrier state will be higher than that expected from that calculated from potency data and compliance to vaccination protocol.

2. Optimal Spacing of Vaccinations

In areas of low endemicity several vaccination schedules differing in both number and spacing of doses have been compared. No significant differences between schedules were observed by Hollinger et al. (36), but Jilg et al. (37) found a substantial and significant improvement in anti-HBs response with a 0,1,12-month schedule compared to a 0,1,6-month schedule. This problem of optimal spacing of doses is of some importance in developing countries since

Table 6 Immune Response as Function of HB Vaccine Doses Received by Infants in Developing Countries

No. vaccine doses	Anti-HBs immune response (%)	
	≥10 mIU/ml	≥1000 mIU/ml
1	24	6
2	75	17
3	94	44
4	97	54

strict compliance with immunization schedules may not be observed in mass immunization programs. Moreover, there are wide variations in the EPI schedules found in different countries and sometimes in different regions of the same country.

In two studies performed in developing countries (26,38) an analysis of the anti-HBs response according to the spacing of doses was investigated. These investigators concluded that vaccinating every 2 months should yield the highest anti-HBs titers. However, precise timing of vaccination should not be critical since it is unlikely that moderate departures from this schedule would lead to substantially lower titers. These studies did not confirm the finding that delaying the third (or fourth) dose leads to higher antibody titers.

3. Intradermal Immunization

Because hepatitis B vaccine may be more costly than other routine childhood vaccines, a number of investigators have examined the immune response to intradermal immunization with very low doses of HB vaccines (Table 7). Four control studies of intradermal hepatitis B vaccine were reported in African newborns (15,39) and in adults from Pakistan (33). Although many of these

Table 7 Intradermal Immunization

Population	Country	Ref.	Type	Dose	Schedule	Route	% seroconv.	GMT
			Vaccine				Anti-HBs response	
Newborns	Gambia	15	Plasma (PM)	5 μg	0,1,6	i.m.	100	—
			Plasma (PM)	1 μg	0,1,6	i.d.[a]	53	—
Newborns	Gambia	15	Plasma (MSD)	10 μg	0,1,6	i.m.	100	461
			Plasma (MSD)	2 μg	0,1,6	i.d.	93	136
			Plasma (MSD)	1 μg	0,1,6	i.d.	100	—
Newborns	Kenya	39	Plasma (PM)	5 μg	0,3,7	i.m.	91	800
			Plasma (PM)	1 μg	0,3,7	i.d.[a]	94	90
Adults	Pakistan	33	Recombinant (MSD)	10 μg	0,1,5	i.m.	94	1094
			Plasma (MSD)	2 μg	0,1,5	i.d.	90	387
			Recombinant (MSD)	1 μg	0,1,5	i.d.	78	43

[a]Without adjuvant.

studies found acceptable levels of seroconversion, the GMT was usually considerably lower than that found with intramuscular immunization with higher doses of vaccine, and efficacy in preventing perinatal transmission was found to be quite low. In addition, many investigators attempting intradermal immunization of infants believe this route to be more painful for the child.

4. Hepatitis B Immunization in Recipients with Schistosomiasis

Because reduction in the immune response to various antigens (40,41) has been reported in subjects infected with schistosomia, the immune response to hepatitis B vaccine has been investigated in this group. Moreover, concurrent hepatitis B infection and schistosomiasis may cause more severe hepatic lesions than either disease alone (42), and transmission of hepatitis B from HBsAg-positive mothers to their infants has been reported to take place more frequently with mothers with schistosomiasis when compared to mothers without this infection (43). Thus, additional protection of this group may be warranted.

Three studies (44–46) performed in Egypt have reported that although the plasma and recombinant hepatitis B vaccines are effective in most patients treated for uncomplicated *Schistosoma mansoni* infection, a weak or failed response was associated with the hepatosplenic schistosomiasis. There was a negative correlation between the anti-HBs response and liver lesions due to *S. mansoni*. However, this poor response in some subjects with *S. mansoni* infection will not impair the overall efficacy of immunization programs against hepatitis B in countries where both HBV and *S. mansoni* are epidemic, since HB immunization will take place in the first months of life, years before the establishment of hepatosplenic schistosomiasis in infected subjects.

B.   Association of HB Vaccine with Other Vaccines

In endemic areas, such as many countries in Africa, South America, and the Middle East, transmission of hepatitis B virus occurs early in life but is predominantly horizontal. However, HBV infections that occur during the perinatal period result in a high proportion of HBV chronic carriage. Thus, optimal protection against hepatitis B infection is obtained when the vaccine is administered at or shortly after birth. This fits with the most recent schedule devised by EPI (47) in which BCG immunization must be performed at birth.

In such HBV-endemic countries, prevention should be carried out early in life through mass immunization. In view of reducing the number of immunization sessions to obtain maximum vaccine coverage, the booster dose of hepatitis B vaccine must be given at 9 months of age simultaneously with measles vaccine, which in some countries is given with yellow fever immunization. Several studies were carried out to determine whether HB vaccine could adversely interact with other EPI vaccines (Table 8).

Table 8   Association of HB Vaccine with Other EPI Vaccines

Immune response	Method	Ref.	Vaccines	% Positive	Mean
BCG (cellular)	Tuberculin skin test	23	BCG	77	8.9 mm
			BCG + HB	74	7.4 mm
Tetanus Ab	Agglutination	48	DTP-Polio	100	1.77 IAU/ml
			DTP-polio + HB	100	1.66 IAU/ml
Diphtheria Ab	Agglutination	48	DTP-Polio	100	1.34 IAU/ml
			DTP-Polio + HB	100	0.90 IAU/ml
Pertussis Ab	Agglutination	48	DTP-Polio	86	35.2
			DTP-Polio + HB	86	25.8
Polio type I Ab	Neutralization	23	DTP-Polio	91	ND
			DTP-Polio + HB	94	ND
Polio type II Ab	Neutralization	23	DTP-Polio	95	ND
			DTP-Polio + HB	88	ND
Polio Type III Ab	Neutralization	23	DTP-Polio	100	ND
			DTP-Polio + HB	96	ND
Yellow Fever Ab	Neutralization	50	YF	94	31.8
			YF + HB	92	21.1
Measles Ab	IAHA	49	Measles	82	1.32 IU/ml
			Measles + HB	85	1.76 IU/ml

1. Simultaneous Injection of Hepatitis B Vaccine with BCG and Killed
    Poliovirus Vaccines

Infants less than 5 days of age were enrolled in the study (23) at the maternity units and EPI centers of the town of Pikine in Senegal. According to the order of arrival, children were given vaccines as follows: BCG at birth and hepatitis B vaccine at age 0, 2, 3, and 9 months; BCG at 4 months of age and hepatitis B vaccine at 0, 2, 3, and 9 months; BCG at birth and hepatitis B vaccine at 2, 3, 4 and 9 months of age. All infants received diphtheria/tetanus/pertussis/polio vaccine (DTP-polio) at age 2, 3, and 4 months of age.

No statistical difference in the presence of vaccinal lesions was observed between infants receiving BCG alone or simultaneously with HB vaccine.

Regional reactions were limited to uncomplicated lymphadenopathy in 6–10% of the infants. Lymphadenopathy was generally at the limit of detection by palpation and not related to the simultaneous administration of HB vaccine.

At 6 months of age, a positive tuberculin reaction was observed in 74% of infants receiving HB vaccine and BCG at birth and in 77% of those receiving BCG alone (Table 8). Mean size of tuberculin reaction was 7.4 and 8.9 mm, respectively. Immunization of newborns with BCG associated with the first dose of hepatitis B vaccine produced an immune response equivalent to that observed with each of the vaccines given separately. In addition, no increase in adverse side effects were observed when these vaccines were given simultaneously.

Immune response to the three types of poliovurus was investigated in these infants at 9 months of age. Neutralizing antibodies were detected in 90–97% of the infants according to the virus serotype. No difference was observed between infants simultaneously receiving hepatitis B vaccine and killed poliovirus vaccine and those receiving only killed poliovirus vaccine. Immune response to all three types of poliovirus were observed in 88 and 79% of infants receiving the two vaccines simultaneously and in 86% of infants receiving only poliovirus vaccine.

Immune response to HB vaccine was investigated at 9 months of age. Eighty-eight percent (88%) of infants receiving HB vaccine at birth with BCG and at 2 and 3 months of age had evidence of protective levels of anti-HBs antibodies, compared to 81% of infants receiving hepatitis B vaccine at birth, 2, and 3 months of age and BCG at 4 months of age. Anti-HBs geometric mean titers were 88 and 93 mIU/ml, respectively.

2. Simultaneous Administration of HB Vaccine and
    Diphtheria/Tetanus/Pertussis (DTP) Vaccine

Senegalese children 3–24 months of age were included in this study (48) and divided into three groups. One group received three HB vaccine doses at 6-month intervals. A second group received DTP-polio plus BCG plus HB vaccine at the first session and DTP-polio and HB vaccines at the second and third sessions. The third group received DTP-polio plus BCG at the first session and DTP-polio vaccine at the two following sessions.

No evidence of general or severe undesirable side effects was observed during the study. At the time of the third injection, anti-HBs antibodies were detected in 96% of the infants receiving HB vaccine alone and in 90% of those receiving both HB vaccine and DTP-polio vaccine. Moreover, no differences were observed in the distribution of anti-HBs antibody levels between infants receiving either HB vaccine alone or HB vaccine simultaneously with DTP-polio vaccine.

Antitoxin titer to diphtheria were determined by the passive hemagglutination technique. Six months after the second dose of vaccine, all infants were found positive for diphtheric antibodies, with geometric mean titers of 1.3 IAU/ml for infants receiving DTP-polio vaccine alone and 0.9 IAU/ml in those receiving HB and DTP-polio vaccine simultaneously. No differences were noted in the distribution pattern of diphtheric antibodies between infants receiving DTP-polio alone or DTP-polio simultaneously with HB vaccine.

Anti-toxin titer to tetanus were also determined by the passive hemagglutination technique. At the time of the third injection, all the infants from both groups receiving DTP-polio vaccine showed evidence of the presence of tetanus antibodies, with their geometric mean titers being 1.6 and 1.8 IAU/ml among those receiving DTP-polio vaccine simultaneously or not to HB vaccine. The distribution pattern of tetanus antibody titers were also similar in infants from both groups.

Pertussis agglutinins were detected in 86% of the infants from both groups. The geometric mean titer, expressed as reciprocals of serum dilution, were 35 and 26 in infants who received DTP-polio vaccine alone or DTP-polio vaccine simultaneously with HB vaccine, respectively. No difference in antibody titer distribution patterns was observed for any of the other antigens studied.

3.   Simultaneous Injection of Hepatitis B and Measles Vaccines

Infants living in the Dakar area (Senegal) were immunized with hepatitis B and DTP-polio vaccine at 2 and 4 months of age (49). Half of them received a 5-μg plasma-derived hepatitis B vaccine (PM) and half a 20-μg recombinant vaccine (PM) produced on mammalian cells.

At 9 months of age a portion of the infants received measles and yellow fever vaccines, and the third dose of hepatitis B vaccine was given at 10 months of age. The remaining infants received hepatitis B vaccine simultaneously with measles and yellow fever vaccines at 9 months of age.

Blood samples were taken at 9 and 10 months of age and antimeasles antibodies titers were measured by the hemagglutination inhibition (H.I.) test. Measles H.I. antibody seroconversion rates one month after measles vaccination range from 82 to 87% with geometric mean titers of 66 to 89 (reciprocal of the endpoint dilution), corresponding to 1320 and 1780 mIU/ml. No statistical difference between all groups was observed with respect to either seroconversion rate or antibody titers. This study shows that simultaneous injection of measles and hepatitis B vaccine did not alter the immune response to measles vaccine.

4.   Simultaneous Administration of Hepatitis B and Yellow Fever Vaccines

A first group of infants was immunized with hepatitis B and DTP-polio vaccines (50). At the third session of vaccination they received hepatitis B vaccine, DTP-polio vaccine, measles vaccine, and yellow fever vaccine. A second group consisted of infants receiving DTP-polio vaccine, yellow fever vaccine, and measles vaccine. No untoward reactions were noted during the study. Yellow fever antibodies were detected in a similar proportion (93%) of infants immunized with yellow fever vaccine and with yellow fever vaccine given with hepatitis B vaccine. However, a lower proportion of high yellow fever antibody levels was observed when the vaccines were injected at the same time. As no evidence of untoward reactions was noted during the study, it can be concluded from the results that hepatitis B vaccine and yellow fever vaccine could be injected at the same time. These results show that hepatitis B vaccine may be introduced into existing recommended EPI schedules without reducing the immune response to any of the currently recommended antigens.

REFERENCES

1. E. Marinier, V. Barrois, B. Larouzé, W. T. London, A. Cofer, L. Diakkate, and B. S. Blumberg, Lack of perinatal transmission of hepatitis B virus infection in Senegal, West Africa. *J. Pediatr.*, *106*:843–847 (1985).

2. P. Coursaget, B. Yvonnet, J. L. Barres, J. Perrin, E. Tortey, B. Diop, P. Kocheleff, B. Duflo, S. M'Boup, I. Diop-Mar, J. E. Bocande, and J. P. Chiron, Hépatite B et cancer primitif du foie en Afrique Intertropicale. *Rev. Epidem. et Santé Publ.*, *33*:267–275 (1985).

3. K. C. Hyams, N. M. Osman, E. M. Khaled, A. A. El Wahab Koraa, I. Z. Imam, N. M. El Ghorab, M. A. Dunn, and J. N. Woody, Maternal-infant transmission of hepatitis B in Egypt. *J. Med. Virol.*, *24*:191–197 (1988).

4. P. Coursaget, B. Yvonnet, J. Chotard, P. Vincelot, M. Sarr, C. Diouf, J. P. Chiron, and I. Diop-Mar, Age- and sex-related study of hepatitis B virus chronic carrier state in infants from an endemic area (Senegal). *J. Med. Virol.*, *22*:1–5 (1987).

5. P. Maupas, P. Coursaget, J. P. Chiron, A. Goudeau, F. Barin, J. Perrin, F. Denis, and I. Diop-Mar, Active immunization against hepatitis B in an area of high endemicity. Part I: Field design. *Prog. Med. Virol.*, *27*:168–184 (1981).

6. P. Maupas, J. P. Chiron, A. Goudeau, P. Coursaget, J. Perrin, F. Barin, F. Denis, and I. Diop-Mar, Active immunization against hepatitis B in an area of high endemicity. Part II: Prevention of early infection of the child. *Prog. Med. Virol.*, *27*:185–201 (1981).

7. P. Maupas, J. P. Chiron, F. Barin, P. Coursaget, A. Goudeau, J. Perrin, F. Denis, and I. Diop-Mar, Efficacy of hepatitis B vaccine in prevention of early HBs Ag carrier state in children. Controlled trial in an endemic area (Senegal). *Lancet*, *i*:289–292 (1981).

8. P. Coursaget, J. P. Chiron, F. Barin, A. Goudeau, B. Yvonnet, F. Denis, P. Correa, R. N'Doye, and I. Diop-Mar, Hepatitis B vaccine: Immunization of children and newborns in an endemic area (Sénégal). *Dev. Biol. Standard*, *54*:245–257 (1983).

9. O. W. Prozesky, C. E. Stevens, W. Szmuness, H. Rolka, E. J. Harley, M. C. Kew, J. E. R. Scholtz, and A. D. Mitchell, Immune response to hepatitis B vaccine in newborns. *J. Infect.*, *7* (suppl. 1):53–55 (1983).

10. B. Yvonnet, P. Coursaget, E. Petat, E. Tortey, C. Diouf, F. Barin, F. Denis, I. Diop-Mar, and J. P. Chiron, Immunogenic effect of hepatitis B vaccine in children: Comparison of two and three doses protocols, *J. Med. Virol.*, *14*:137–139 (1984).

11. B. Yvonnet, P. Coursaget, F. Denis, F. Digoutte, E. Petat, F. Barin, A. Goudeau, P. Correa, I. Diop-Mar, and J. P. Chiron, Immune response to hepatitis B vaccination at birth, *Ann. Virol. (Inst. Pasteur)*, *136E*:151–160 (1985).

12. E. A. Ayoola, and A. O. K. Johnson, Hepatitis B vaccine in pregnancy: Immunogenicity, safety and transfer of antibodies to infants. *Int. J. Gynaecol. Obstet.*, *25*:297–301 (1985).

13. J. Perrin, P. Coursaget, F. Ntarème, and J. P. Chiron, Hepatitis B immunization of newborns according to a two dose protocol. *Vaccine*, *4*:241–244 (1986).

14. C. Greenfield, V. O. Osidiana, P. M. Tukei, R. Musoke, J. Mati, C. Loucq, B. Fritzell, and H. C. Thomas, Cheaper immunisation against hepatitis B. *East Afr. Med. J.*, *63*:3–12 (1986).

15. H. C. Whittle, W. H. Lamb, and R. W. Ryder, Trials of intradermal hepatitis B vaccines in Gambian children. *Ann. Trop. Paediatrics*, *7*:6–9 (1987).

16. B. Yvonnet, P. Coursaget, F. Deciron, P. Vincelot, M. Sarr, C. Diouf, J. P. Chiron, and I. Diop-Mar, Hepatitis B immunization of infants with a reduced number of injections: Study of a schedule of three injection at three-months intervals. *Trans. Roy. Soc. Trop. Med. Hyg.*, *81*:165–166 (1987).

17. B. Yvonnet, P. Coursaget, D. Leboulleux, J. L. Barres, B. Fritzell, G. Sarr, J. P. Chiron, and I. Diop-Mar, Low-dose hepatitis B vaccine immunization in children. *Lancet*, *i*:169 (1987).

18. B. Yvonnet, P. Coursaget, J. Chotard, M. Sarr, R. N'Doye, J. P. Chiron, and I. Diop-Mar, Hepatitis B vaccine in infants from an endemic area: Long-term anti-HBs persistence and revaccination. *J. Med. Virol.*, *22*:315–321 (1987).

19. H. Bahakim, S. Ramia, and K. Karbaan, Combined immunoprophylaxis in the prevention of perinatal transmission of hepatitis B and hepatitis D virus infections in Saudi children. *Ann. Trop. Paediatrics*, *10*:139–143 (1990).

20. E. Tsega, B. Tafesse, E. Nordenfelt, G. Wolde-Hawariat, B. G. Hansson, and J. Lindberg, Immunogenicity of hepatitis B vaccine simultaneously administered with the Expanded Programme on Immunisation (EPI). *J. Med. Virol.*, *32*:232–235 (1990).

21. E. Tabor, R. Gerety, J. Cairns and A. C. Bayley, Antibody responses of adults, adolescents and children to a plasma-derived hepatitis B vaccine in a rural African setting. *J. Med. Virol.*, *32*:134–138 (1990).

22. J. Chotard, A. J. Hall, H. M. Inskip, F. Loik, M. Jawara, M. Vall Mayans, B. M. Greenwood, H. Whittle, A. B. H. Njie, K. Cham, F. X. Bosch, and C. S. Muir, The Gambia Intervention study: Preliminary results of the two year follow-up. *Progress in Hepatitis B Immunization* (P. Coursaget and M. J. Tong, eds.), Colloque INSERM/John Libbey Eurotext No. 194, Paris, pp. 501–508 (1990).

23. P. Coursaget, E. Relyveld, A. Brizard, M. P. Frenkiel, B. Fritzell, L. Teulieres, C. Bourdil, B. Yvonnet, J. P. Chiron, E. Jeannee, S. Guindo, and I. Diop-Mar, Simultaneous injection of hepatitis B vaccine with BCG and killed poliovirus vaccine. *Vaccine*, *10*:379–382 (1992).

24. H. C. Whittle, H. Inskip, A. J. Hall, M. Mendy, R. Downes, and S. Hoare, Vaccination against hepatitis B and protection against chronic viral carriage in the Gambia. *Lancet*, *337*:747–750 (1991).

25. B. D. Schoub, S. Johnson, J. M. McAnerney, N. Blackburn, M. C. Kew, J. P.

McCutcheon, and N. D. Carlier, Integration of hepatitis B vaccination into African primary health care programmes. *Br. Med. J.*, *302*:313–316 (1991).

26. S. C. Hadler, M. A. de Monzon, D. R. Lugo, and M. Perez, Effect of timing of hepatitis B vaccine doses on response to vaccine in Yucpa indians. *Vaccine*, 7:106–110 (1989).

27. The Gambia Hepatitis Intervention Study. Annual report 1990.

28. P. Coursaget, B. Yvonnet, J. Chotard, M. Sarr, A. Samb, R. N'Doye, I. Diop-Mar, and J. P. Chiron, Long-term efficacy of hepatitis B vaccine in infants from an endemic area. *Progress in Hepatitis B Immunization* (P. Coursaget, M. J. Tong, eds.) Colloque INSERM/John Libbey Eurotext Paris, pp. 287–300 (1990).

29. A. Ayoola, Vaccination against hepatitis B in Nigerian children: Trials of reduced dose and intradermal vaccine. *J. Trop. Pediatr.*, *31*:253–256 (1985).

30. A. J. Hall and the hepatitis study group, The Gambian Hepatitis B Control Programme. *Viral hepatitis and liver disease* (F. B. Hollinger, S. M. Lemon, H. S. Margolis, eds.). Williams and Wilkins, Baltimore, 712–716 (1991).

31. S. A. Ouattara, M. Meite, and Y. Aron, Vaccination contre l'hépatite B en Côte-D'Ivoire: étude de la réponse anti-HBs chez des sujets adultes sains porteurs uniquement de l'anticorps anti-HBc avant la vaccination. *Bull. Soc. Path. Ex.*, 79:27–38 (1986).

32. A. Sehgal, K. Pavri, V. Arankalle, C. I. Jhala, S. P. Dhorje, and C. L. Ramamoorthy, Antibody response to hepatitis B vaccine in medical and paramedical personnel in India. *Indian J. Med. Res.*, *85*:231–234 (1987).

33. P. J. Bryan, M. Sjogren, M. Iqbal, A. R. Khattak, S. Nabi, A. Ahmed, B. Cox, A. Morton, J. Shuck, P. Macarthy, P. Perine, I. Malik, and L. J. Legters, Comparative trial of low-dose, intradermal, recombinant and plasma-derived hepatitis B vaccines. *J. Infect. Dis.*, *162*:789–793 (1990).

34. M. L. G. Ferraz, R. X. Guimaraes, A. E. B. Silva, M. P. Castilho, M. M. Yamamoto, and M. P. Vilela, Prophylaxis of hepatitis type B: Results of a study in health care personnel in a university hospital. *Progress in Hepatitis B Immunization* (P. Coursaget and M. J. Tong, eds.), Colloque INSERM/John Libbey Eurotext No. 194, Paris, pp. 274–275 (1990).

35. P. Coursaget, J. P. Chiron, B. Yvonnet, F. Barin, A. Goudeau, F. Denis, J. Perrin, R. N'Doye, and I. Diop-Mar, Hepatitis B immunization in pregnancy: Maternal immune response and transmission of anti-HBs antibodies to infants. *Int. J. Microbiol.*, *1*:27–34 (1983).

36. F. B. Hollinger, E. Adam, D. Heiberg, and J. L. Melnick, Response to hepatitis B vaccine in a young adult population. *Viral Hepatitis*: *1981 International Symposium* (W. Szmuness, H. J. Alter, J. E. Maynard, eds.) Franklin Institute Press, Philadelphia, pp. 451–456 (1982).

37. W. Jilg, M. Schmidt, and F. Deinhardt, Immune response to late booster dose of hepatitis B vaccine. *J. Med. Virol.*, *17*:240–254 (1985).

38. W. R. Gilks, N. E. Day, P. Coursaget, B. Yvonnet, A. J. Hall, J. Chotard, J. P. Chiron, and I. Diop-Mar, Response to hepatitis B vaccinations: Some new insights. *Progress in Hepatitis B Immunization* (P. Coursaget and M. J. Tong, eds.), Colloque INSERM/John Libbey Eurotext No. 194, Paris, pp. 409–418 (1990).

39. C. Greenfield, V. O. Osidiana, P. M. Tukei, R. Musoke, J. Mati, C. Loucq, B.

Fritzell, and H. C. Thomas, Cheaper immunisation against hepatitis B. *East Afr. Med. J.*, *63*:3–12 (1986).

40. I. V. Brito, M. M. Peel, and G. H. Ree, Immunological response to tetanus toxoid during a schistosomal infection in mice. *J. Trop. Med. Hyg.*, *79*:161–163 (1976).

41. N. E. Reiner, R. Kamel, G. I. Higashi, A. El-Naggar, M. Aguib, J. J. Ellner, and A. A. F. Mahmoud, Concurrent responses of peripheral blood and splenic mononuclear cells to antigenic and mitogenic stimulation in human hepatosplenic schistosomiasis. *J. Inf. Dis.*, *140*:162–168 (1979).

42. L. G. Lyra, G. Reboucas, and Z. A. Andrade, Hepatitis B surface antigen carrier state in hepatosplenic schistosomiasis. *Gastroenterology*, *71*:641–645 (1976).

43. Y. A. Ghaffar, M. K. El Sobky, A. A. Raouf, and L. S. Dorgham, Mother-to-child transmission of hepatitis B virus in a semirural population in Egypt. *J. Trop. Med. Hyg.*, *92*:20–26 (1989).

44. S. Bassily, K. C. Hyams, N. M. El-Ghorab, M. M. Mansour, N. A. El-Masry, and M. A. Dunn, Immunogenicity of hepatitis B vaccine in patients infected with schistosoma mansoni. *J. Trop. Med. Hyg.*, *36*:549–553 (1987).

45. S. Bassily, K. C. Hyams, N. El-Ghorab, and N. A. El-Masry, Safety and immunogenicity of a recombinant hepatitis B vaccine in patients infected with schistosoma mansoni. *Ann. J. Trop. Med. Hyg.*, *42*:449–452 (1990).

46. Y. A. Ghaffar, M. Kamel, M. F. Abdel Wahab, L. S. Dorgham, M. S. Saleh, and A. S. El Deeb, Hepatitis B vaccination in children infected with schistosoma mansoni: correlation with ultrasonographic data. *Am. J. Trop. Med. Hyg.*, *43*:516–519 (1990).

47. Vaccination of newborns; EPI Geneva, WHO report No. TB/86147 (1986).

48. P. Coursaget, B. Yvonnet, E. H. Relyveld, J. L. Barres, I. Diop-Mar, and J. P. Chiron, Simultaneous administration of diphtheria/tetanus/pertussis/polio vaccine and hepatitis B vaccine in a simplified immunization programme: Immune response to diphtheria toxoid, tetanus toxoid, pertussis and hepatitis B surface antigen. *Infect. Immun.*, *51*:784–787 (1986).

49. P. Coursaget, L. Bringer, C. Bourdil, B. Yvonnet, J. P. Chiron, G. Sarr, E. Jeannee, S. Guindo, I. Diop-Mar, and B. Fritzell, Simultaneous injection of hepatitis B and measles vaccines. *Proc. Roy. Soc. Trop. Med. Hyg.*, *85*:788 (1991).

50. B. Yvonnet, P. Coursaget, V. Deubel, I. Diop-Mar, J. P. Digoutte, and J. P. Chiron, Simultaneous administration of hepatitis B and yellow fever vaccines *J. Med. Virol.*, *19*:307–311 (1986).

51. P. Coursaget, L. Bringer, G. Sarr, C. Bourdil, B. Fritzell, C. Blondeau, B. Yvonnet, J. P. Chiron, E. Jeannee, S. Guindo, I. Diop-Mar, Comparative immunogenicity in children of mammalian cell-derived recombinant hepatitis B vaccine and plasma derived hepatitis B vaccine, *Vaccine*, *10*:379–382 (1992).

11

Hepatitis B Vaccination: Overview of Clinical Studies in the Far East

E. K. Yeoh

Hospital Authority,
Hong Kong

Betty Young

Queen Elizabeth Hospital,
Kowloon, Hong Kong

Hepatitis B virus (HBV) is estimated to be carried by about 300 million people worldwide, with over 250,000 persons dying annually from hepatitis B–associated acute and chronic liver disease (1). The carrier rate of hepatitis B surface antigen (HBsAg) varies widely, from 0.1% in Scandinavia, the United Kingdom, and the United States to 3–5% around the Mediterranean basin to 10–15% in Africa and the Far East. In high carrier–rate areas such as the Far East, infection is probably acquired by perinatal transmission, in contrast to childhood infection in Africa and the Mediterranean region and infection of high-risk adults in low carrier–rate countries. Clinical studies on HBV infection in the Far East have thus focused on its epidemiological pattern, the important contribution of neonatal and early childhood transmission, its relationship with chronic hepatitis, cirrhosis, and hepatocellular carcinoma and means of prevention of the infection.

I. EPIDEMIOLOGY

The prevalence of HBV infection and related diseases such as chronic hepatitis, cirrhosis, and primary hepatocellular carcinoma (PHC) vary widely in the Far East (Table 1). Ethnic origin appears to be an important factor for this difference in prevalence. Ethnic Chinese have a higher carrier rate than other ethnic groups, such as Indonesians (9), Malays (10), Indians (11), and Japanese (12). This is well illustrated in Singapore, where ethnic Chinese have a significantly higher

Table 1 Prevalence of HBsAg in the
Far East

Group	HBsAg$^+$ (%)	Ref.
Ethnic Chinese		
Taiwan	14.6	2
China	11.7	3
Hong Kong	9.6	4
Singapore	6.9	5
Filipino	12.0	6
Korean	12.3	7
Thai	8–10	8
Indonesian	5.5	9
Malay		
Malaysia	3.1–5.5	10
Singapore	1.6	5
Indian		
India	5.0	11
Singapore	1.5	5
Japanese	1.3	12

HBsAg prevalence rate (6.9%) than Malays (1.6%) and Indians (1.5%) (5). This has been attributed to genetically determined differences in immunological responsiveness to HBV infection (13).

The prevalence of HBV infection in the Far East increases with age. In Hong Kong (4), the HBsAg carrier rate rises from 3.3% in the 1–5 year age group to 9.4% in the 11–15 age group and to a maximum of 11.4% in the 21–30 age group. The prevalence of HBV infection, as determined by the presence of HBsAg and anti-HBs in the serum, also rises from 13.6% in the 1–5 age group, to 37.7% in the 11–15 age group, to 45.8% in the 21–30 age group and 77.5% in those over 51 years of age.

In Taiwan, the positive rate of anti-HBc was 16.6% between 0 and 1 year of age and rose steadily and remained over 88% after age 40 (14), and the prevalence rate of HBsAg was 5.1% in infancy, increased to 10.7% between 1 and 2 years of age, and then remained constant at about 10% thereafter (15). The rising prevalence of HBV infection with age was similarly observed in Thailand (8) and Philippines (6). These results showed that HBV infection in the Far East developed very early in life, by vertical transmission of the infection from carrier mothers to their offspring in the neonatal period and subsequently by intrafamily and horizontal transmission from playmates in early childhood.

In the Far East, mother-to-infant transmission is the major mode of transmission and can occur in utero, in the peripartum period, or later in the postnatal period. Infection in utero has been well documented. Transplacental leakage of infected maternal blood, induced by uterine contractions during pregnancy and the disruption of placental barriers, plays an important role in the antepartum transmission of the infection (16). Li et al. also demonstrated that 4 (8%) out of 48 fetuses aborted from HBsAg-positive women at gestational age of 20–32 weeks showed evidence of transplacental infection (17).

Transmission of the infection during the peripartum period is important in the Far East, in particular among the Chinese population. Lee et al. demonstrated that in healthy carrier mothers, HBsAg was detected in 33% of amniotic fluid samples, 50% of cord blood samples, 71% of breast milk samples, and 95.3% of gastric aspirates from their newborns (18). Transmission of the infection could result from swallowing of the infective fluid by the baby during delivery, and from materno-fetal transfusion during labor.

Postnatal infectivity of carrier mothers was well demonstrated by Beasley and Hwang (19), who reported that in 105 children born to HBsAg-positive mothers and given hepatitis B immunoglobulin (HBIG) at birth and in some instances at 3 and 6 months, 38.1% of the infants became infected over an average of 17.5 months of follow-up. The annual incidence rate was 26.0% and was highest (57.1%) for children whose mothers were positive for hepatitis B e antigen (HBeAg), moderate (20.4%) for those whose mothers were negative for both HBeAg and antibody to HBeAg (anti-HBe), and lowest (11.3%) for those whose mothers were positive for anti-HBe. This relationship of maternal HBeAg to vertical transmission of the infection was already documented in 1976 in a study in Japan (20) where all 10 infants born to HBeAg-positive mothers became HBsAg carriers and in a similar study in 1977 in Taiwan (21), where 17 out of 20 (85%) such infants became HBsAg carriers.

Among the Chinese population, it was estimated that antepartum transmission occurred in at least 10% of births and intrapartum transmission in about 40%, and person-to-person transmission after delivery played a relatively minor role (22). This may be explained by the fact that in most areas in the Far East, 5–12% of parturient women are HBsAg positive, and 30–50% of these have high levels of circulating virus indicated by the presence of hepatitis B e antigen (HBeAg) or HBV DNA (23–25). This contrasts with other areas of high HBV endemicity, such as Africa, where infection in childhood is more frequent than perinatal transmission because less than 20% of HBsAg-positive mothers are HBeAg-positive (26,27).

Intrafamily spread of the HBV is important in perpetuating the infection. Lok et al. (28) demonstrated that among 731 family members of 240 HBsAg carriers, 28.3% were positive for HBsAg and 43.1% positive for anti-HBs or anti-HBc. The carrier rate was higher among siblings (53%) and offspring (50.5%) of female carriers, but similar to that of the age-matched general population for spouses (10.8%). Hence, maternal transmission was the most important mode of spread of the infection within the family.

However, in Taiwan (29), among 337 spouses tested for HBV markers, the frequency of HBV seropositivity among husbands was 100% if their wives carried HBeAg. In contrast, HBV infection rate of wives did not show an association with the husbands' HBsAg or HBeAg carrier status. Hence, female-to-male transmission of HBV between spouses appears to be more efficient.

Early childhood HBV infection in the Far East is of great importance. In Taiwan (30), Beasley reported that among 1110 preschool children with an average length of follow-up of 2.1 years, the annual incidence of HBV infection was 5.0%. Among the 98 children who experienced HBV infections during the study, 23% became HBsAg carriers, and HBsAg persistence was age-related, with most carriers being among the youngest children infected.

It was estimated that the probability of chronic HBV carriage, given an acute HBV infection, increases dramatically in infancy and early childhood (1). Seventy to 90% of children infected in the first year of life will result in persistent HBV carriage, compared to 40–70% when infected between 2 and 3 years, 10–40% at 4–6 years, and 6–10% when infected after the age of 7. The early age of induction of chronic carriage also increases HBV-induced mortality because of the longer survival period of these chronic carriers. Hence, clinical studies on the prevention of hepatitis B infection in the Far East have focused on such high-risk groups, in particular, infants born to HBsAg-positive mothers.

II. PREVENTION OF HEPATITIS B INFECTION

A. Passive Immunization Against Hepatitis B

Hepatitis B immunoglobulin (HBIG) is prepared from pooled plasma with high titer of hepatitis B surface antibody, and it may confer temporary passive immunity in certain pre- and postexposure situations. The most important indication for the use of HBIG is for infants born to HBsAg carrier mothers. In 1978 the results of a placebo-controlled study in Taiwan indicated that 0.2 ml of HBIG given within the first 7 days of life to infants of HBeAg carrier mothers did not prevent the persistent HBsAg carrier states in these children (31).

In 1981, Beasley et al. (32) compared the use of three doses of 0.5 ml HBIG given at birth, 3 months, and 6 months to a single dose of 1.0 ml HBIG at birth and the use of placebo in infants born to e antigen–positive HBsAg carrier mothers. At 15 months, the carrier rate in the placebo-treated infants was 91% compared to 23% among those who received three doses and 45% among those who received a single dose of HBIG. The efficacy was 75 and 45%, respectively, for the two treatment schedules.

Ko et al. (33) later showed that reduced dose of 0.25 ml HBIG given at birth,

3 months, and 6 months produced similar protection to those given the standard dose of 0.5 ml. Since HBIG has to be given repeatedly and is relatively expensive, passive immunization alone to such high-risk infants was not recommended.

B. Active and Passive-Active Immunization Against Hepatitis B

After a decade of research, hepatitis B vaccines were licensed and marketed in 1981, and they provide the most effective means of prevention of the infection. The safety, immunogenicity, and efficacy of such vaccines have been widely tested in adults and high-risk individuals such as intravenous drug abusers and homosexuals in Western countries. Since the Far East has a different epidemiological pattern, clinical studies have thus concentrated on vaccination of infants born to carrier mothers, children and family contacts of HBsAg carriers, and health-care personnel.

In the Far East, the immunogenicity of hepatitis B vaccine was well established in adult health-care workers in Malaysia (34), in healthy Chinese children (35) and neonates (36) in Taiwan, and in nursery school children in Japan (37). They all developed satisfactory antibody levels after the course of vaccination. Children were found to develop a better immune response to the vaccine than adults in a study in Thailand (38). Although the seroconversion rates were similar after three monthly injections of 5 μg of a plasma-derived vaccine (Hevac B) to a group of healthy Thai adults and children (92.0 and 96.3%, respectively), children developed significantly higher anti-HBs levels (800 mIU/ml) than adults (353 mIU/ml). Since children have a much better immune response to hepatitis B vaccine than adults, the prevention of horizontal transmission of hepatitis B virus should be done by vaccination in children.

In postexposure prophylaxis in high-risk individuals such as those exposed to needlestick contaminated with infectious serum and infants born to HBsAg carrier mothers, comparisons were made in the use of vaccine alone, HBIG alone, and the combined administration of vaccine and HBIG. In Japan (39), a group of staff in a hemodialysis unit were exposed to needlestick contaminated with blood containing HBsAg, HBeAg, and high levels of DNA polymerase activity. They received hepatitis B vaccine (20 μg) simultaneously with HBIG within 48 hours after the exposure, and the vaccination was repeated at 1 and 3 months. Twelve months after the accident, only one (4%) out of the 23 vaccinated members contracted HBV infection, a frequency significantly lower than 11 (33%) of the 33 historical controls who were given HBIG alone.

In Hong Kong, Wong et al. (40) compared four groups of infants of HBeAg carrier mothers. Group I received four doses of 3 μg heat-inactivated hepatitis B vaccine produced by Netherlands Red Cross Transfusion Service given at birth,

1, 2, and 6 months, in conjunction with seven monthly HBIG injections. Group II received the same vaccine schedule but received only one HBIG injection at birth. Group III received only the vaccine at birth, 1, 2, and 6 months. Group IV received only placebos. The development of the persistent carrier state in the three treatment groups was significantly less frequent than in controls (2.9, 6.8, and 21.0% versus 73.2%). The protective efficacy rates in the 2 groups of infants receiving both hepatitis B vaccine and HBIG (96 and 91%) were significantly higher than the vaccine alone group (71%).

Similar results were observed in Taiwan (41), where vaccine alone given at 2, 6, and 10 weeks of life resulted in a protective efficacy of 73.7%, compared to 87.7 and 94.1% when the same schedule of vaccination was combined with a single dose of HBIG at birth and two doses of HBIG at birth and 1 month of age, respectively. In Korea (42), it was demonstrated that passive-active immunization in the form of a single dose of 0.5 ml HBIG at birth in conjunction with three doses of 10 μg hepatitis B vaccine at 1, 2, and 6 months resulted in better long-term protection than passive immunization alone, i.e., three doses of 0.5 ml HBIG at birth, 3 months, and 6 months in infants born to HBsAg carrier mothers. Hence, passive-active immunization against hepatitis B offers better postexposure prophylaxis against the infection in high-risk individuals than the use of HBIG or hepatitis B vaccine alone.

C. Issues of Hepatitis B Vaccination

There is no doubt that hepatitis B vaccine is the single most important tool for the prevention of hepatitis B, but there are other issues of hepatitis B vaccination that need to be addressed. These include the dosage, schedule, and timing of vaccination, type of hepatitis B vaccine, the need for a booster dose and the dosage of HBIG in postexposure prophylaxis, particularly in infants born to carrier mothers.

In Taiwan, Beasley et al. (43) studied the efficacy of a single dose versus two doses of HBIG and the effect of time of commencement of vaccination in infants of e antigen–positive HBsAg carrier mothers. Group A infants received 0.5 ml HBIG at birth and 3 months, at which time vaccination (20 μg MSD plasma-derived vaccine) was initiated and repeated 1 and 6 months later. Group B infants received HBIG only at birth and the same schedule of vaccination was initiated within the first week of life. Group C infants received HBIG at birth only, and vaccination was initiated at 1 month of age. No difference in efficacy between a single dose of HBIG at birth and 2 doses at birth and 3 months was found. With HBIG coverage from birth, the timing of the start of vaccination does not seem to be of importance within the first month of life. It was suggested that to maximize compliance and minimize costs, hepatitis B vaccination should be initiated during the confinement.

In Hong Kong, Yeoh et al. studied the determinants of immunogenicity and efficacy of hepatitis B vaccination in infants born to HBsAg carrier mothers. The standard three-dose schedule of 10 μg of plasma-derived MSD vaccine given at birth, 1, and 6 months was compared to a schedule when the vaccine was given at birth, 1, and 2 months. The time of commencement of the standard three-dose vaccination regimen was evaluated by initiating vaccination at birth and at 2 months of age. Vaccination was also combined with different dosaging of HBIG: single dose of 0.5 ml at birth, single dose of 1 ml at birth, two doses of 0.5 ml at birth and 2 months, and three doses at birth, 2, and 4 months. It was observed that the efficacy of vaccination was dependent only on the maternal HBeAg status. The immunogenicity was determined by the age at which vaccination was commenced, as the group of infants who commenced vaccination at 2 months had a significantly higher antibody titer (797 mIU/ml at 1 year) than those vaccinated at birth (136–206 mIU/ml). The dosage and schedule of vaccination and of HBIG appeared to be less important determinants of immunogenicity. Nonresponsiveness to the course of vaccine was observed in 2.9% of vaccinees. 2.5% had titers less than 10 IU/ml, and 20.4% had titers of 10–99 mIU/ml. The effect of a single booster dose at 15 months of age was evaluated in nonresponders and hyporesponders (anti-HBs titer less than 100 mIU/ml), and it was observed that there were modest elevations of GMT soon after the booster dose, however, these fell to levels close to those of the controls by 3 years. At 3 years, 19% of infants who initially responded to vaccination lost detectable anti-HBs. They were randomized to booster and control groups. A booster dose produced anamnestic responses with anti-HBs rising to 800 mIU/ml 2 weeks after the booster, but at 5 years of age, GMT had fallen to only 50 mIU/ml. There was also no HBsAg breakthrough observed in either the booster or control groups. Hence, booster doses of vaccine before the age of 5 do not appear to be necessary.

Differences in procedures of preparation and inactivation of the hepatitis B vaccines may result in differences in vaccine efficacies. In China (44), two plasma-derived vaccines were compared. One group of infants born to HBsAg carrier mothers were given 16 μg of National Institute of Allergy and Infectious Diseases (NIAID) vaccine and the other group 20 μg of Beijing Institute of Vaccine and Serum (BIVS) vaccine at birth, 1, and 6 months of age. The seroconversions to the vaccines at 1 year were 95 and 75% and vaccine efficacy 88 and 51%, respectively. The lower immunogenicity and efficacy of the BIVS vaccine as compared to the NIAID vaccine may be explained by the differences in preparation and inactivation. The NIAID vaccine was only in activated with formalin, whereas the BIVS vaccine were heat inactivated (60°C, 10 hours) and formalin concentrations used were higher.

The Pasteur vaccine was compared with the Green Cross Corporation (GCC) vaccine in adults in Hong Kong (45,46). There are differences in the production of these two vaccines, with an added step of heat inactivation and longer formaldehyde treatment for the GCC vaccine. Results showed that both vaccines had comparable immunogenicity and safety, although the GCC vaccine gave a significantly lower but still "protective" anti-HBs level at 3–18 months. Similar to the study in China (44), the added steps of inactivation in its production may account for the difference in immunogenicity.

The immunogenicity of four plasma-derived vaccines were compared in Thai young adults (47) given 20 μg per dose of vaccine at 0, 1, and 6 months. Only the Merck and Pasteur vaccines could achieve more than 90% seroconversion (anti-HBs titer greater than 10 mIU/ml), whereas the Dutch CLB and Korean Cheil-Sugar vaccines needed a fourth dose to achieve this level of seroconversion.

The introduction in 1987 of a second-generation hepatitis B vaccine derived from recombinant yeast containing the gene for HBsAg (the S gene) has prompted researchers to compare the immunogenicity and efficacy of plasma-derived and recombinant yeast vaccines. In Thailand (48), 5 μg of recombinant hepatitis B vaccine (HB VAX II, MSD) was investigated for efficacy in the prevention of perinatal HBV transmission in high-risk neonates born from HBeAg–positive HBsAg carrier mothers as compared to 10 μg of plasma-derived hepatitis B vaccine (HB VAX, MSD). Both groups of infants received HBIG at birth. There were no statistically significant differences in the efficacy and seroconversion rate of these two vaccines with the protective efficacy being 89.2 and 94.6% for the two groups of infants. However, the geometric mean titers in the plasma-derived vaccine group (179.55 mIU/ml) were significantly higher than those in the recombinant vaccine group (42.2 mIU/ml), but the anti HBs titer was still above the protective level (10 mIU/ml) in most of the infants.

However, a similar study in Hong Kong (49) showed that the geometric mean titer was higher in the recombinant vaccine group, and it also confirmed that the yeast-derived recombinant hepatitis vaccine is safe, immunogenic, and at least as effective as the plasma-derived vaccine in preventing the HBsAg carrier state in infants born to HBsAg-positive women. In Japanese nursery school children (50), 5 μg of the recombinant vaccine resulted in higher seroconversion rates and higher antibody titers than 10 μg of the plasma-derived vaccine.

Since most commercially available plasma-derived and yeast-derived recombinant vaccines are equally immunogenic and efficacious, most countries in the Far East with a high carrier rate have implemented vaccination programs for such high-risk neonates. Implementation of a nationwide vaccination program depends heavily on cost, particularly in the developing world. Hence, reduced doses of the vaccines were tested.

The use of reduced dose of vaccine was tested in healthy adults in Singapore (51). Reduced dose of 5 μg of a yeast-derived recombinant DNA vaccine

(B-Hepavac II) was as effective as the standard 10-μg dose with similar seroconversion rate (91 and 95%, respectively) and geometric mean titers (836 mIU/ml and 811 mIU/ml, respectively) 2 months after the last dose.

Further reduction in the vaccine dose was studied in Singapore children (52) and ranged well below the currently recommended levels at 0.6, 1.25, 2.5, and 5.0 μg. All these children received three doses of vaccine at 0, 1, and 5 months. Early immunogenic response appeared dose-related with a higher response occurring with increasing dosage; the GMT among the groups, however, was similar, especially at and after 9 months. Although these data indicate that vaccine dosage as low as 0.6 μg can elicit a good antibody response in the majority of children, care must be taken not to generalize too much beyond this group.

In Thailand (53), a reduced dose of plasma-derived vaccine (Hevac B) was tested for efficacy in infants of e antigen–positive HBsAg carrier mothers. One group received the standard dose (5 μg), and the other group the reduced dose (2 μg) of vaccine at birth, 1, 2, and 12 months of age. Both groups were given HBIG at birth. There was no statistically significant difference in the efficacy and antibody responses of these two regimens. The protective efficacy rate was 94.0 and 93.2% in infants receiving the standard dose and reduced dose regimens, respectively. At 12 months, the anti-HBs seroconversion rates were 80.0 and 86.7%, with geometric mean titers of 84.57 and 78.56 mIU/ml, respectively. It is thus concluded in this study that a reduced dose (2 μg) of vaccine could be used as effectively as the standard dose (5 μg) in the prevention of perinatal HBV transmission in high-risk neonates.

Various issue of hepatitis B vaccination have been addressed. The vaccine is thus the most important tool in the control of the infection. Policies and strategies for vaccination depend on the local epidemiological data, socioeconomic condition, cultural background, logistics, territorial geography, and the health-care delivery system. Many countries in the Far East have already developed a vaccination program for those at risk. A nationwide program was first developed to vaccinate newborns of carrier mothers. Integration of this program into the Expanded Programme on Immunization (EPI) was subsequently developed in some countries, and newborns are immunized irrespective of their maternal HBsAg status. Vaccination of all preschool children should now be the goal in the Far East.

III. THE FUTURE

Current research in hepatitis B is now focused on molecular biology. Our knowledge of its transmission, infection, pathophysiology, sequelae, and prevention may evolve. It is hoped that it will soon be possible to successfully treat and eradicate the infection.

REFERENCES

1. Maynard, J. E. Hepatitis B: global importance and need for control. Vaccine 1990, 8 (suppl): 18s–20s.
2. Sung, J. L., Chen, D. S., Lai, M. Y., et al. Epidemiological study on hepatitis B virus infection in Taiwan. Chinese J Gastroenterol 1964, 1: 1.
3. Zhao, K. Epidemiology of hepatitis B in China. In: Viral Hepatitis B Infection in the Western Pacific Region: Vaccine and Control (Eds. Lam, S. K., Lai, C. L., Yeoh, E. K.), World Scientific Press, Hong Kong, 1984: 23–28.
4. Yeoh, E. K., Chang, W. K., Kwan, J. P. W. Epidemiology of viral hepatitis B infection in Hong Kong. In: Viral Hepatitis B Infection in the Western Pacific Region: Vaccine and Control (Eds. Lam, S. K., Lai, C. L., Yeoh, E. K.), World Scientific Press, Hong Kong, 1984: 33–41.
5. Goh, K. T. Epidemiology of Hepatitis B Virus Infection in Asian Countries: Outlook in Singapore. Asian Journal of Clinical Sciences (Suppl) Hepatitis B Virus Infections: Current Status and Recent Developments 1990 Monograph No. 11: 87–98.
6. Domingo, E. O., Lingao, A. L., Lansang, M. A. D. Seroepidemiology of hepatitis B virus in the general population and in patients with chronic liver disease in the Philippines. In: Asian Symposium on Strategies for Large Scale Hepatitis B Immunisation (Ed. Goulli, N.), Science Press, Hong Kong, 1986: 49–54.
7. Hong, W. S., Kim, C. Y. Seroepidemiology of hepatitis type A and type B in Seoul, Korea. Korean J Intern Med 1982, 25: 19.
8. Sumakorn, B., Chunsittiwat, S. Epidemiology of hepatitis B in Thailand. In: Asian Symposium on Strategies for Large Scale Hepatitis B Immunisation (Ed. Goulli, N.), Science Press, Hong Kong, 1986: 21–26.
9. Sulaiman, A., Akbar, N., Noer, H. M. S., et al. Hepatitis B antigen and antibody in Indonesia In: Viral Hepatitis and Its Related Diseases (Ed. Suzuki, H.), Kishimoto Printings and Publishing, Kobe, 1982.
10. Manaff, S. A., Sarvananthan, R. Report on the prevalence and characteristics of hepatitis B infection in Malaysia. In: Asian Symposium on Strategies for Large Scale Hepatitis B Immunisation (Ed. Goulli, N.), Science Press, Hong Kong, 1986: 43–47.
11. Tandon, B. N., Gandhi, B. M., Voshi, Y. K. Etiological spectrum of viral hepatitis and prevalence of markers of hepatitis A and B virus infection in North India. Bull WHO 1984: 62, 67.
12. Department of Blood Affairs of Japanese Red Cross. The Present Status of Blood Affairs 1980–85.
13. Yap, E. H., Ong, Y. W., Simons, M. J., et al. Australia antigen in Singapore II: differential frequency in Chinese, Malays and Indians. Vox Sang 1972, 22: 371–375.
14. Sung, J. L., Chen, D. S., Lai, M. Y., et al. Epidemiology study of hepatitis B virus infection in Taiwan. In: Viral Hepatitis B Infection in the Western Pacific Region: Vaccine and Control (Eds. Lam, S. K., Lai, C. L., Yeoh, E. K.), World Scientific Press, Hong Kong, 1984: 55–65.
15. Hsu, J. Y., Chang, M. H., Chen, D. S., Lee, C. Y., Sung, J. L. Baseline

seroepidemiology of hepatitis B virus infection in children in Taipei, 1984: A study just before mass hepatitis B vaccination program in Taiwan. J Medical Virol 1986, 18: 301–307.

16. Lin, H. H., Lee, T. Y., Chen, D. S., et al. Transplacental leakage of HBeAg-positive maternal blood as the most likely route in causing intrauterine infection with hepatitis B virus. J Pediatr 1987, 111: 877–881.

17. Li, L., Sheng, M. H., Tong, S. P., Chen, H. Z., Wen, Y. M. Transplacental transmission of hepatitis B virus. Lancet 1986, II: 872.

18. Lee, A. K. Y., Ip, H. M. H., Wong, V. C. W. Mechanisms of maternal-fetal transmission of hepatitis B virus. J Infect Dis 1978, 138: 668–671.

19. Beasley, R. P., Hwang, L. Y. Postnatal infectivity of hepatitis B surface antigen-carrier mothers. J Infect Dis 1983, 147: 185–190.

20. Okada, K., Kamiyama, I, Inomata, M., et al. e Antigen and anti-e in the serum of asymptomatic carrier mothers as indicators of positive and negative transmission of hepatitis B virus to their infants. N Engl J Med 1976, 294: 746–749.

21. Beasley, R. P., Trepo, C., Stevens, C. E., Szmuness, W. The e antigen and vertical transmission of hepatitis B surface antigen. Am J Epidemiol 1977, 105: 94–98.

22. Wong, V. C. M., Lee, A. K. Y., Ip, H. M. H. Transmission of hepatitis B antigens from symptom free carrier mothers to the fetus and the infant. Br J Obstet Gynaecol 1980, 87: 958–965.

23. Stevens, C. E., Neurath, R. A., Beasley, R. P., et al. HBeAg and anti-HBs detection by radioimmunoassay. Correlation with vertical transmission of hepatitis B virus in Taiwan. J. Med Virol 1979, 3: 237–241.

24. Xu, Z. Y., Liu, C. B., Francis, D. P., et al. Prevention of perinatal acquisition of hepatitis B virus carriage using vaccine: preliminary report of a randomized, double-blind placebo-controlled and comparative trial. Pediatrics 1985, 76: 713–718.

25. Lee, S. D., Lo, K. J., Wu, J. C., et al. Prevention of maternal-infant hepatitis B transmission by immunization: the role of serum hepatitis B virus DNA. Hepatology 1986, 6: 369–373.

26. Marinier, E., Barrois, V., Larouze, B., et al. Lack of perinatal transmission of hepatitis B virus infection in Senegal, West Africa. J Pediatr 1985, 106: 843–849.

27. Hyams, K. C., Osman, N. M., Khaled, E. M., et al. Maternal-infant transmission of hepatitis B in Egypt. J Med Virol 1988, 24: 191–97.

28. Lok ASF, Lai Cl, Wu PC, et al. Hepatitis B virus infection in Chinese families in Hong Kong. Am J Epidemiol 1987, 126: 191–97.

29. Ko, Y. C., Yen, Y. Y., Yeh, S. M., Lan, S. J. Female to male transmission of hepatitis B virus between Chinese spouses. J Med Virol 1989, 27: 142–144.

30. Beasley, R. P., Hwang, L. Y., Lin, C. C., et al. Incidence of hepatitis B virus infections in preschool children in Taiwan. J Infect Dis 1982, 146: 198–204.

31. Beasley, R. P., Stevens, C. E. Vertical transmission of HBV and interruption with globulin. In: Viral Hepatitis (Eds. Vyas, G. N., Cohen, S. N., Schmid, R.), Franklin Institute Press, Philadelphia, 1978: 333–345.

32. Beasley, R. P., Hwang, L. Y., Lin, C. C., et al. Hepatitis B immunoglobulin (HBIG) efficacy in the interruption of perinatally transmitted hepatitis B virus carrier state. Lancet 1981, 2: 388–393.

33. Ko, T. M., Lin, K. H., Ho, M. M., et al. Reduced doses of hepatitis B immune globulin in the prevention of perinatal transmission of hepatitis B. J Med Virol 1987, 21: 301–309.

34. Ton, S. H., Noriah, R., Duraisamy, G. Immunogenicity of hepatitis B vaccine in healthy Malaysian adults. Indian J Med Res 1988, 87: 542–544.

35. Hwang, L. Y., Beasley, R. P., Stevens, C. E., Szmuness, W. Immunogenicity of HBV vaccine in healthy Chinese children. Vaccine 1983, 1: 10–12.

36. Lee, G. C. Y., Hwang, L. Y., Beasley, R. P., Chen, S. H., Lee, T. Y. Immunogenicity of hepatitis B virus vaccine in healthy Chinese neonates. J Infect Dis 1983, 148: 526–529.

37. Hayashi, J., Kashiwagi, S., Nomura, H., Kajiyama, W., Ikematsu, H. The control of hepatitis B virus infection with vaccine in Japanese nursery schools. Am J Epidemiol 1987, 126: 474–479.

38. Pongpipat, D., Suvatte, V., Assateerawatts, A., Bhethraratt, S. Active pre-exposure immunisation against hepatitis B virus: immunogenicity of hepatitis B vaccine in healthy Thai adults and children. Asian Pacific J Allergy Immunol 1987, 5: 63–65.

39. Mitsui, T., Iwano, K., Suzuki, S., et al. Combined hepatitis B immune globulin and vaccine for postexposure prophylaxis of accidental hepatitis B virus infection in hemodialysis staff members: comparison with immune globulin without vaccine in historical control. Hepatology 1989, 10: 324–327.

40. Wong, V. C. W., Ip, H. M. H., Reesink, H. W., et al. Prevention of the HBsAg carrier state in newborn infants of mothers who are chronic carriers of HBsAg and HBeAg by administration of hepatitis-B-vaccine and hepatitis-B immunoglobulin. Lancet 1984, i: 921–926.

41. Lo, K. J., Tsai, Y. T., Lee, S. D., et al. Combined passive and active immunization for interruption of perinatal transmission of hepatitis B virus in Taiwan. Hepato-gastroenterol 1985, 32: 65–68.

42. Chung, W. K., Yoo, J. Y., Sun, H. S., et al. Prevention of perinatal transmission of hepatitis B virus: a comparison between the efficacy of passive and passive-active immunization in Korea. J Infect Dis 1985, 151: 280–286.

43. Beasley, R. P., Hwang, L. Y., Lee, G. C. Y., et al. Prevention of perinatally transmitted hepatitis B virus infections with hepatitis B immune globulin and hepatitis B vaccine. Lancet 1983, ii: 1099–1102.

44. Xu, Z. Y., Liu, C. B., Francis, D. P., et al. Prevention of perinatal acquisition of hepatitis B virus carriage using vaccine: preliminary report of a randomized, double-blind placebo-controlled and comparative trial. Pediat 1985, 76: 713–718.

45. Lau, J. Y. N., Lai, C. L., Wu, P. C., Lin, H. J. Comparison of two plasma-derived hepatitis B vaccines: long term report of a prospective, randomized trial. J Gastroenterol Hepatol 1989, 4: 331–337.

46. Lok, A. S. F., Lai, C. L., Wu, P. C., Ng, M. M. T. Response to hepatitis B vaccine in family members of HBsAg carriers. J Med Virol 1986, 19: 33–39.

47. Phanuphak, P., Phanpanich, T., Wongurai, S., et al. Comparative immunogenicity study of four plasma-derived hepatitis B vaccines in Thai young adults. Vaccine 1989, 7: 253–256.

48. Pongpipat, D., Suvatte, V., Assateerawatts, A. Hepatitis B immunization in high

risk neonates born from HBsAg positive mothers: comparison between plasma derived and recombinant DNA vaccine. Asian Pac J Allergy Immunol 1989, 7: 37–40.

49. Yeoh, E. K., Chang, W. K., Ip, P., et al. Efficacy and safety of recombinant hepatitis B vaccine in infants born to HBsAg-positive mothers. J Infect 1986, 13 (suppl A): 15–18.

50. Hayashi, J., Kashiwagi, S., Kajiyama, W., et al. Comparison of results of recombinant and plasma-derived hepatitis B vaccines in Japanese nursery-school children. J Infect 1988, 17: 49–55.

51. Guan, R., Tay, H. H., Yap, I, Smith, R., Tan, L. H. Immunogenicity of a low dose recombinant DNA hepatitis B vaccine in healthy adults in Singapore. Asian Pacific J Allergy Immunol 1989, 7: 85–88.

52. Tan, K. L., Oon, C. J., Goh, K. T., Wong, L. Y. M., Chan, S. H. Immunogenicity and safety of low doses of recombinant yeast-derived hepatitis B vaccine. Acta Paediatr Scand 1990, 79: 593–598.

53. Pongpipat, D., Suvatte, V., Assateerawatts, A. Hepatitis B immunization in high risk neonates born from HBsAg and HBeAg positive mothers: comparison of standard and low dose regimens. Asian Pac J Allergy Immunol 1988, 6: 107–110.

12

Protective Efficacy of Hepatitis B Vaccines in Infants, Children, and Adults

Brian J. McMahon

Alaska Native Medical Center,
Anchorage, Alaska

Robert B. Wainwright

Centers for Disease Control,
Anchorage, Alaska

I. INTRODUCTION

Hepatitis B virus (HBV) infection is a major health problem throughout the world (1). HBV not only causes acute hepatitis B, but also can result in chronic infection, which can subsequently lead to the development of cirrhosis and hepatocellular carcinoma (2). The development of vaccines against hepatitis B (HB) has presented the opportunity to interrupt the spread of this infection. Several elegantly designed efficacy trials that clearly demonstrated that the vaccine protected high-risk adults and infants from HBV infection have been successfully conducted. The purpose of this chapter is to review the efficacy studies that led to licensure and subsequent widespread usage of HB vaccine (see also Chapters 10 and 11).

II. DEVELOPMENT OF HEPATITIS B VACCINE

In the 1960s, Dr. Saul Krugman and coworkers demonstrated that there were two distinct types of viral hepatitis (3). One (MS-1) could be transmitted by feces from infected persons. Another (MS-2) could be transmitted by the inoculation of infectious sera. In the early 1970s, Krugman and coworkers found that boiling infectious sera containing the MS-2 strain for one minute could inactivate this virus (4). In addition, boiling did not interfere with the antigenicity of the MS-2 strain since a 1 : 10 dilution of boiled infectious sera prevented HBV infection in most recipients who were later challenged with infectious sera. These early studies by Krugman paved the way for the development of the plasma-derived HB vaccine utilizing sera from chronic carriers of hepatitis B surface antigen (HBsAg).

The plasma-derived vaccine was produced by ultracentrifugation of sera from HBsAg-positive carriers. The ultracentrifugation concentrated the 22-nanometer (nm) HBsAg particles, which consist of excess, noninfectious surface antigen protein (5). The particles were then heated and in some vaccines treated with one or more chemicals including 5M urea, pepsin at low pH, and formalin to inactivate any infectious material in the preparation. Aluminum hydroxide (alum) is added as an adjuvant. Later these same 22-nm HBsAg particles were successfully produced utilizing recombinant technology in yeast (6).

III. EFFICACY TRIALS IN NEONATES AND CHILDREN

A. Efficacy Trials in Neonates Using Plasma-Derived Vaccine

Neonates whose mothers are positive for HBsAg as well as hepatitis B e antigen (HBeAg) have an 80–90% risk of developing the HBsAg chronic carrier state. A randomized double-blind, placebo-controlled efficacy trial of hepatitis B immunoglobulin (HBIG) was conducted by Beasley and coworkers in Taiwan between 1978 and 1982 (7). In that study of infants of HBsAg/HBeAg-positive mothers, the HBsAg carrier rate was 92% among 61 placebo recipients versus 26% among 57 infants who received three doses of HBIG and 54% of infants who received one dose of HBIG.

The first study using passive/active immunization of infants born of HBsAg/HBeAg-positive mothers was reported in 1983 by Beasley and coworkers (8). In this study, 159 infants were randomized to receive one of three active/passive prophylaxis schedules using HBIG and plasma-derived HB vaccine manufactured by Merck Sharp & Dohme (MSD). These immunized infants were compared with 84 untreated controls: 61 from the previously described HBIG placebo/control trial, and 23 infants whose parents declined immunization (Table 1). In the treatment groups combined, only 5.7% (range 2–8.6%) of the infants became chronic HBsAg carriers compared with 88% of the control group. Average efficacy was 93.6% (range 90.2–97.8%).

In 1984, a large randomized placebo-control trial involving 189 infants of HBsAg/HBeAg-positive mothers was reported from Hong Kong (9). All infants were randomized to a placebo group or one of three treatment groups, and each received 3 μg of heat-inactivated plasma-derived HB vaccine (Netherlands Red Cross Transfusion Service) at birth, 1, 2, and 6 months of age. In addition, two groups received HBIG, one at birth and the other monthly through the first 6

Table 1 Efficacy Trials of HBIG and Plasma-Derived Hepatitis B Vaccine in Infants of HBsAg/HBeAg-Positive Mothers

Study site (Ref.)	Vaccine used	Groups studied (no. participants)		Age of Subject (months)		HBsAg carrier rate (%)	Protective efficacy (%)
				HBIG	HB vaccine		
Taiwan (8)	MSD (20 μg)	HBIG/Vx	(51)	0,3	3,4,9	2	97.8
		HBIG/Vx	(50)	0	0,1,6	6	93.2
		HBIG/Vx	(58)	0	1,2,7	8.6	90.2
		Control	(84)	—	—	88.1	—
Hong Kong (9)	Dutch Red Cross (3 μg)	HBIG/Vx	(36)	0,1,2,3,4,5,6	0,1,2,6	2.9	96
		HBIG/Vx	(35)	0	0,1,2,6	6.8	90.7
		Vaccine Only	(35)	—	0,1,2,6	21	71.3
		Placebo	(34)	—	—	73.2	—
United States (10)	MSD (20 μg)	HBIG/Vx	(25)	0	0,1,6	20	
		HBIG/Vx	(88)	0	1,2,6	12.5	
Taiwan (11)	Pasteur (5 μg)	Vaccine Only	(38)	—	0,1,2,12	19.4	75.3
		HBIG/Vx	(36)	0	0,1,2,12	11.4	85.5
		HBIG/Vx	(38)	0.1	0,1,2,12	8.1	89.7
		Control	(29)	—	—	78.4	
Shanghai (12)	NIAID (16 μg)	Placebo	(29)	—	—	65.5	
		NIAID	(27)	—	0,1,6	7.4	88.7
	BIVS (20 μg)	BIVS	(28)	—	0,1,6	28.5	45.5–67.3[a]
		HBIG/BIVS	(16)	0	0,1,6	6.2	90.5

MSD, Merck Sharp & Dohme; NIAID, National Institute of Allergy and Infectious Diseases; BIVS, Beijing Institute of Vaccine and Serum.
[a]Two different vaccine lots were used.

months of life. Subsequent carrier rates were 6.8 and 2.9% in the two groups of infants receiving HBIG plus vaccine, 21% in the infants receiving vaccine alone, and 73.2% in the placebo group. Protective efficacy was 90.7, 96, and 71.3%, respectively (Table 1). In 1985, Stevens and coworkers reported the results of an unblinded passive-active immunization study of 113 infants of HBsAg/HBeAg-positive Asian-American mothers in the United States. The infants received one dose of HBIG and three doses of 20 μg of plasma-derived HB vaccine (MSD) (10). While only 14.2% became chronic carriers, this was higher than the 5.7% in the study in Taiwan using the same vaccine (Table 1). There has been no explanation of this difference in chronic carrier rates.

Several other efficacy trials of plasma-derived HB vaccine took place in the early to mid-1980s, mainly in Asia. Some of these large trials are summarized in Table 1 (11,12). The protective efficacy of HBIG and vaccine ranged from 89.7 to 97.8%. These and other efficacy trials in infants will be covered in further detail in other chapters of this book. In addition, a large-scale immunization program in Taiwan that included 78% of infants born to HBsAg-positive mothers in that country found that the estimated efficacy of HBIG and vaccine was 85% in 786 infants of HBeAg-positive mothers (13).

Three of the above studies addressed the efficacy of using plasma-derived HB vaccine alone starting at birth in infants of HBsAg/HBeAg-positive mothers. Efficacy in these studies has ranged from 45.5 to 75.3% (Table 1) (9,11,12). In addition, a randomized study using vaccine alone versus HBIG plus vaccine at birth in infants of HBsAg/HBeAg-positive mothers demonstrated that 23% of the vaccine alone group became carriers versus 5% in the vaccine and HBIG group (14).

Infants of HBsAg-positive mothers who are negative for HBeAg are at a much lower risk of becoming chronic carriers, probably less than 10% (15). However, there are several case reports of severe or fulminant acute icteric hepatitis B occurring in infants of carrier mothers who are negative for HBeAg but positive for anti-HBe (16,17). Few trials of infants of HBsAg-positive/anti-HBe positive mothers have been reported, but HB vaccine plus HBIG appears to be 100% efficacious in preventing vertical transmission resulting in either the chronic carrier state or acute icteric hepatitis (18,19). In addition, one study has shown that the use of plasma-derived HB vaccine alone (MSD) was 100% efficacious in preventing the development of the carrier state in infants of HBsAg-positive mothers who were negative for HBeAg (20).

B. Efficacy Trials in Neonates Using Recombinant Vaccine

Formal efficacy trials of recombinant HB vaccines were not conducted for ethical reasons since licensed plasma-derived vaccines were so effective. However, trials of recombinant-derived HB vaccines were designed for infants of HBsAg/ HBeAg mothers using placebo controls from several of the previously cited plasma-derived vaccine trials. Table 2 shows the results of three of these trials. In two of these trials infants received either plasma-derived or recombinant vaccine (MSD) along with HBIG (21,22). The carrier rate for those infants who received plasma-derived vaccine was 10.2 and 5%, respectively, compared to 4.8 and 10% for those who received recombinant vaccines. These differences were not statistically significant. In another trial, infants of HBsAg/ HBeAg-positive mothers received four doses of Smith Kline (SK) recombinant vaccine without HBIG, and only 3.6% became chronic HBsAg carriers (23).

C. Efficacy Trials in Children

While in some areas hyperendemic for HBV infection, about 50% of HBsAg-positive pregnant women are also HBeAg positive (8), in many other hyperendemic areas such as Africa and Alaska, less than 25% of pregnant HBsAg-positive females are also HBeAg positive (19,24). In these latter areas, 80–90% of persons who become chronic carriers are not infected perinatally, but rather horizontally after birth. Even in the former areas, at least 50% of persons who became chronic carriers are infected after birth. Three studies examined the risk of becoming a chronic carrier in children infected with HBV early in life. In one prospective study from Senegal, 50% of infants infected under the age of 2 years became chronic carriers (25). In a prospective study of 1201 seronegative Alaska Natives, 6 of 21 (28.6%) persons under 5 years of age who were infected with HBV became chronic HBsAg carriers (26). In a prospective study from Taiwan, an estimated 23% of children infected under 5 years of age became chronic carriers (27). These studies illustrated the need to evaluate the efficacy of hepatitis B vaccine in preventing horizontal transmission of HBV early in life.

In 1981, the late Dr. Pierre Maupus and associates reported on a controlled efficacy trial of a plasma-derived (Pasteur) HB vaccine in children in Senegal (28). Children under 2 years of age were randomized to receive four doses of HB vaccine at 0, 1, 2, and 12 months or DPT on the same schedule. Only 4 of 238 (1.7%) initially seronegative children in the vaccine group became chronic carriers versus 14 of 195 (7.2%) in the control group, yielding a protective efficacy rate of 76%. In a study in Alaskan Eskimo children under 10 years of age, none of 563 children became HBsAg-carriers after three doses of HB plasma-derived vaccine (MSD) (29). In a small study of 30 children living in an institutionalized community for drug users where the carrier rate was 8.7%, none of the children (ages 1–14) became infected with HBV after receiving three doses of a recombinant (SKF) vaccine (30).

Table 2 Efficacy of HBIG and Recombinant Hepatitis B Vaccine in Infants of HBsAg/HBeAg-Positive Mothers

Study site (Ref.)	Vaccine used	Groups studied (no. participants)	Age of subject (months)		HBsAg carrier rate (%)	Estimated protection efficacy (%)
			HBIG	HB vaccine		
United States (21)	MSD (10 μg plasma, 5 μg recombinant)	HBIG/Plasma vx (39)	0	0,1,6	10.2	ND
		HBIG/Recombinant vx (83)	0	0,1,6	4.8	>90 (estimated)
Bangkok (22)	MSD (10 μg plasma, 5 μg recombinant)	HBIG/Plasma vx (20)	0	0,1,6	5	94.6
		HBIG/Recombinant vx (20)	0	0,1,6	10	89.2
Bangkok (23)	SK (10 μg)	Recombinant vx (55)	—	0,1,2,12	3.6	95

MSD, Merck Sharp & Dohme; SK, Smith Kline.

IV. EFFICACY TRIALS IN ADULTS

As plasma-derived hepatitis B vaccines were developed in the mid-1970s, a search began for suitable populations with a high enough incidence of HBV infection that a manageable number of patients could be recruited into controlled trials. Groups found to have a high incidence of HBV infection in the United States and Europe included homosexual males, patients on hemodialysis, healthcare workers, and patients institutionalized for mental retardation (31).

A. Efficacy Trials in Homosexual Males Using Plasma-Derived Vaccine

Homosexual males had been found to have an extremely high risk of HBV infection. In a five-city study of gay men, HBsAg was found in 6.3% and the total prevalence of HBV markers was 61% (32). Two large randomized double-blind control trials of HB vaccine in homosexual men were conducted in the United States. In New York City, Szmuness and colleagues conducted a randomized placebo-controlled, double-blind HB vaccine trial in 1083 HBV seronegative homosexual men, 549 of whom received 40 μg of HB plasma-derived vaccine (MSD) and 534 placebo (33). During the study, 45 (18.1%) of the placebo recipients versus 7 (1.4%) of the vaccine recipients developed clinical hepatitis B. In addition, in the placebo group, 70 (24.4%) acquired HBsAg and 93 (35%) acquired anti-HBc compared with 14 (3.5%) and 29 (7.6%), respectively, in the vaccine group. The efficacy of HB vaccine was 92.3% for prevention of clinical hepatitis B, 87.7% for preventing HBsAg positivity, and 78.3% for preventing any serological evidence of HBV infection. In the vaccine group, 96% developed anti-HBs levels greater than 2.1 sample radioimmunoassay units (SRU) after three doses of HB vaccine. No HBsAg-positive events occurred after three doses of HB vaccine in recipients who developed anti-HBs.

A second randomized, double-blind, placebo-controlled trial of 1402 homosexual men was conducted in five American cities used 20 μg of plasma-derived vaccine (MSD) given at 0, 1, and 6 months (34). Anti-HBs was found in 85% of vaccine recipients after three doses of HB vaccine. This was lower than the 95% response seen in the study by Szmuness and coworkers, conducted in a similar population given 40 μg of vaccine and in other studies comparing 40-μg and 20-μg doses (35,36). It was later speculated that the lower response could have resulted from some vaccine being inadvertently frozen, resulting in decreased vaccine potency (37). Regardless of this, the vaccine was highly efficacious. Vaccine recipients had a significant decrease in both symptomatic and asymptomatic HBV infection than controls, as evidenced by acquisition of anti-HBc, 110 versus 58 ($p < 0.00001$). Between 3 and 15 months after immunization, an HBsAg-positive infection was seen in 56 of the placebo recipients versus only one infection in vaccine recipients who achieved an anti-HBs level of >10 SRU. The incidence of HBV events was 0.126% in the placebo group versus 0.0025% in the vaccine recipients. The studies by Francis and by Szmuness both suggested that one or two doses of HB vaccine had a modifying effect on the severity of HBV infection in recipients who had evidence of infection in the first 3 months after initiation of the series. In the Francis study, all of the 28 persons in the placebo group who had an HBV infection in the first 3 months after the first dose were HBsAg-positive compared with 17 of 27 in the vaccine group ($p = 0.0029$).

B. Efficacy Trials in Hemodialysis Patients Using Plasma-Derived Vaccine

Three controlled trials of plasma-derived HB vaccine were performed using patients and staff in hemodialysis centers. In one study, a placebo-controlled randomized double-blind trial in 138 hemodialysis patients using Pasteur plasma-derived vaccine, 60% of the vaccine group achieved anti-HBs levels of >10 MIU (38). After the first injection, 21% of the vaccine group and 45% of the placebo group had an HBV infection ($p < 0.02$). Only two vaccine recipients compared with 12 of the placebo group had an HBV infection 60 days after the first injection, when two doses of vaccine had been given. Six months or more after all three doses had been administered, two persons in the vaccine group became infected, but none became HBsAg carriers. However, of the 10 patients in the control group who became infected, 5 became carriers. In a second randomized, double-blind, placebo-controlled trial from New York in 1311 hemodialysis patients who received 40 μg of plasma-derived vaccine (MSD), efficacy could not be demonstrated due to a low incidence of HBV infection in both the placebo and vaccine recipients (5.4 and 6.4%, respectively) (39). The lack of efficacy was attributed to (a) a low antibody response with only 50.3% of participants achieving anti-HBs levels $\geq$ 10 SRU, and (b) improvements in the United States to control HBV transmission in dialysis units resulting in a lower than anticipated infection rate. Another double-blind, placebo-controlled trial was conducted in the Netherlands in hemodialysis patients using 3 μg of heat-inactivated plasma-derived vaccine of the Dutch Red Cross (40). Anti-HBs was detected in 88% of the patients after four doses. HBV infection occurred in 30 of the placebo and 7 of the vaccine recipients for a life table attack rate of 4 and 17.8%, respectively ($p = 0.0001$). The protective efficacy was 78% from the first inoculation and 86% after 3 months.

C. Efficacy Trials in Health-Care Workers Using Plasma-Derived Vaccine

Three controlled trials using plasma-derived vaccines were conducted in health-care workers. A randomized, placebo-controlled, double-blind trial conducted in

865 staff members from 43 dialysis units in the United States demonstrated that 96% of the recipients of plasma-derived vaccine (MSD) developed anti-HBs (41). Of the placebo recipients, 25 (9.9%) had an HBV infection, compared with 9 (2.2%) of the vaccine recipients ($p < 0.01$). More important, only one HBV infection, an anti-HBc-only seroconversion, occurred in the vaccine recipients receiving three doses of vaccine. The protective efficacy of HB vaccine in the study was 76.8%. In a second randomized, placebo-controlled study in staff of hemodialysis units in the Netherlands, HBV infection occurred in only 2 of 73 recipients of Dutch Red Cross heat-inactivated vaccine, none being HBsAg positive, versus 6 of 75 placebo recipients, 5 being HBsAg positive ($p < 0.05$) (40).

In a third double-blind trial in 1330 health-care workers that was terminated after 13 months due to vaccine licensure, HBV infection occurred in five of the placebo recipients compared with one of the vaccine recipients ($p = 0.1$) (42). These studies indicated that HB vaccine was efficacious in health-care workers in addition to other high-risk groups.

D.   Studies on Postexposure Prophylaxis Using Plasma-Derived Vaccine

A few studies of active immunoprophylaxis of adults exposed to HBV utilizing HB vaccine with or without HBIG have been conducted. Two of these studies involved health-care workers who received accidental needlestick exposures from patients who were HBsAg positive. In a nonrandomized study of persons who had a needlestick exposure, 56 persons received HBIG only at 0 and one month, 28 persons received HBIG plus Pasteur plasma-derived vaccine, and 47 persons received no prophylaxis (43). No persons followed for 10 months in the passive or passive-active immunization group developed an HBV infection, as compared to 4 of 47 (8%) in the nonprophylaxed group ($p = 0.02$). In another study from Japan, 23 staff members in a hemodialysis unit who received HBIG plus plasma-derived vaccine after needlestick exposure with blood containing both HBsAg and HBeAg were compared with 33 similarly exposed staff members who received only HBIG in a previous study (44). HBV infection occurred in only one (4%) of the 23 staff members receiving passive-active immunization versus 11 (33%) staff members who received only passive prophylaxis ($p < 0.02$). In addition to health-care workers with needlestick exposure, one randomized double-blind, placebo-controlled, HB plasma–derived (MSD) vaccine trial was conducted in spouses of patients with acute HBV infection in Greece (45). After 9 months of follow-up, HBV infection had occurred in 16% of the group who received vaccine and 18.3% of the control group, a difference that was not significant. However, the vaccine group had fewer clinical infections (2.7%) than the control group (7%) and fewer infections one month after vaccination (8.7 vs. 14.7%). In a subsequent study from the same group, 143 spouses of patients with acute HBV infection were randomized to receive HBIG alone or HBIG plus vaccine (MSD) (46). There was a trend toward better protection with passive-active immunization, compared to passive prophylaxis alone, as 8 of 71 (11.3%) of the combined group versus 13 of 72 (18.1%) of the passive group alone had an HBV infection. In addition, none of the combined group had an HBV infection 3 months after prophylaxis versus five persons in the HBIG alone group.

E.   Efficacy Trials Using Recombinant Vaccines in Adults

Although placebo-controlled trials of recombinant HB vaccines in adults were not conducted, three studies of recombinant HB vaccines were performed where efficacy was calculated using historical controls. In one study among institutionalized mentally handicapped persons from Belgium, 275 seronegative persons received three doses of recombinant vaccine (SK), and anti-HBs was found in 97% of the recipients after the third dose (47). The incidence of new HBV infection was 5% during the first 8 months after the first inoculation, and no additional HBV infections took place between 8 and 24 months. This was compared to an 8.7% annual incidence in historical controls. A study to determine the efficacy of recombinant HB vaccine (SK) was performed in 278 homosexual males in Antwerp, Belgium (48). In this population group, the annual incidence of HBV infection previously had been shown to be 12%. After three doses of either 20 μg or 40 μg of vaccine, 98% of both groups developed adequate anti-HBs levels. Between the first and third dose, only two participants developed an HBV infection (anti-HBc without HBsAg), and between 6 and 36 months no other HBV infection occurred. Two factors may have contributed to the success rate of HB vaccine in this study. First, only 2% of participants were positive for HIV antibodies at the start of the study. It has been well documented that persons positive for HIV antibodies have a decreased response to HB vaccines (49,50). This may explain the higher rate of response to HB vaccine in this study than in previous studies among homosexual males. Second, surveillance of the participants indicated that during the study period there was an increased use of condoms in this cohort and a decrease in some sexually transmitted diseases, implying that behavioral changes could have been responsible for some of the decline in HBV transmission rates after vaccination.

V.   OTHER EFFICACY STUDIES

Two studies that indirectly determine efficacy have been performed in Alaska. The first study was an HB vaccine demonstration project conducted in the

Yukon-Kuskokwim Delta of southwest Alaska in a population of Yupik Eskimos shown to be at high risk of HBV infection (29,51). In this study, 3988 residents of 17 villages were tested, and 33.7% were found to have evidence of HBV infection with 8.2% being HBsAg-positive. Three doses of plasma-derived vaccine (MSD) were administered to 1581 persons, and 95% achieved anti-HBs levels of 10 SRU or greater. Since a 6-month period occurred between the initial screening and first dose of vaccine, it was possible to calculate the incidence of HBV infection during this period based on seroconversion rates and compare this incidence to the incidence after three doses of HB vaccine. The annual incidence was 50 HBV infections per 1000 persons during the 6 months prior to immunization, 19 HBV infections per 1000 persons ($p = 0.002$) during the first year after the first dose of vaccine was initiated and 0.45 per 1000 persons in the first 5 years after completion of the series.

In a second study conducted in the same area, the results of mass immunization of 90% of the area's serosusceptible population on the incidence of acute symptomatic HBV infection was assessed (52). In the area, 16,034 Alaska Natives were screened for HBV seromarkers and 9840 received three doses of vaccine. In addition, all newborns were offered HB vaccine beginning at birth. The annual incidence of acute symptomatic HBV infection fell from 215 cases per 100,000 prior to immunization to 14 per 100,000 after immunization. Since then the annual incidence has remained between 7 and 14 per 100,000 (Fig. 1).

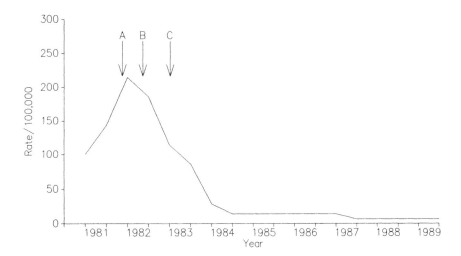

Figure 1   Incidence of acute symptomatic hepatitis B in Alaska natives living in Southwest Alaska, 1981–1989. (A) Immunization demonstration project in 17 villages begun (November 1981). (B) Immunization demonstration project completed (May 1982). (C) Mass immunization in all villages begun (March 1983).

Mass immunization of 95% of the serosusceptible residents in this area hyperendemic for HBV infection coupled with routine immunization of newborns has
dramatically reduced transmission of HBV infection.

VI. LONG-TERM EFFICACY OF HEPATITIS
B VACCINES

A few studies have been able to demonstrate that long-term protection from HBV
infection is provided in persons who respond to HB vaccines. Persons who
respond to HB vaccines have a gradual decline of anti-HBs levels over time (53).
Although the peak anti-HBs level achieved is inversely related to the age of the
vaccine, the rate of decline in anti-HBs levels over time appears to be similar in
all age groups (51). Even after anti-HBs levels become nondetectable in responders, a booster dose of HB vaccine will result in amnestic response in most
persons who have lost anti-HBs. In a study of 54 persons who had received three
doses of plasma-derived HB vaccine (MSD) 5–7 years earlier and achieved
initial anti-HB levels above 2.1 SRU, 47 of 50 had an amnestic response (53). Of
the three patients who failed to respond to a booster dose, all but one had initial
anti-HBs levels below 10 SRU. This suggests that protection from HB vaccine
outlasts the disappearance of anti-HBs.

Hadler and coworkers followed 773 male homosexuals for 5 years after
completion of the HB vaccination series (37). Anti-HBs levels were undetectable
in 15% and below 10 SRU in another 27%. In the placebo group described earlier
(34), the rate of HBV infection was 21.1 cases per 100 patient-years of follow-up
compared with only 7.9 in persons who received three doses of HB vaccine and
were followed for 5 years. The incidence of HBV infection was related to the
peak anti-HBs response after vaccination. The incidence was 16.7 cases per 100
patient-years in nonresponders, a rate similar to the control group, and 8.9 in
persons with a peak anti-HBs level below 10 SRU. In persons with an anti-HBs
level above 10 SRU, the rate varied from 8.9 to less than 3 in persons with less
than and greater than 50 SRUs, respectively (Table 3). Only two HBsAg-positive
infections occurred in vaccinees who achieved peak anti-HBs levels of 10 SRU
or greater, and both of these were mild infections with subsequent clearance of
HBsAg.

At 7–8 years postvaccination in the same homosexual cohort, only 142 of the
participants were available for follow-up (54). The proportion of persons with
anti-HBs levels above 2.1 and 10 SRU was approximately the same as in the
5-year follow-up. After 8 years of follow-up, 70 of the original 634 responders
(>10 SRU anti-HBs) had an HBV infection, but only two (3%) were HBsAg-
positive and had become chronic carriers. One of the two patients with viremia
had elevated transaminase levels, and both were positive for HIV infection.
Analysis of participants who had an excellent response to HB vaccine (>100

Table 3 HBV Infection Rates (Per 100 Person-Years of Follow-up) in Homosexual Males 5 Years After Initial Vaccination

Group	Peak anti-HBs level/SRU after 3 doses	Total HBV infection rate	HBsAg-positive rate	% Carriers
Placebo (historical)	—	21.1	13.3	8.7
Vaccinated	0	16.7	6.1	1.4
	2.1–9.9	8.9	3.0	1.4
	10–49	8.9	0.41	0
	50–99	2.7	—	0
	>100	0.74	0.08	0

Source: Ref. 37.

SRU) showed that a significantly greater proportion of persons who either were HIV positive or acquired HIV infection after starting vaccine had anti-HBs levels below 10 SRU at 5 years (63–86%) compared with participants who remained HIV negative (36%, $p < 0.01$). Despite this, long-term protection was excellent up to 8 years in high-risk homosexual males.

Another long-term follow-up study is currently being conducted in 1600 Alaska natives living in an area hyperendemic for HBV infection (51,55–57). The initial response rates to HB vaccine were discussed earlier. This population has been followed yearly, and the preliminary results through year 8 have been analyzed (Table 4). At 5 years, 79% of responders had anti-HBs levels of 10 SRU or greater. Only four breakthrough infections had occurred: three in responders and one in a person with a peak anti-HBs level of 4 SRU. All

Table 4 Long-Term Efficacy of Hepatitis B Vaccine in Alaska Natives

Group (Ref.)	% Responder with anti-HBs>10 MIU	No. breakthrough HBV infections		Total HBV infection rate per 1000
		Anti-HBc	HBsAg	
Control group	—	13	30	50
Vaccine group				
5-year f/u (51)	81%	4	0	0.45
6-year f/u (55)	—	5	0	0.36
7-year f/u (56)	74%	8	0	0.85
8-year f/u (57)	74%	10	0	—

f/u, Follow-up.

breakthrough infections were characterized by acquisition of anti-HBc with a boost in anti-HBs titer. The annual incidence of new HBV infections fell from 50 per 1000 prior to vaccination to 0.45 per 1000, a 110-fold decline. No new HBV infections occurred in vaccinated persons living in households with HBsAg-positive carriers. At 6 years, only five (one additional) breakthrough infections had occurred (55). At 7 years and at 8 years, anti-HBs levels were calculated in MIU and 74% of responders had anti-HBs levels above 10 MIU (56,57). By 8 years, 10 breakthrough infections had occurred—all asymptomatic without HBsAg. All developed anti-HBc and a boost in anti-HBs. In this high-risk population, HB vaccine is protective for at least 8 years, and no booster doses are needed at that time.

Only a few long-term studies of the efficacy of HB vaccine have been performed in infants who were vaccinated under one year of age. Coursaget et al. followed 143 children from Senegal who received their first dose of Pasteur plasma–derived vaccine at 6 weeks of age for 6 years and compared them to 135 children who were not immunized (58). The protective efficacy of HB vaccine was 87% during the 6 years after the 12-month booster dose. Between the 5th and 6th year after immunization, four infants in the vaccine group became HBsAg positive. Another study from Hong Kong also showed that some immunized infants can acquire HBsAg between 6 and 36 months after vaccination (59). Of 183 infants of HBsAg⁻/HBeAg-positive mothers who were HBsAg negative at 6 months, 8 (4%) were found to be HBsAg positive by 36 months. In a second large study of 1112 infants of HBsAg-positive mothers from Hong Kong followed up to 5 years of age, only one infant became HBsAg positive after one year of age (60). There is no mention in the two above studies from Hong Kong whether the infants who became HBsAg positive had initially responded to HB vaccine with protective levels of anti-HBs.

Three other studies showed no HBsAg-positive infections in infants of HBsAg/HBeAg-positive mothers who responded to HB vaccine and were followed for 3–6 years. In studies of 199 infants from Taiwan (61), 41 infants from the United States (62), and 80 infants from Beijing (63), no HBsAg-positive infections were observed in infants who responded to HB vaccine from 3 to 6 years postvaccination. A fourth study in 132 infants of HBsAg-positive mothers, 32 of whom were also HBeAg-positive, conducted in Montreal also demonstrated that no infants became HBsAg-positive after 9 months of age (64).

The studies in infants suggest that while HB vaccine provides excellent long-term protection for 4–6 years, HBsAg-positive breakthrough infections in vaccine responders may have occurred. It is not evident in most of these studies whether or not the infants who became HBsAg-positive during follow-up did indeed respond to HB vaccine. Nevertheless, protection for infants may not last as long as it does for children immunized at over one year of age and for adults, where no HBsAg infections have been reported, except in HIV-positive individuals, during the first 8 years of follow-up (37,51,55–57). Further evidence that booster doses may be necessary in persons immunized in infancy is provided by data that indicate that the levels of anti-HBs are significantly lower in this group when compared to persons immunized at over one year of age (51).

VII.   CONCLUSION

Both plasma-derived and recombinant HB vaccines are highly efficacious in preventing acute HBV infection. Randomized, placebo-controlled, double-blind trials using plasma-derived vaccine in high-risk infants and adults have demonstrated significant efficacy for HB vaccine. In addition, studies using recombinant-derived HB vaccine in adults and especially in infants have shown significant protective efficacy when compared to historical controls. Large-scale vaccination-demonstration projects have demonstrated dramatic drops in the incidence of HBV infection in hyperendemic areas. Finally, long-term evaluations have shown HB vaccine to be efficacious for at least 8 years in children and adults, and for 4–5 years in infants. The continuation of these long-term studies should provide information over the next few years as to when protection wanes and when booster doses may be needed.

REFERENCES

1.   Soveslavsky, O. HBV as a global problem. In Vyas, G. N., Cohen, S. N., Schmid, R., eds. Viral Hepatitis. Franklin Institute Press, Philadelphia, 1978; 347–356.
2.   Beasley, R. P. The major etiology of hepatocellular carcinoma. Cancer, 1988; 61: 1942–1956.
3.   Krugman, S., Giles, S. P., Hammond, J. Infectious hepatitis: Evidence for two distinct clinical, epidemiological and immunological types of infection. JAMA, 1967; 200: 365–373.
4.   Krugman, S., Giles, J. P., Hammond, J. Viral hepatitis type B (MS-2 strain): Studies on active immunization. JAMA, 1971; 217: 41–45.
5.   Hilleman, M. R., Bertland, A. U., Buynak, E. B., et al. Clinical and laboratory studies of HBsAg vaccine. In Vyas, G., Cohen, S. N., Schmid, R., eds. Viral Hepatitis. Franklin Institute Press, Philadelphia, 1978; 525–537.
6.   Emini, E. A., Ellis, R. W., Miller, M. J., et al. Production and immunological analysis of recombinant hepatitis B vaccine. J Infect Dis, 1986; 13 (suppl A): 3–9.
7.   Beasley, R. P., Hwang, L. Y., Stevens, C. E., et al. Efficacy of hepatitis B immune globulin for prevention of perinatal transmission of the hepatitis B carrier state: Final report of a randomized double-blind, placebo-controlled trial. Hepatology, 1983; 3: 135–141.
8.   Beasley, R. P., Hwang, L. Y., Lee, G. C. Y., et al. Prevention of perinatally transmitted hepatitis B virus infection with hepatitis B immune globulin and hepatitis B vaccine. Lancet, 1983; ii: 1099–1102.
9.   Wong, V. C. W., Ip, H. M. H., Reesink, H. W., et al.. Prevention of the HBsAg

carrier state in newborn infants of mothers who are chronic carriers of HBsAg and HBeAg by administration of hepatitis B vaccine and hepatitis B immune globulin. Lancet, 1984; i: 921–926.

10. Stevens, C. E., Toy, P. T., Tong, M. J., et al. Perinatal hepatitis B virus transmission in the United States: Prevention by passive-active immunization. JAMA, 1985; 253: 1740–1745.

11. Lo, K. J., Tsai, Y. T., Lee, S. D., et al. Immunoprophylaxis of infection with hepatitis B virus in infants born to hepatitis B surface antigen-positive carrier mothers. J Infect Dis, 1985; 152: 817–822.

12. Xu, Z. Y., Lin, C. B., Francis, D. P., et al. Prevention of perinatal acquisition of hepatiti B virus carriage using vaccine: Preliminary report of a randomized, double-blind placebo-controlled and comparative trial. Pediatrics, 1985; 5: 713–718.

13. Hsu, H. M., Chen, D. S., Chuang, C. H., et al. Efficacy of a mass hepatitis B vaccination program in Taiwan: Studies on 3464 infants of hepatiti B surface antigen-carrier mothers. JAMA, 1980; 260: 2231–2235.

14. Hwang, L. Y., Beasley, R. B., Lee, G. C. Y., et al. Prevention of perinatally transmitted hepatitis B virus infection with hepatitis B immune globulin and/or HB vaccine. In Vyas, G. N., Dienstag, J. L., Hoofnagle, J. H., eds. Viral Hepatitis and Liver Disease. Grune & Stratton, Orlando, FL, 1984; 678–679.

15. Stevens, C. E., Neurath, R. H., Beasley, R. P., Szmuness, W. HBeAg and anti-HBe detection by radioimmunoassay: Correlation with vertical transmission of hepatitis B virus in Taiwan. J Med Virol, 1979; 3: 237–241.

16. Sinatra, F. R., Shah, P., Weissman, J. Y., Thomas, D. W., Merritt, R. J., Tong, M. J. Perinatal transmitted acute icteric hepatitis B in infants born to hepatitis B surface antigen-positive and anti-hepatitis Be-positive carrier mothers. Pediatrics, 1982; 70: 557–559.

17. Tong, M. J., Sinatra, F. R., Thomas, D. W., Nair, P. V., Merritt, R. J., Wang, D. W. Need for immunoprophylaxis in infants born to HBsAg-positive carrier mothers who are HBeAg negative. J Pediatrics, 1984; 105: 945–947.

18. Schalm, S. W., Mazek, J. A., DeGast, B. C., et al. Prevention of hepatitis B infection in newborns through mass screening and delayed vaccination of all infants of mothers with hepatitis B surface antigen. Pediatrics, 1989; 83: 1041–1048.

19. Helminiak, C., McMahon, B. J., Parkinson, A. J., et al. Prevention of perinatal transmission of hepatitis B virus (HBV) in Alaska native newborns of HBsAg-positive mothers. In Coursaget, P., Tong, M. J., eds. Progress in Hepatitis B Immunization. Colloque Inserm/John Libbey Eurotext Ltd., London, 1990; 194: 389.

20. Theppisai, U., Thanuntaseth, C., Chiewsilp, P., Siripoonya, P. Long-term immunoprophylaxis of hepatitis B surface antigen carrier in infants born to hepatitis B surface antigen-positive mothers using a plasma derived vaccine. Asia—Oceania J Gynaecol, 1989; 15: 111–115.

21. Stevens, C. E., Taylor, P. E., Tong, M. J., et al. Yeast-recombinant hepatitis B vaccine: Efficacy with hepatitis B immune globulin in prevention of perinatal hepatitis B virus transmission. JAMA, 1987; 257: 2612–2616.

22. Pongpiput, D., Suvatte, V., Assateerawatts, A. Hepatitis B immunization in high risk neonates born from HBsAg-positive mothers: Comparison between plasma

derived and recombinant DNA vaccine. Asian Pac J Allergy Immunol, 1989; 7: 37–40.

23. Poovorawan, Y., Sanpavat, S., Pongpunlert, W., Chumdermpadetsuk, S., Sentrakul, P., Safary, A. Protective efficacy of a recombinant DNA hepatitis B vaccine in neonates of HBe antigen-positive mothers. JAMA, 1989; 261: 3278–3281.

24. Botha, J. F., Ritchie, M. J. J., Dusheiko, G. M., et al. Hepatitis B virus carrier state in black children in Ovamboland: Role of perinatal and horizontal infection. Lancet, 1984; i: 1210–1212.

25. Coursaget, P., Yvonnet, B., Chotard, J., et al. Age- and sex-related study of hepatitis B virus chronic carrier state in infants from an endemic area (Senegal). J Med Virol, 1987; 22: 1–5.

26. McMahon, B. J., Alward, W. L. M., Hall, D. B., et al. Acute hepatitis B infection: Relationship of age to the clinical expression of disease and the subsequent development of the carrier state. J Infect Dis, 1985; 151: 599–603.

27. Beasley, R. P., Hwang, L. Y., Lin, C. C., et al. Incidence of hepatitis B virus in preschool children in Taiwan. J Infect Dis, 1982; 146: 198–204.

28. Maupas, P., Chiron, J. P., Barin, F., Coursaget, P., Goudeau, A. Efficacy of hepatitis B vaccine in prevention of early HBsAg carrier state in children. Lancet, 1981; i: 289–292.

29. Heyward, W. L., Bender, T. R., McMahon, B. J., et al. The control of hepatitis B virus infection with vaccine in Yupik Eskimos: Demonstration of safety, immunogenicity and efficacy under field conditions. Am J Epidemiol, 1985; 121: 914–923.

30. Rumi, M. G., Romeo, R., Bortolini, M., et al. Immunogenicity of a yeast-recombinant hepatitis B vaccine in high risk children. J Med Virol, 1989; 27: 48–51.

31. Szmuness, W., Harley, E. J., Ibram, H., et al. Sociodemographic aspects of the epidemiology of hepatitis B. In Vyas, G., Cohen, S. N., Schmid, R., eds. Viral Hepatitis. Franklin Institute Press, Philadelphia, 1978: 297–320.

32. Schreeder, M. T., Thompson, S. E., Hadler, S. C., et al. Epidemiology of Hepatitis B infection in gay men. J Homosex, 1980; 5: 307–310.

33. Szmuness, W., Stevens, C. E., Harley, E. J., et al. Hepatitis B vaccine: Demonstration of efficacy in a controlled clinical trial in a high-risk population in the United States. N Engl J Med, 1980; 303: 833–841.

34. Francis, D. P., Hadler, S. C., Thompson, S. E., et al. The prevention of hepatitis B with vaccine: Report of the Center for Disease Control Multi-Center Efficacy Trial among homosexual men. Ann Intern Med, 1982; 97: 362–366.

35. Krugman, S., Holley, H. P., Jr., Davidson, M., et al. Immunogenic effect of inactivated hepatitis B vaccine: Comparison of 20 μg and 40 μg doses. J Med Virol, 1981; 8: 119–121.

36. Szmuness, W., Stevens, C. E., Harley, E. J., et al. The immune response of healthy adults to a reduced dose of hepatitis B vaccine. J Med Virol, 1981; 8: 123–129.

37. Hadler, S. C., Francis, D. P., Maynard, J. E., et al. Long-term immunogenicity and efficacy of hepatitis B vaccine in homosexual men. N Engl J Med, 1986; 315: 209–214.

38. Crosnier, J., Jungers, P., Courouce, A. M., et al. Randomized placebo-controlled trial of hepatitis B surface antigen vaccine in French hemodialysis units: II, Hemodialysis patients. Lancet, 1981; i: 797–800.

39. Stevens, C. E., Allen, H. J., Taylor, P. E., Zang, E. A., Harley, E. J., Szmuness, W. Hepatitis B vaccine in patients receiving hemodialysis: Immunogenicity and efficacy. N Engl J Med, 1984; 311: 496–501.

40. Desmyter, J., Colaert, J., DeGroote, G., et al. Efficacy of heat-inactivated hepatitis B vaccine in haemodialysis patients and staff: Double-blind placebo-controlled trail. Lancet, 1983; ii: 1323–1327.

41. Szmuness, W., Stevens, C. E., Harley, E. J., et al. Hepatitis B vaccine in medical staff of hemodialysis units: Efficacy and sub-type cross-protection. N Engl J Med, 1982; 307: 1481–1486.

42. Dienstag, J. L., Werner, B. G., Polk, B. F., et al. Hepatitis B vaccine in health care personnel: Safety, immunogenicity, and indication of efficacy. Ann Int Med, 1984; 101: 34–40.

43. Palmovic, D. Prevention of hepatitis B infection in health care workers after accidental exposure. J Infect, 1987; 15: 221–224.

44. Mitsui, T., Iwano, K., Suzuki, S., et al. Combined hepatitis B immune globulin and vaccine for post exposure prophylaxis of accidental hepatitis B virus infection in hemodialysis staff members: Comparison with immune globulin without vaccine in historical controls. Hepatology, 1989; 10: 324–327.

45. Roumeliotou-Karayannis, A., Papaevangelou, G., Tassopoulos, N., Richardson, S. C., Krugman, S. Post-exposure active immunoprophylaxis of spouses of acute viral hepatitis B patients. Vaccine, 1985; 3: 31–34.

46. Papaevangelou, G., Roumeliotou-Karayannis, A., Richardson, S. C., Nikolakakis, P., Kalafatas, P. Post exposure immunoprophylaxis of spouses of patients with acute viral hepatitis B. In Zuckerman, A. J., ed. Viral Hepatitis and Liver Disease. Alan R. Liss Inc., New York, 1980;

47. VanDamme, P., Uranckx, R., Safary, A., Andre, F. E., Meheus, A. Protective efficacy of a recombinant Deoxyribonucleic acid hepatitis B vaccine in institutionalized mentally handicapped clients. Am J Med, 1989; 87(3A): 265–295.

48. Goilav, C., Prinsen, H., Piot, P. Protective efficacy of a recombinant DNA vaccine against hepatitis B in male homosexuals: Results at 36 months. Vaccine, 1990; 8: 50–52.

49. Collier, A. C., Corey, L., Murphy, V. L., Handsfield, H. H. Antibody to human immunodeficiency virus and suboptimal response to hepatitis B vaccination. Ann Intern Med, 1988; 109: 101–105.

50. Hadler, S. C., Judson, F. N., O'Malley, P. M., et al. Outcome of hepatitis B virus infection in homosexual men and its relation to prior human immunodeficiency virus infection. J Infect Dis, 1991; 163: 454–459.

51. Wainwright, R. B., McMahon, B. J., Bulkow, L. R., et al. Duration of immunogenicity and efficacy of hepatitis B vaccine in a Yupik Eskimo population. JAMA, 1989; 261: 2362–2366.

52. McMahon, B. J., Rhoades, E. R., Heyward, W. L., et al. A comprehensive program to reduce the incidence of hepatitis B virus infection and its sequelae in Alaskan Natives. Lancet, 1987; ii: 1134–1136.

53. Krugman, S., Davidson, M. Hepatitis B vaccine: Prospects for duration of immunity. Yale J Biol Med, 1987: 333–338.

54. Hadler, S. C., Judson, P. M., O'Malley, N. L., et al. Studies of hepatitis B vaccine in homosexual men. In Coursaget, P., Tong, M. J., eds. Progress in Hepatitis B Immunization. Colloque Inserm/John Libbey Eurotext Ltd., London, 1990; 194: 165–175.

55. Wainwright, R. B., McMahon, B. Protection provided by hepatitis B vaccine in a Yupik Eskimo population. In Coursaget P and Tong, M. J., eds. Progress in Hepatitis B Immunization. Colloque Inserm/John Libbey Eurotext Ltd., London, 1990; 194: 537–538.

56. Wainwright, R. B., McMahon, B. J., Bulkow, L. R., Parkinson, A. J., Harpster, A. P. Protection provided by hepatitis B vaccine in a Yupik Eskimo population—7-year results. Arch Int Med, 1991 151: 1634–1636.

57. Wainwright, R. B., McMahon, B. J., Bulkow, L. R., Parkinson, A. J., Harpster, A. P., Hadler, S. C. Duration of immunogenicity and efficacy of hepatitis B vaccine in a Yupik Eskimo population—preliminary results of an 8-year study. In Hollinger, F. B., Lemon, S. M., Margolis, H., eds. Viral Hepatitis and Liver Disease. Williams and Wilkins, Baltimore. 1991: pp. 762–766.

58. Coursaget, P., Yvonnet, B., Chotard, J., et al. Seven year study of hepatitis B vaccine efficacy in infants from an endemic area (Senegal). Lancet, 1986; ii: 1143–1145.

59. Reesink, H. W., Henrietta, M. H., Lelie, P. N., Wong V. C. W., Kuhns, M. Prevention of the HBV carrier state in infants of HBsAg positive mothers with HB vaccine and HBIG. A three year follow-up. In Coursaget, P., and Tong, M. J., eds. Progress in Hepatitis B Immunization. Colloque Inserm/John Libbey Eurotext Ltd., London, 1990; 194: 363–370.

60. Yeoh, E. K., Young, B., Chang, W. K., Chan, Y. Y., Chau, A. Determinant of long-term efficacy and immunogenicity of hepatitis B vaccine in infants born of HBsAg carrier mothers. Hepatology, 1988; 8: 1390.

61. Lo, K. J., Lee, S. O., Tsai, Y. T., et al. Long-term immunogenicity and efficacy of hepatitis B vaccine in infants born to HBeAg-positive HBsAg-positive carrier mothers. Hepatology, 1988; 8: 1647–1650.

62. Tong, M. J., Stevens, C. E., Taylor, P. E., Toy, P. T., Vyas, G., Krugman, S. Prevention of hepatitis B infection in infants born to HBeAg positive HBsAg positive carrier mothers in the United States. An update 1989. In Coursaget, P., Tong, M. J., eds. Progress in Hepatitis B Immunization. Colloque Inserm/John Libbey Eurotext Ltd., London, 1990; 194: 339–345.

63. Liu, L. H., Wang, H. X., Wang, X. L., et al. 3 and 4 year follow-up on the efficacy of HBV vaccine combined with HBIG versus vaccine alone in the interruption of perinatal transmission. In Coursaget, P., Tong, M. J., eds. Progress in Hepatitis B Immunization. Colloque Inserm/John Libbey Eurotext Ltd., London, 1990; 194: 396–397.

64. Delage, G., Remy-Prince, S., Ducic, S., et al. Combined passive-active immunization against the hepatitis B virus of 132 newborns of chronic carrier mothers: Long term results. Pediatric Infectious Dis J. 1988; 7: 769–776.

13

Prevention of Hepatocellular Carcinoma

Juei-Low Sung, Ding-Shinn Chen, and Chin-Yun Lee

National Taiwan University, Taiwan, Republic of China

Hsu-Mei Hsu

Executive Yuan, Republic of China

Kwang-Juei Low

Veteran Administration, General Hospital, Taiwan, Republic of China

I. INTRODUCTION

Primary hepatocellular carcinoma (PHC) is one of the most common causes of cancer mortality in the world, accounting for 250,000–1,000,000 deaths per year, although there exist some geographical and racial variations in the incidence with male preponderance (1,2). A publication of the International Union Against Cancer (UICC) shows certain countries and populations, including China, Southeast Asia, and South African blacks, to have very high PHC incidences—more than 20 per every 100,000 males each year. Those areas with moderately high rates—10–20 per 100,000 males each year—include Japan, southern Europe, Switzerland, and Bulgaria (2). The incidence of PHC increases linearly with age throughout life (3). The incidence of PHC may be increasing with time in many populations (2,4).

II. ETIOLOGY OF HEPATOCELLULAR CARCINOMA

In most parts of the world, PHC is associated with cirrhosis, especially of the mixed macro-micronodular type (2,5). In Asia it is associated with 80–90% of the PHC cases (2). Most investigators believe that malignant changes arise in the regenerating nodules (6a,b).

High prevalence rates of hepatitis B surface antigen (HBsAg) were first reported in sera of patients with PHC in Taiwan in 1971 (7) and 1972 (8) using

263

less sensitive tests. After radioimmunoassay (RIA) became available, the HBsAg-positive rate was shown to be 88%, and it was also high in patients with cirrhosis (89.7%) and chronic active hepatitis (93%), far in excess of rates found in healthy persons (18%) and patients with cholangiocarcinoma (8%) and metastatic cancer of the liver (19%) (9).

Studies around the world have shown that there is a worldwide correlation between the incidence of PHC and the prevalence of the HBsAg carrier state. The incidence of both is high in the sub-Saharan African region, China, Southeast Asia, and Oceania (2,10).

In the follow-up study of HBsAg-positive chronic active hepatitis in Taiwan, 36.9% of them developed cirrhosis, and 8% of these cirrhotics terminated into PHC. In a prospective study of early detection of small PHCs by periodic real-time ultrasonography (US), the annual incidence of PHC in HBsAg-positive patients with cirrhosis was 3.4% during mean follow-up of 20.0 months (11).

A prospective study done in Taiwan by Beasley et al. showed that there exists a remarkably high risk for PHC among males positive for HBsAg; 113 cases of PHC developed among the 3454 HBsAg carrier males and 3 cases of PHC among 19,253 HBsAg-negative males, a relative risk of 217 (10). These clinical, seroimmunological, and epidemiological studies have clearly shown the importance of chronic hepatitis B virus (HBV) infection in the development of PHC. HBV markers such as HBsAg, hepatitis B core antigen (HBcAg), and HBV DNA can be demonstrated in the liver cells of PHC patients (12).

At least three viruses containing double-stranded DNA similar to human HBV DNA are found in animals: woodchuck (*Marmota monax*), Beechy ground squirrel (*Spermophilus beecheyi*), and Peking duck (*Anas domesticus*). In woodchuck the infections are transmitted vertically, and PHC develop in many chronic carriers (13,14). Additional evidence linking HBV and PHC comes from the woodchuck hepatitis virus (WHV)/woodchuck model (15). Among 41 woodchucks infected by inoculation of WHV at birth, 32% became chronic carriers. After 48 months, 92% of chronic carriers developed PHC. During the same period, none of the 46 uninfected developed PHC (16). This study suggests that WHV is carcinogenic without an exogenous carcinogen, and probably the same applies to HBV.

In the past 10 years to search the direct oncogenesis of HBV, clonally integrated HBV DNA sequences has been studied. Integration of HBV DNA into the host cell lines is detected in many PHC cell lines, and in most of the PHC tissues from HBsAg-positive patients up to 92.5% or more (17). However, integration of HBV DNA does not seem to be necessary to maintain the neoplastic state, although it could be necessary to initiate neoplasia. A transfoming gene, *Lca*, was isolated from an PHC DNA by NIH 3T3 transformation assay, but needs to be confirmed and further characterized (18).

In transgenic mice which overproduce HBV large envelope polypeptide, severe and prolonged hepatocellular injury develops that initiates a programmed response within the liver, characterized by inflammation, regenerative hyperplasia, transcriptional deregulation, and aneuploidy. This response progresses to neoplasia (19).

Recently, the recombination of a truncated *C-myc* gene with a cellular gene for W64 PHC was demonstrated. *C-myc* alterations might occur after a long preneoplastic period with chronic stimulation, provoked in some cases by HBV, which favors chromosomal breaks, and finally leads to oncogene activation and to the development of PHC in woodchuck and humans (20).

Although molecular biology studies have so far not provided any definitive explanation for the role of HBV in liver oncogenesis, very intimate association between chronic HBV infection and development of PHC has been demonstrated. Therefore, it is very likely that control of HBV infection, especially chronic infection, will reduce the incidence of cirrhosis of the liver as well as PHC dramatically in hyperendemic area of HBV infection. In the nonendemic areas of HBV, other factors, particularly alcoholism (21) and possibly mycotoxin, i.e., aflatoxin (22), appear to be incriminated.

It was suggested that non-A, non-B viruses may act to trigger development of PHC (23). It has now been shown that many patients with chronic cryptogenic and posttransfusion non-A, non-B hepatitis, HBsAg-negative cirrhosis, and HBsAg-negative PHC have antibodies (anti-C 100-3) against recently the identified hepatitis C virus (HCV). In HBsAg-negative patients with cirrhosis and PHC, anti-C 100-3 was positive in 81.4% in Spain (24), in 70% in Italy (25), in 62.5% in Taiwan (26), and in 76.2% in Japan (27), strongly suggesting that HCV might also cause PHC.

III. IMPROVEMENT OF PROGNOSIS OF PRIMARY HEPATOCELLULAR CARCINOMA

The prognosis of this malignancy is thought to be extremely poor, with a mean survival of several months. The preexistence of cirrhosis and the difficulty of early detection are recognized as major contributing factors. With the discovery of new devices, improvements of methods of operation, and better preoperative and postoperative care, operation mortality has been reduced from 25% in the 1960s to less than 10% (28).

After the value of alpha fetal protein (AFP) in the diagnosis of PHC was recognized, rather small and small PHCs began to be detected (28–30). Since then several groups of investigators have tried to use serum AFP determination for screening and regular follow-up of high-risk populations to detect small PHC (29,30). In the high-risk area of the Qidong district of eastern China, many asymptomatic PHCs were discovered by such a screening. Among 475 PHCs detected in this screening, 35.2% of the tumors were less than 5 cm in diameter, and the 2-year survival rate was 69% (31).

However, in our own experience, among 33 cases of PHC detected using

AFP surveillance, 41% had tumors larger than 5 cm in diameter, and in 128 cases of PHCs with tumors smaller than 5 cm in diameter, 28.9% had a serum AFP less than 20 ng/ml. Of the 39 cases with tumors smaller than 2 cm in diameter, serum AFP presented in 35.9% (11). The results indicate that AFP has inadequate sensitivity as a tool for early detection of PHC. In addition, elevation of AFP is not diagnostic and cannot be used to locate tumors.

With the advent of high-resolution linear array and convex real-time scanner in US, a hepatic tumor as small as 1 cm in diameter can be detected within 15 minutes, and the diagnosis can be confirmed by US-guided aspiration cytology or biopsy (32,33). Extrapolated from the data obtained in our study on the doubling time of tumors, the suitable screening interval for early detection of small PHC was set at 4–5 months (34).

In our prospective study of early detection of PHC by periodic real-time US, which started in April 1981 and was comprised of 1313 subjects, including some regarded as at high risk or moderate risk of PHC, the initial screening showed a total of 45 patients to have PHCs. In the subsequent US follow-ups repeated every 4–6 months for 348.3 man-years (average 1.8 years), another 24 cases of PHC (2.1%) were found among the remaining 1128 patients, 23 (4.7%) among the 494 cirrhotics, and 1 (0.2%) of the 427 HBsAg carriers. Among them, 37.6% of tumors were smaller than 2 cm in diameter, 66.7% were smaller than 3 cm, 29.2% were between 3 and 5 cm, and only one was larger than 5 cm (11,30).

Concerning the treatment of PHC, surgical resection is still the treatment of choice at the present time if the tumor is small enough for resection and the liver can tolerate operation. In cases where hepatic resection is not suitable or acceptable, percutaneous transcatheter arterial embolization (TAE) with anticancer drugs has been applied with good effect, especially with Lipiodol-chemoembolization (11,35–37). Recently several investigators treated small PHC by US-guided percutaneous intratumor absolute ethanol injection (PEI) with good response (11,37–40), especially in PHCs less than 2 cm in diameter, with a 4-year survival rate of 74% out of 50 cases (40).

In the series of PHCs admitted to Zhong Shan Hospital in Shanghai from January 1971 to December 1982, the 5-year survival rate was 43.9% among 100 subclinical PHCs, in sharp contrast to 4.2% in the whole series and 16.1% in the resection group among 477 clinical PHCs. The resection rate was 60.0% in the subclinical group and 24.7% in the clinical group (31). The Liver Cancer Study Group in Japan issued a report on a follow-up survey of PHCs between the years 1984 and 1985, done in 507 hospitals, involving 7320 cases. The operation rate was 19.5%, and the 5-year survival rate was 28.5% (38).

In the survival rate calculation using life table analysis in 190 patients with PHCs smaller than 5 cm in diameter in Taiwan, the 5-year survival rate was 42.7% in the resection group and 43.6% in the TAE group, and the 4-year survival rate was 20.8% in the PEI group, showing a drastic difference from the nontreated group, which had a 4-year survival rate of only 3% (11,37). However, during follow-ups of 100 patients with PHC who received surgical resection, recurrence developed in 57% within 6 years, showing a high rate of recurrence not only due to metastasis but also possibly due to multicentric origins of PHC.

In addition, for the above-mentioned improvement of prognosis, great efforts were made and a substantial amount of money was spent. The methods applied may not be acceptable in many developed countries because of the low incidence of PHC or in developing areas because of high cost and lack of technology. Therefore, a safe, effective, and less expensive prevention method for PHC is needed.

IV.   PREVENTION OF HBV INFECTION

Transmission of HBV occurs vertically from HBV-infected persons, especially from hepatitis B e antigen (HBeAg) positive mothers. Horizontal infection plays a large part in HBV dissemination. However, in the Asian-Pacific region, the primary mode of transmission is vertical, from HBeAg-positive mothers to their newborn babies (41–45) (see also Chapter 11). Such maternal transmission plays a very important role in the number of chronic HBsAg carriers in ethnic groups such as Chinese (41,43–45), where a large proportion of the women of childbearing age are HBeAg positive (46).

Since the initial licensure in 1981 for plasma-derived hepatitis B vaccine, more than 12 commercial producers have marketed the vaccine globally. Experiences with these products have demonstrated that they are safe and highly efficacious. For maternal transmission from HBeAg-positive women, the combination of hepatitis B immunoglobulin (HBIG) and hepatitis B vaccine is more effective than either alone, resulting in an HBsAg carrier rate of only 5–10% (49–51).

There have been few long-term follow-up studies with a limited number of vaccinees reported that antibodies to HBsAg (anti-HBs) dropped gradually as the infants grew up, but a substantial level of anti-HBs persists in the majority of vaccinees, and HBV infection was almost unknown during the first 4–5 years (52–55). The natural booster phenomenon was seen, and none had seroconverted to HBsAg or anti-HBc (53). Therefore, it is likely that no booster vaccination is needed during preschool age only if primary vaccination is complete (53,55).

In 1986 yeast-derived hepatitis B vaccines by two manufacturers made by recombinant DNA technologies were licensed. More recently, mammalian cells have been used to express hepatitis B surface antigens, and the products are undergoing human clinical trials.

Several studies have reported that both the immunogenicity and protective efficacy of yeast-recombinant hepatitis B vaccine are comparable with plasma-derived vaccine (54,56–58). Following prophylaxis, the HBsAg carrier rate in infants of HBeAg⁻/HBsAg-positive mothers who received immunoprophylaxis with HBIG plus vaccine was 3.8% in the yeast-recombinant vaccine group and 13.9% in the plasma-derived vaccine group, and the anti-HBc positivity was 1.6% in the former and 5.6% in the latter group (54). Therefore, yeast-recombinant hepatitis B vaccine is equivalent in preventing chronic antigenemia in newborns and in preventing HBV infection.

V. PRELIMINARY STUDY OF THE EFFICACY OF MASS IMMUNIZATION FOR CONTROL OF HBV INFECTION AND ITS SEQUELAE—CIRRHOSIS OF LIVER AND HEPATOCELLULAR CARCINOMA

In Taiwan, cancer is the leading cause of death, and within cancer deaths PHC ranks number 1 in terms of mortality rate, especially in males. The adjusted death rate among males is 31.68 per 100,000. Cirrhosis of the liver is also prevalent, ranking number 6 among the leading causes of death (3). In these two diseases, HBsAg is positive in 85% and anti-HBc in 98% of cases (9,59).

On the other hand, HBV infection as well as HBsAg carriage are prevalent. The first mode of HBV transmission is from HBeAg-positive HBsAg carrier mothers to their infants, with a 95% chance of infection and an 85% chance of infected infants becoming chronic carriers (60), and that is followed by horizontal transmission, making the HBV infection rate more than 80% and HBsAg carrier rate 19% of the population before the fourth decade of life and 12% after the third decade of life. The estimated number of HBsAg carriers in Taiwan in 1979 was 2.9 million out of 17.5 million population (44).

Most of the HBsAg carriers and HBsAg-positive patients with PHC develop HBV infection maternally or horizontally during childhood (44,47,48,61). The rate of positivity of HBeAg in asymptomatic HBsAg carriers in Taiwan is shown to be higher than that in Caucasians (46), and the HBeAg positivity in pregnant women is 8% (59). This phenomenon contributes to the high HBsAg-positivity rates in Taiwan. It has been estimated that as many as 25–30% of individuals who became chronic HBV carriers and have an estimated life expectancy of at least 30 years at the time of infection will die of HBV-induced cirrhosis or HCC (10).

After studies in Taiwan showed that one dose of intramuscular HBIG at birth plus vaccination using a plasma-derived vaccine (Merck Sharp & Dohme or Pasteur Institute) is safe and highly effective in preventing perinatal infection from HBeAg-positive mothers in 96% (50) and 88% (51) of cases, a nationwide mass vaccination program against HBV infection was planned. The Pasteur Institute agreed to provide technical assistance to found a plant for the production of plasma-derived hepatitis B vaccine in Taiwan.

The priorities of nationwide mass hepatitis B immunization were determined by the relative risk of HBV infection and the likelihood of the development of chronic HBsAg carriage after infection (Table 1) (61).

All newborn infants are given a plasma-derived vaccine (HEVAC B, Institute Pasteur Production), 5 μg intramuscularly at 1, 5, and 9 weeks with a booster at 12 months. Those infants born to highly infectious carrier mothers receive an additional 0.5 ml of HBIG (HyperHep, Cutter Laboratories) intramuscularly no later than 24 hours after birth (62).

To identify highly infectious pregnant women, HBsAg is screened for at the third trimester, and all HBsAg-positive serum samples are tested for HBeAg by enzyme immunoassay or RIA; when an HBeAg test is unavailable, serum HBsAg is titrated by the reversed passive hemagglutination (RPHA) at a dilution of 2560. HBsAg-positive women with HBeAg-positivity or a reciprocal HBsAg RPHA titer $\geq$ 2560 are classified as highly infectious (62).

Cost/benefit calculations show that nationwide mass hepatitis B immunization to newborns is cost-effective; the cost of nationwide mass immunization to newborns for 10 years is $222,000,000, which is much less expensive than the cost of medical care and lost income—$318,000,000—for patients suffering from chronic HBV infection for 10 years (59). This program was started in 1984 after a preparation period of 3 years.

Table 1 Priorities and Timetable of Mass Hepatitis B Vaccination Program in Taiwan

Priority of vaccination	Year Schedule									
	1984	1985	1986	1987	1988	1989	1990	1991	1992	1993
Newborns of HBsAg[a] carrier mothers	X	X								
All newborns[b]			X	X	X	X	X	X	X	X
All children ≤ 5 years old				X	X	X				
Susceptible medical personnel				X						
Susceptible household of HBsAg carriers					X	X	X			
Susceptible persons										
6–9 years old					X	X	X			
10–19 years old						X	X	X		
20–39 years old							X	X	X	
≥40 years old								X	X	X

[a]HBsAg indicates hepatitis B surface antigen.
[b]Screening of highly infectious HBsAg-carrier mothers will continue.

For evaluation of the efficacy of the nationwide hepatitis B immunization program, a 5-year follow-up study was planned, which was later extended to 10 years. Infants who finished the immunization program were selected from different areas and divided into four groups according to maternal HBV status, such as highly infectious (HBeAg-positive or HBsAg RPHA-positive at 1:2560 dilution) and less infectious (HBeAg-negative or HBsAg-negative at 1:2560 dilution), and further divided into 10 subgroups according to immunization status as follows: among infants born to highly infectious mothers, some received the scheduled HBIG and vaccine on time, some received HBIG and vaccine but not on time, and some received the vaccine on time but omitted the scheduled HBIG; among infants born to less infectious mothers, some received vaccine on time and some received vaccine but not on time.

To cover the loss of persons in follow-up, more subjects (508) were selected by simple random sampling from each stratified group. Local public health nurses visited each randomly selected infant, filled out a simple home-visit questionnaire, and drew 3 ml of venous blood 18 months after birth and then every year for 5 years. All serological tests were performed at the Hepatitis Standard Laboratory of the National Institute of Preventive Medicine, including HBsAg, anti-HBs, and anti-HBc by RIA and levels of anti-HBs were expressed in mIU/ml (63).

According to the schedule, the evaluation program was started on July 1, 1984. During the first 5 years, 1,657,640 infants were born; the annual rate of screening of HBV markers was 77.2% (76.6–77.8%), the HBsAg positivity rate 16.6% (16.1–17.7%), the positivity rate of HBeAg and its equivalent among HBsAg-positives 47.2% (44.3–50.6%). The coverage rate of HBIG was 72.6% (65.4–82.8%), and the coverage rates of vaccine were 93.3% (92.3–95.1%) for the first, 90.5% (89.3–90.9%) for the second, 87.7% (86.3–89.5%) for the third, and 75.8% (75.1–81.6%) for the fourth dose. For analysis of the efficacy of this nationwide mass hepatitis B immunization program, 4163 infants born to HBsAg-positive mothers were randomly selected from the 10 subgroups according to the protocol and were bled at 18, 24, 36, and 48 months of age (66).

Among 20,047 infant vaccinees born to highly infectious HBsAg-positive mothers, the HBsAg positivity rates and the efficacy rates of protection from yielding chronic HBsAg carrier state at the age of 48 months were 13.6 and 84.9% in those who received HBIG plus vaccine on schedule as expected according to the trial studies; 18.2 and 79.8% in those who received vaccine but omitted HBIG; and 18.8 and 79.1% in those off schedule (Table 2). The HBsAg positivity rate was lower and the efficacy rates were higher in those who received HBIG plus vaccine than in those who omitted HBIG ($p < 0.005$), supporting the usefulness of the addition of HBIG to vaccine observed in small-scale studies of similar high-risk infants (49–51,53,54).

Among the remaining 22,425 infant vaccinees born to less infectious HBsAg-

Table 2 Protective Efficacy of Immunization Among 20,047 Infants Born to Highly Infectious Mothers by Different Compliance of Immunization and by Age in Nationwide Mass Hepatitis B Immunoprophylaxis in Taiwan

July 1984– June 1988	18 mo. (%)		24 mo. (%)		36 mo. (%)		48 mo. (%)	
	HBsAg	Efficacy	HBsAg	Efficacy	HBsAg	Efficacy	HBsAg	Efficacy
HBIG + vaccine	14.2	84.4	14.7	83.7	14.0	84.4	13.6	84.9
Vaccine only, no HBIG	19.7	78.1	23.4	74.0	19.6	78.2	18.2	79.8
Off schedule	17.0	81.1	19.1	78.8	18.9	79.0	18.8	79.1

positive mothers, HBsAg positivity rates at 18 and 48 months of age were 3.0 and 3.7% for those who received vaccine on schedule and 6.4 and 5.0% for those who did not receive vaccine on time. The anti-HBs positivity rates at 18 and 48 months of age were 85.4 and 85.9% for the former group and 83.4 and 84.8% for the latter. Nonresponse to hepatitis B vaccine appeared in 3.0–3.7% of those on schedule and in 5.0–6.4% of those off schedule.

The titers of anti-HBs have been shown to be related to the time of persistence of anti-HBs (53,54). The distribution of anti-HBs titers at age 18, 24, 36, and 48 months showed that an anti-HBs titer higher than 10 mIU/ml (the effective titer for prevention) appeared in 78.9% at age 18 months and decreased to 70.1% at 48 months of age with GMT $\pm$ SD of 255 $\pm$ 8 at 18 months decreasing to 87 $\pm$ 7 at 48 months of age (Table 3).

There were no definite changes in prevalence rates of HBsAg or anti-HBs during the 4 years after immunization. However, there were gradual increases, though slight, in the prevalence rates of anti-HBc, from 25.5–27.1% at 18 months of age to 28.6–32.3% at 48 months of age in those born to highly infectious HBsAg-positive mothers, and from 5.9–8.3% at 18 months of age to 7.4–10.1% at 48 months of age in those born to less infectious HBsAg-positive mothers, suggesting that new HBV infections developed in 4% of the former group and 2% in the latter group between 18 and 48 months but healed, leaving no increase of the HBsAg positivity rate.

Among 235 HBsAg-positive 18-month-old infants, 87.2% continued to be positive for HBsAg, 10.5% showed seroconversion to anti-HBs, 0.5% showed anti-HBc alone, and 1.7% turned seronegative at the age of 48 months (Table 4).

In 1545 anti-HBs-positive and anti-HBc-negative vaccinees who were followed regularly for 36 months, annual incidence of HBV infection was 2.2–3.8%. However among those with new HBV infection, seroconversion to anti-HBs appeared in 82.8–78.0% and HBsAg positivity in 11.5–18.6%, making the increase of HBsAg positivity only 0.6–0.9% (Table 5).

Table 3 Prevalence Rates of Anti-HBs, Anti-HBs Higher Than 10 mIU/ml, HBsAg, Anti-HBc, and Nonresponder in 22,425 Newborn Infant Vaccinees Born to Less Infectious, HBeAg-negative HBsAg-positive Mothers by Age in Nationwide Mass Vaccination in Taiwan

July 1984–June 1988	18 mo.	24 mo.	36 mo.	48 mo.
Anti-HBs+ (%)				
On schedule	85.4	92.4	89.0	85.9
Off schedule	83.2	85.7	85.8	84.8
Anti-HBs > 10 mIU/ml (%)				
On schedule	78.9	81.5	78.1	70.1
Off schedule	70.2	79.3	76.7	71.0
HBsAg+ (%)				
On schedule	3.0	3.7	3.5	3.7
Off schedule	6.4	5.4	5.4	5.0
Nonresponder (%)				
On schedule	3.0	3.7	3.5	3.7
Off schedule	6.4	5.4	5.4	5.0

Using data obtained from the above-mentioned evaluation studies on the efficacy of the nationwide mass hepatitis B immunization and some historical data, the HBsAg positivity rate in people born in the first several years after 1986 when all newborn infants were intended to be recruited in the program, according to the calculation listed in Table 6, is estimated to be 2.3%. This rate decreased to 0.2% several years later, in accordance with the steady decrease in the number of carriers, in infants as well as in students (the main infectious sources of horizontal transmission).

Table 4 Persistence of Anti-HBs in Vaccine Responders Observed at Age of 48 months

HBV status at 48 mo.	Time when anti-HBs+					
	18 mo.		24 mo.		36 mo.	
	No.	%	No.	%	No.	%
HBsAg+	11	0.6	15	0.9	13	0.8
Anti-HBs+	1649	95.9	1616	96.6	1657	96.2
Anti-HBc alone	6	0.4	5	0.3	6	0.4
Seronegative	54	3.1	37	2.2	46	2.7
Total	1720	100	1643	100	1722	100

Table 5 Occurrence of HBV Infection in Anti-HBs-Positive, Anti-HBc-Negative Vaccinees Regularly Followed for 48 Months

	Time anti-HBs+, anti-HBc–					
	18 mo. (n = 1582)		24 mo. (n = 1582)		36 mo. (n = 1582)	
HBV status at 48 mo.	No.	%	No.	%	No.	%
HBsAg	10	11.5	14	14.6	11	18.6
Anti-HBs	72	82.8	79	82.3	46	78.0
Anti-HBc alone	5	5.7	3	3.1	2	33.4
Total	87	100.0	96	100.0	59	100.0
Annual incidence (%)[a]		5.5		6.1		3.1

[a]HBV infection defined as HBsAg or anti-HBc seroconversion in a vaccinee.

Table 6 Calculation of HBsAg Prevalence Rate After Nationwide Mass Hepatitis B Immunoprophylaxis to All Newborn Infants in Taiwan

			HBsAg positivity	
			%	Number
Annual birth number between July 1984 and June 1989:		331,528		
Screening of HBsAg	77.2%	255,854		
HBsAg+	16.6%	42,472		
HBeAg+ or equivalent	42.2%	20,047		
HBIG + vaccine on schedule	72.6%	14,554	14%	2,038
Vaccine only or off schedule	27.4%	5,493	19%	1,044
HBeAg– or equivalent	52.8%	22,425		
On schedule	46.5%	10,428	3.7%	395
Off schedule	53.4%	11,997	5%	600
HBsAg–				
With vaccine		161,744	0.2%	349
No vaccine		51,638	18%	929
Escape screening	22.8%	75,574		
With vaccine	78.8%	57,285	0.2%	115
No vaccine	24.2%	18,389	18%	3,313
Total		331,528	2.3%	7,505

Source: Refs. 44, 53.

VI. DISCUSSION AND CONCLUSION

A nationwide mass HBV immunoprophylaxis for newborn infants has been shown to be feasible and effective in hyperendemic areas, such as Taiwan. This should be a significant step toward the control of HBV infection and will result in a dramatic decrease in incidence of cirrhosis of the liver and PHC.

However, this program is costly and requires great effort in the areas of education, testing, and registration for screening and frequent injection. Therefore, a program not using HBIG should be considered. Although the efficacy rate may drop from 84 to 79% in those who only receive vaccine, much of the cost, work, and hazards can be eliminated.

In our program, four doses of vaccine were given, and the coverage rate of vaccine decreased from 93.3% for the first dose to 87.7% for the third to 75.8% for the fourth. Experience, including in Taiwan, has shown three doses of vaccine to have the same efficacy rate (49,50,54). Therefore, one can use a three-dose schedule and follow WHO's recommendation to include hepatitis B vaccine in the Expanded Program on Immunization (EPI) as the seventh universal immunogen. We expect to have available more recombinant-derived immunogenic hepatitis B vaccine, which could reduce the vaccination to two doses in the future.

Excellent immunogenicity and efficacy of the licensed recombinant DNA, yeast-derived hepatitis B vaccine (54,56) were also demonstrated in Taiwan (57,58). We believe that the recombinant hepatitis B vaccine may decrease the cost of vaccination considerably and lead to an effective program of global prevention and control of HBV infection as well as its sequelae, including chronic hepatitis, cirrhosis of the liver, and PHC.

REFERENCES

1.   A. J. Zuckerman, Report of a W.H.O. scientific group, *Lancet*, 1:463 (1983).
2.   K. Okuda and R. P. Beasley, Epidemiology of hepatocellular carcinoma, *Hepatocellular Carcinoma* (K. Okuda and I. Mackay, eds.), UICC Report 17, Geneva, p. 9 (1982).
3.   M. W. Yu, S. F. Tsai, K. H. Hsu, S. L. You, S. S. Lee, T. M. Lin, and C. J. Chen, Epidemiologic characteristics of malignant neoplasms in Taiwan: II. Liver cancer, *J. Natl. Public Health Assoc. (R.O.C.)*, 8:125 (1988).
4.   K. Okuda, I. Fujimoto, A. Hanai, and Y. Urano, Changing incidence of hepatocellular carcinoma in Japan, *Cancer Res.*, 47:4967 (1987).
5.   H. M. Cameron, The pathology of liver cancer, *Liver Cell Cancer* (H. M. Cameron, D. A. Linsell, and G. P. Warwick, eds.) Elsevier, Amsterdam, p. 17 (1976).
6a. P. P. Anthony, C. L. Vogel, and L. F. Baker, Liver cell dyplasia: A premalignant condition, *J. Clin. Pathol.*, 26:217 (1973).
6b. P. P. Anthony, Precursor lesions for liver cancer in humans, *Cancer Res.*, 36:2579 (1976).

7. M. J. Tong, S. C. M. Sun, B. T. Schaefer, N. K. Chang, K. J. Lo, and R. L. Peters, Hepatitis-associated antigen and hepatocellular carcinoma in Taiwan, *Ann. Int. Med.*, *75*:687 (1971).

8. J. L. Sung, T. Sekine, T. M. Lin, K. Nishioka, M. Mayumi, Y. F. Liaw, and C. H. Liu, Hepatitis-associated antigen in hepatocellular carcinoma, *J. Formosan Med. Assoc.*, *71*:505 (1972).

9. J. L. Sung and D. S. Chen, Hepatitis B surface antigen and antibody in liver disease in Taiwan, *Proceedings of the 5th Asian Pacific Congress of Gastroenterology*, Singapore, p. 265 (1976).

10. R. P. Beasley and L. Y. Huang, Epidemiology of hepatocellular carcinoma, *Viral Hepatitis and Liver Disease* (G. N. Vyans, J. L. Dienstag, and J. H. Hoofnagle, eds.), Grune & Stratton, Orlando, FL, p. 209 (1984).

11. J. L. Sung, D. S. Chen, J. C. Shen, G. T. Huang, M. Y. Lai, P. M. Yang, J. T. Lin, T. H. Wang, C. Y. Wang, C. S. Lee, Y. M. Tsang, and H. C. Hsu, Hepatocellular carcinoma: Early detection and treatment, *Viral Hepatitis and Liver Disease* (F. B. Hollinger, S. M. Lemon, and H. S. Margolis, eds.), Williams & Wilkins, Baltimore (in press).

12. M. D. Kew, Hepatoma and HBV, *Viral Hepatitis* (G. N. Vyas, S. N. Cohen, and R. Schmidt, eds.) Franklin Institute Press, p. 439 (1978).

13. W. S. Manson, G. Seal, and J. Summers, Virus of Peking duck with structural and biological relatedness to human hepatitis B virus, *J. Virol*, *36*:829 (1980).

14. W. S. Robinson, P. C. Marion, and M. Feinston, The hepadna virus group: Hepatitis and related viruses, *Viral Hepatitis* (W. Szmuness, H. J. Alter, and J. E. Maynard, eds.) Franklin Institute Press, Philadelphia, p. 57 (1982).

15. H. Popper, L. Roth, R. H. Purcell, B. C. Tennant, and J. L. Gerin, Hepatocarcinogenicity of the woodchuck hepatitis virus, *Proc. Nat. Acad. Sci. U.S.A.*, *84*:866 (1987).

16. B. C. Tennant, W. E. Hornbuckle, J. M. King, P. J. Cote, H. Popper, and J. L. Gerin, HCC following experimental woodchuck hepatitis virus infection, *Viral Hepatitis and Hepatocellular Carcinoma* (J. L. Sung and D. S. Chen, eds.), Excerpta Medica, Current Clinical Practice Series 57, Hong Kong, p. 678 (1990).

17. M. Y. Lai, D. S. Chen, P. J. Chen, S. C. Lee, J. C. Sheu, G. T. Huang, T. C. Wei, C. S. Lee, S. C. Yu, H. C. Hsu, and J. L. Sung, Status of hepatitis B virus DNA in hepatocellular carcinoma: A study based on paired tumor and nontumor liver tissues, *J. Med. Virol.*, *25*:249 (1990).

18. T. Ochiya, A. Fujiyama, S. Fukushige, I. Hatada, and K. Matsubara, Molecular cloning of an oncogene from human hepatocarcinoma cells, *Proc. Nat. Acad. Sci. U.S.A.* p. 4993 (1986).

19. F. V. Chisari, K. Klopchin, T. Moriyama, C. Pasquinelli, H. A. Dunsford, S. Sell, C. A. Pinkert, R. L. Brinster, and R. D. Palmiter, Molecular pathogenesis of hepatocellular carcinoma in hepatitis B virus transgenic mice, *Cell*, *59*:1145 (1989).

20. T. Moroy, A. Marchio, J. Ttiemble, H. De The, M.-A. Buendia, P. Tiollais, and A. Dejean, Two different mechanisms for hepatitis B virus-induced hepatocellular carcinoma, *Viral Hepatitis and Liver Disease* (A. J. Zuckerman, ed.), Alan R. Liss, Inc., New York, p. 737 (1988).

21. C. S. Lieber, H. K. Seitz, and J. A. Garro, Alcohol-related diseases and carcinogenesis, *Cancer Res.*, *39*:2863 (1979).

22. G. N. Wogan. Aflatoxins and their relationship to hepatocellular carcinoma, *Hepatocellular Carcinoma* (K. Okuda and R. L. Peters, eds.), John Wiley & Sons, New York, p. 25 (1976).

23. J. Gilman, J. R. Geisinger, and J. E. Richter, Primary hepatocellular carcinoma, *Ann. Intern Med.*, *101*:794 (1984).

24. J. Bruix, J. M. Barrhea, X. Calvet, G. Ercilla, J. Costa, J. M. Sanchez-Tapias, M. Ventura, M. Vall, M. Bruguera, C. Bru, R. Castillo, and J. Rodes, Prevalence of antibodies to hepatitis C virus in Spanish patients with hepatocellular carcinoma and hepatic cirrhosis, *Lancet*, *2*:1004 (1989).

25. M. Colombo, G. Kuo, Q. L. Choo, M. F. Donato, E. Del Ninno, M. A. Tommasini, N. Dioguardi, and M. Honghton, Prevalence of antibodies to hepatitis C virus in Italian patients with hepatocellular carcinoma, *Lancet*, *2*:1006 (1989).

26. D. S. Chen, G. C. Kuo, J. L. Sung, M. Y. Lai, J. C. Shen, P. J. Chen, P. M. Yang, H. M. Hsu, M. H. Chang, C. J. Chen, L. C. Hahn, Q. L. Choo, T. H. Wang, and M. Honghton, Hepatitis C virus infection in an area hyperendemic for hepatitis B and chronic liver disease: The Taiwan experience, *J. Infect. Dis.*, *162*:817 (1990).

27. K. Nishioka, J. Watanabe, S. Furuta, E. Tanaka, S. Iino, H. Suzuki, T. Tsuji, M. Yano, G. Kuo, Q. L. Choo, M. Houghton, and T. Oda, A high prevalence of antibody to the hepatitis C virus in patients with hepatocellular carcinoma, *Cancer*, *67*:429 (1991).

28. T. Y. Lin, C. S. Lee, K. M. Chen and C. C. Chen, Role of surgery in the treatment of primary carcinoma of the liver: A 31-year experience. *Br. J. Surg.*, *74*:839 (1987).

29. Z. Y. Tang, Screening and early treatment of primary liver cancer—with special reference to the east part of China, *Ann. Acad. Med. Singapore*, *9*:234 (1980).

30. J. C. Hsu, J. L. Sung, D. S. Chen, M. Y. Lai, T. H. Wang, J. Y. Yie, P. M. Yang, C. N. Chuang, P. C. Yang, C. S. Lee, H. C. Hsu and S. W. How, Early detection of hepatocellular carcinoma by real-time ultrasonography, *Cancer*, *56*:660 (1985).

31. Z. Y. Tang, Surgical treatment of subclinical hepatocellular carcinoma, *Subclinical Hepatocellular Carcinoma* (Z. Y. Tang, ed.), Springer-Verlag, Berlin, p. 54 (1985).

32. K. Okuda, Advances in hepatobiliary ultrasonography, *Hepatology*, *1*:662 (1981).

33. J. C. Sheu, J. L. Sung, D. S. Chen, J. Y. Yu, T. H. Wang, C. T. Su, Y. M. Tsang, Ultrasonography of small hepatic tumors using high-resolution linear array real-time instruments. *Radiology*, *150*:797 (1984).

34. J. C. Hsu, J. L. Sung, D. S. Chen, P. M. Yang, M. Y. Lai, C. S. Lee, H. C. Hsu, C. N. Chuang, P. C. Yang, T. H. Wang, J. T. Lin, and C. Z. Lee, Growth rate of asymptomatic hepatocellular carcinoma and its clinical implications. *Gastroenterology*, *89*:259 (1985).

35. R. Yamada, M. Sato, M. Kawabata, H. Nakatsuka, K. Nakamura, and S. Takashima, Hepatic artery embolization in 120 patients with unresectable hepatoma, *Radiology*, *148*:397 (1983).

36. Y. Sasaki, S. Imaoka, S. Nakamori, O. Ishikawa, H. Ohigashi, H. Koyama, K. Taniguchi, T. Iwanaga, M. Fujita, K. Kasugai, J. Kojima, S. Tanaka, and S.

Ishiguro, Effect of intra-arterial injection of lipiodol-adriamycin suspension combined with arterial embolization on hepatocellular carcinoma, *J. Jpn. Soc. Cancer Ther.*, *20*:1357 (1985) (in Japanese).

37. G. T. Huang, J. C. Sheu, D. S. Chen, P. M. Yang, M. Y. Lai, C. Z. Lee, C. S. Lee, and J. L. Sung, Follow-up of treated and untreated asymptomatic HCC (< 5cm) in Taiwan, *Viral Hepatitis and Hepatocellular Carcinoma* (J. L. Sung and D. S. Chen, eds.), Excerpta Medica Current Clinical Practice Series 57, Hong Kong, p. 659 (1990).

38. The Liver Cancer Study Group of Japan, Follow-up survey of primary liver cancer—Report 8, *Hepatologia Jpn.*, *49*:1619 (1988).

39. J. C. Sheu, G. T. Huang, D. S. Chen, J. L. Sung, P. M. Yang, T. C. Wei, M. Y. Lai, C. T. Su, K. M. Tsang, H. C. Hsu, I. J. Su, T. T. Wu, J. T. Lin, and C. N. Chuang, Small hepatocellular carcinoma: Intratumor ethanol treatment using new needle and guidance systems, *Radiology*, *163*:43 (1987).

40. Y. Majima, T. Fukimoto, I. Iwai, M. Tanaka, K. Hirai, and K. Tanikawa, Percutaneous ethanol injection therapy for HCC < 20mm in diameter, *Viral Hepatitis and Hepatocellular Carcinoma* (J. L. Sung and D. S. Chen, eds.), Excerpta Medica, Current Clinical Practice Series 57, Hong Kong, p. 646 (1990).

41. C. E. Stevens, R. P. Beasley, J. Tsui, and W. C. Lee, Vertical transmission of hepatitis B antigen in Taiwan, *N. Engl. J. Med.*, *292*:771 (1975).

42. K. Okada, I. Kamiyama, M. Inomata, M. Imai, Y. Miyakawa, and M. Mayumi, e Antigen and anti-e in the serum of asymptomatic carrier mothers as indicator of positive and negative transmission of hepatitis B virus to their infants. *N. Engl. J. Med.*, *294*:746 (1976).

43. R. P. Beasley, C. Treppo, C. E. Stevens, and W. Szmuness, The e antigen and vertical transmission of hepatitis B surface antigen, *Am. J. Epidemiol.*, *105*:94 (1977).

44. J. L. Sung, D. S. Chen, M. Y. Lai, J. Y. Yu, T. H. Wang, C. Y. Wang, C. Y. Lee, S. H. Chen, and T. M. Ko, Epidemiological study on hepatitis B virus infection in Taiwan, *Chin. J. Gastroenterol.*, *1*:1 (1984).

45. J. L. Sung, Hepatitis B virus eradication strategy for Asia, *Vaccine*, *8* (Suppl.):S95 (1990).

46. J. L. Sung, D. S. Chen, M. Y. Lai, T. H. Wang, C. Y. Wang, J. Y. Yu, and C. Y. Lee, Hepatitis B e antigen and antibody in asymptomatic Chinese with hepatitis B surface antigenemia in Taiwan, *Gastroenterol. Jpn.*, *17*:34 (1982).

47. R. P. Beasley, L. Y. Hwang, C. C. Lin, M. L. Leu, C. E. Stevens, W. Szmuness, and K. P. Chen, Incidence of hepatitis B virus infections in preschool children in Taiwan, *J. Infect. Dis.*, *146*:198 (1982).

48. R. P. Beasley, L. Y. Hwang, C. C. Lin, Y. C. Ko, and S. J. Twu, Incidence of hepatitis among students at a university, *Am. J. Epidemiol.*, *117*:213 (1983).

49. R. P. Beasley, L. Y. Hwang, C. E. Stevens, C. C. Lin, F. J. Hsieh, K. Y. Wang, F. S. Sun, and W. Szmness, Efficacy of hepatitis B immune globulin for prevention of perinatal transmission of the hepatitis B carrier state. Final report of a randomized double-blind, placebo-controlled trial, *Hepatology*, *3*:135 (1983).

50. R. P. Beasley, L. Y. Hwang, G. C.-Y. Lee, C.-C. Lan, C.-H. Roan, F.-Y. Huang, and C.-L. Chen, Prevention of perinatally transmitted hepatitis B virus infections with hepatitis B immune globulin and hepatitis B vaccine, *Lancet*, *2*:1099 (1983).

51. K.-J. Lo, Y.-T. Tsai, S.-D. Lee, T.-C. Wu, J.-Y. Wang, G.-H. Chen, C.-L. Yeh, B. N. Chiang, S. H. Yeh, A. Goudeau, P. Cousaget, and M. J. Tong, Immunoprophylaxis of infection with hepatitis B virus in infants born to hepatitis B surface antigen-positive carrier mothers, *J. Infect. Dis.*, *152*:817 (1985).

52. P. Cousaget, B. Yvonnet, J. Chotard, M. San, P. Vincelot, R. N. Doye, I. Diop-Mar I, and J. P. Chiron, Seven-year study of hepatitis B vaccine efficacy from an endemic area (Senegal), *Lancet*, *2*:1143 (1986).

53. K. J. Lo, S. D. Lee, Y. T. Tsai, T. C. Wu, C. Y. Chan, G. H. Chen, and C. L. Yeh, Long-term immunogenicity and efficacy of hepatitis B vaccine in infants born to HBeAg-positive HBsAg-carrier mothers, *Hepatology*, *8*:1647 (1988).

54. C. E. Stevens, P. E. Taylor, M. J. Tong, P. I. Toy, G. N. Vyas, E. A. Zang, and S. Krugman, Prevention of perinatal hepatitis B virus infection with hepatitis B immune globulin and hepatitis B vaccine, *Viral Hepatitis and Liver Disease* (A. Zuckerman, ed.), Alan R. Liss, Inc., London, p. 982 (1988).

55. C.-Y. Lee, R. P. Beasley, and L.-W. Hwang, Long-term follow-up of immunogenicity and efficacy of hepatitis B vaccination in high-risk infants, *Viral Hepatitis and Hepatocellular Carcinoma* (J. L. Sung and D. S. Chen, eds.), Excerpta Medica, Current Clinical Practice Series 75, Hong Kong, p. 427 (1990).

56. F. E. Andre, Overview of a 5-year clinical experience with a yeast-derived hepatitis B vaccine, *Vaccine*, *8*(Suppl.): S74 (1990).

57. C. Y. Lee, L. M. Huang, M. H. Chang, C. Y. Hsu, S. J. Wu, and J. L. Sung, The protective efficacy of recombinant hepatitis B vaccine in infants of HBeAg-positive HBsAg carrier mothers, *Pediatr. Infect. Dis.*, *10*: (in press).

58. M. S. Lai, J. L. Sung, and D. S. Chen, Immunogenicity of a yeast-recombinant hepatitis B vaccine in healthy children—a comparison of two different vaccination schedules, *Viral Hepatitis and Hepatocellular Carcinoma* (J. L. Sung and D. S. Chen, eds.), Excerpta Medica, Current Clinical Practice Series 57, Hong Kong, p. 414 (1990).

59. J. L. Sung, Control of hepatitis B in Taiwan, *Viral Hepatitis and Hepatocellular Carcinoma* (J. L. Sung and D. S. Chen, eds.), Excerpta Medica, Current Clinical Practice Series 57, Hong Kong, p. 435 (1990).

60. C. E. Stevens, R. A. Neurath, R. P. Beasley, and W. Szmuness, HBeAg and anti-HBe detection by radioimmunoassay: Correlation with vertical transmission of hepatitis B virus in Taiwan, *J. Med. Virol. 3*:237 (1979).

61. J. L. Sung and D. S. Chen, Maternal transmission of hepatitis B surface antigen in patients with hepatocellular carcinoma in Taiwan, *Scand. J. Gastroenterol. 15*:321 (1980).

62. D. S. Chen, N. H. M. Hsu, J. L. Sung, T. C. Hsu, S. T. Hsu, Y. T. Kuo, K. J. Lo, and Y. T. Shih, A mass vaccination program in Taiwan against hepatitis B virus infection in infants of hepatitis B surface antigen-carrier mothers, *JAMA, 257*:2597 (1987).

63. H. M. Hsu, D. S. Chen, C. H. Chuang, J. C. F. Lu, D. M. Jwo, C. C. Lee, H. C. Lu, S. H. Cheng, Y. F. Wang, C. C. Wang, K. J. Lo, C. J. Shih, and J. L. Sung, Efficacy of a mass hepatitis B vaccination program in Taiwan. Studies on 3464 infants of hepatitis B surface antigen-carrier mothers, *JAMA, 260*:2231 (1988).

14

Hepatitis B Vaccination of Children in Endemic Areas

Alexander Milne and Christopher D. Moyes

Hepatitis Control Centre, Whakatane, New Zealand

I. THE PROBLEM

All workers in hepatitis B virus (HBV) control know that in general the virus is most prevalent in those countries that can least afford to implement control measures. In some hyperendemic countries, such as Vanuatu, carrier rates as high as 30% are found in children, and most of the population is infected during their early lives.

In the South Pacific, where HBV is endemic, more than half of the 22 South Pacific Commission states have introduced vaccination programs for newborns. In other high-risk states in the area and in most poorer countries globally, universal infant vaccination has yet to be achieved, and for some the prospects of intervention are bleak.

Until the late 1980s the high cost of vaccination was the greatest impediment to the introduction of control programs. The position has changed, and where there is a will, a way may be found whereby most nations can implement a practical hepatitis B control program for children.

In many countries the first priority has been to prevent the perinatal transmission of HBV from infectious carrier mothers to their infants. These infants are a great risk to household and other contacts for many years, and there is circumstantial evidence (1,2) that they are at a risk of chronic sequelae from HBV infection higher than that of children who become carriers in later years. However, in most countries 50–85% of carriers result from postnatal infection, often

279

from other children, and generalized infant vaccination is required to prevent this.

In some countries, HBsAg carrier rates can double between about 1 and 4 years (see also Chapter 7). A vaccination program directed to older children, as well as to infants, will thus be of benefit to the children and the community.

It is important that some basic information be available on the epidemiology of hepatitis B before immunization programs are implemented in a country, if only to evaluate the outcome of such a program, and the following outline may be helpful.

Preventative strategies require knowledge of the epidemiology of infection, which differs between populations. The questions that must be answered are:

1. How common is hepatitis B infection (especially in childhood where chronic carriage is more likely to follow)?
2. How large is the pool of carriers?
3. Are ethnic differences sufficient to justify selective policies of vaccination?
4. How common is perinatal transmission?

Except for communities where the virus is dying out, the bulk of infection in endemic areas occurs in childhood, and acquisition of the carrier state is largely confined to these years. Older schoolchildren are a readily accessible and reasonably complete sample of the population in most countries, and simple seroprevalence studies of this group will give answers to the first three questions (Fig. 1). Anti-HBc and HBsAg rates approximate to total infection and carrier prevalence, respectively, and can be easily performed in most countries using enzyme immunoassay (EIA) methods. More precise information regarding the age of infection can be acquired by extending these studies to younger children. However, it should be appreciated that there may be very wide differences between geographically close communities (3,4) and between ethnic groups (5,6); the sample population should therefore cover as wide a geographic base as possible (including both urban and rural communities) and include adequate numbers of each major ethnic group to allow separate marker prevalence rates to be calculated. In general, at least 100 children are required from each sex of each ethnic group to obtain reasonable confidence intervals.

It is also advisable to determine the contribution of perinatal infection to the carrier pool; in parts of Southeast Asia this may be as much as 35–50% (7,8). This is in contrast to most of Africa and Oceania, where usually less than 20% of carriers have been infected by their mothers (9, 10), the carrier state resulting predominantly from cross-infection from other children; in some this is common in the first months of life and early protection is important (11); in others the bulk of infection occurs during mixing at schools and preschools (12), although the individual risk of becoming a carrier following infection is much higher in the first year or two of life (13).

Where women can be tested antenatally, a single test for HBsAg with HBeAg

PERINATAL TRANSMISSION

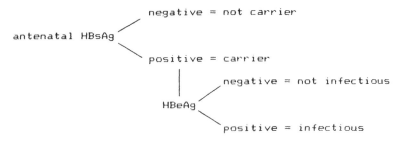

85% x HBeAg prevalence = approx. prevalence of carrier state from perinatal transmission.

HORIZONTAL TRANSMISSION

Schoolchildren near upper age for universal schooling

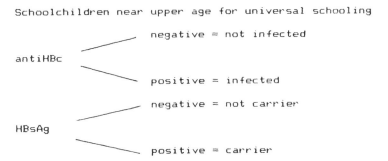

Figure 1 Economical assessment of HBV infection in an endemic area (using approximations). Sample should cover all major geographic areas and include a minimum of 100 of each sex from each major ethnic group. Prevalence of carrier state = approx. HBsAg rate. Incidence of infection = approx. anti-HBc rate.

on those found positive will allow an estimate of perinatal transmission, taken as 85% of the HBeAg positivity rate (14). Care should be taken, however, in selection of such cases—for example, women resident in urban areas may be available for testing, but there may be considerably higher prevalence of infection and carriage in rural areas (15,16), and there may be differences between socioeconomic groups.

A. Delta Infection

Delta virus (HDV) is a major factor in determining ultimate morbidity of carriers and is assessed by testing carrier sera; this test is usually available through World

Health Organization (WHO) reference laboratories. Testing for delta virus is not necessary for determining priorities for prevention, but its presence in a population adds to the urgency of establishing control.

B. Morbidity

Ideally the human and economic cost of HBV infection should be estimated from a knowledge of incidence of HBV-positive cases of acute hepatitis, chronic hepatitis, hepatocellular carcinoma, and polyarteritis. Unfortunately such data are often impossible to determine, even in developed countries such as New Zealand where, despite a statutory requirement to notify of acute hepatitis B, only one third of proven cases were correctly notified (17). Failure to check HBV markers in cases of disease and lack of autopsy data for economic or cultural reasons can lead to a gross underestimate of morbidity from the virus.

C. Priorities

Once the problem of HBV in children in a country or region has been delineated, a plan can be drawn up for prompt implementation if the health-care infrastructure and funding are in place. In New Zealand a major community-funded immunization program in one high-risk area was introduced in 4 weeks. The national program took more than 6 months to organize.

II. STRATEGIES FOR DELIVERY OF HBV VACCINE

A. Infant Vaccination

Priorities should be determined on the basis of seroprevalence data and should be focused on the prevention of the carrier state, therefore on the control of perinatal and early childhood infection. The only practical method of achieving this end is by vaccination. In most endemic societies *universal infant vaccination* must be the aim (see also Chapter 16).

Prevention of perinatal infection is optimal if mothers are routinely screened antenatally for the carrier state and hepatitis B immune globulin (HBIG) given at birth in addition to vaccination (18). However, in many societies such a policy is impracticable or unaffordable. The use of vaccine alone has a protective efficacy of 75–90% (18,19); thus universal infant vaccination without screening will prevent the great majority of infants from becoming carriers and is a practicable option for many countries.

The timing and delivery of vaccine will vary with local practice, but in any case should be *integrated to the normal EPI schedule*. HBV vaccine can be given at the same time as all the standard EPI innoculations except measles (20,21). Although the infant's immune response to vaccine improves with age, there are considerable advantages in completing the schedule expeditiously, as early protection is achieved (this is vital for prevention of carriage from perinatal infection) and compliance with vaccines is usually much better for those doses given in the first months of life. The much higher antibody level attained in adults by delaying the third dose of vaccine for several months is much less evident following infant vaccination, where there is little difference in eventual antibody levels between a short and long schedule (22) (Fig. 2), and is of minor importance compared to the need to achieve compliance. In most countries therefore, *HBV vaccine should be given at birth and two further doses with DPT vaccines in the first 6 months.*

B. Catch-Up Programs

Where funds allow, control can be speeded by "one-off" catch-up programs to vaccinate susceptibles. The aim is to prevent new carriers of HBV and is therefore most efficient when focused on young children (less than 5 years old). Vaccination of children over 10 years is a much lower priority, and in endemic societies it is preferable to test for prior infection to enable follow-up of identified carriers, if this is affordable.

Vaccination of adults in endemic communities is not justified except for susceptible health-care workers in high-risk categories.

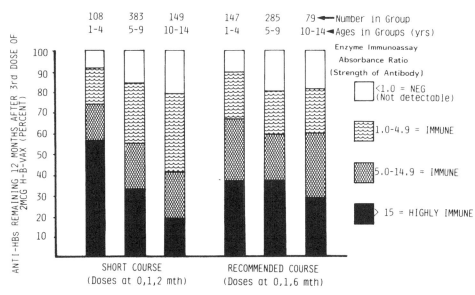

Figure 2 Anti-HBs levels by immunoassay in anti-HBc–negative children given three × 2μg H-B-VAX on a 2- or 6-month schedule (tested 10–12 months after dose 3).

C. Boosters

Occasional breakthrough HBV infections have been reported from West Africa more than 5 years after vaccination (23), indicating that booster doses may be advisable in long-term control. Our own studies have not detected any such events up to 6 years after infant vaccination, and we have reported an anamnestic response to low doses of vaccine after 4 years in all subjects who had shown any response to infantile vaccination, even though some had received very small doses and in many there was no detectable antibody immediately prior to the booster (24). Five-year booster studies in older children were equally reassuring (25). This indicates that, even after infantile vaccination, immunity against disease much outlasts detectable anti-HBs. As the risk of becoming a carrier is relatively small in the older child, infantile vaccination alone should be effective in eliminating the carrier pool. Thus a booster dose at school entry may be ideal, but is not of primary importance in disease control.

D. Public Education

Hepatitis B infection and its relationship to disease is complex, and this confuses medical professionals as well as members of the public. It is important, therefore, to have a well-funded education program for both the medical profession and the population. Material should be simply expressed with a few clear ideas and must be consistent. It also needs to be reinforced and repeated over a period of time before the general public can be considered informed. The delivery will vary from country to country, but should reach most parents in some form, whether by mass media or oral contact: in general a national awareness campaign is best reinforced by local meetings and educational initiatives.

Good leadership is vital. If frontline staff or their controlling officers are not committed to the program, or aware of the benefits, or are unable to communicate effectively with other staff or with mothers, then the program could fail. It is important that staff at all levels understand that HBV is a serious virus, which can be controlled more readily than many other health problems. Managers who do not understand the program or who are not convinced of the need for intervention need to be educated to the reasons for and benefits of immunization.

E. Economic Aspects of Hepatitis B Control

Until very recently, the greatest impediment to the introduction of hepatitis B vaccination for children has been the cost of vaccines. This need no longer be the case, and there are several strategies by which poorer countries can overcome this.

1. Seeking or Accepting Donor Vaccine or Funding from Wealthier
    Countries to Purchase the Vaccine

Various organizations, for example, the International Task Force on Hepatitis B
Immunization (Seattle, WA) and the WHO can advise on the availability of low cost
or donor vaccine. The Kitasato Institute in Tokyo provides free vaccine to Fiji,
Tonga, Western Samoa, Papua New Guinea, Philippines, Cook Islands, Vanuatu,
and the Solomon Islands in exchange for specified HBsAg-positive blood donor
plasma. Generally the onus is on the government of each nation to provide funds or
obtain funds from wealthier countries or organizations, but service clubs can assist in
fundraising to purchase vaccine.

2. Combining Orders for Vaccine

Substantial cost savings can be affected if several countries or states or communities
combine orders to allow bulk purchase of vaccine at a rate that would be affordable
for many poorer countries. For example, the International Task Force was able to
obtain supplies of a plasma-derived hepatitis B vaccine for less than $1 per pediatric
dose. The New Zealand Department of Health was able to obtain supplies of a
recombinant DNA (rDNA) hepatitis B vaccine at about the same price per pediatric
dose. A major manufacturing company has assured us that rDNA vaccine could be
available for less than $1.00 per dose provided the order was large enough. A
combined tender and bid process may thus be the single most effective means of
ensuring that children in endemic areas get the protection they need. However, even
$1.00 per dose is too costly for some poorer countries. In Kiribati, for example,
hepatitis B is a serious problem, but as recently as 1987 it was 28th on the list of
health-care priorities. Wealthier nations must help.

3. The Use of Reduced Doses of Vaccine

Hepatitis B vaccines in general are highly immunogenic, and they have been
used successfully in neonates and children in doses much lower than recommended (26–28). In younger children, in whom the risk of becoming a carrier is
greatest, some *but not all* vaccines may be used in much reduced doses (29). In
fact, studies in New Zealand have shown (30–32) that the recommended doses of
some vaccines are wasteful and an inappropriate use of an expensive treatment. It
is much more cost-effective to give large numbers of children reduced doses of
potent vaccines than to give fewer children larger doses. However, it is most
important that the dose and vaccine in use has been evaluated in the population
involved, as it may be that nutritional factors, parasitic infections, or other
factors may compromise immunogenicity and efficacy. Workers should therefore know their subjects and their vaccines, or seek advice from resource centers.

Figure 3 presents an example of a dose-response study in which age-matched
12- to 14-year-old children were given one of three dosage regimens using Merck
Sharp & Dohme rDNA vaccine. The geometric mean titer (GMT) of antibody
to HBsAg (anti-HBs) was greater using larger doses, but seroconversion was

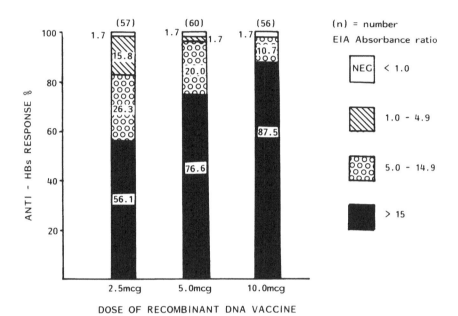

Figure 3   Anti-HBs seroconversion and levels of antibody by enzyme immunoassay in children given MSD recombinant DNA hepatitis B vaccine at 0, 1, and 6 months (tested 2 months after dose 3).

identical. Challenge (booster) studies done on large numbers of low-level responders in our laboratory show that immune memory persists for at least 3 years in approximately 98% of vaccinees (33). Furthermore, a current 5-year follow-up of children aged up to 13 years at the time of low-dose primary vaccination reveals that 97% raised an anamnestic response to a low-dose booster with levels of antibody greater than 10 mIU/ml, which is arbitrarily accepted as protective. The GMT of anti-HBs was almost 5000. Thus, 2-μg doses of this rDNA vaccine was protective.

4.   The Use of Fewer Doses of Vaccine

A major disadvantage of hepatitis B vaccines generally is that at least three doses are advised to achieve a reliable immune response and thus, hopefully, immune memory. In many countries where transport is a problem or delivery of health care difficult, a four-dose regimen can be a strain on busy staff. Some staff consider the need for multiple doses to be a convenient justification to see babies again for other matters, but generally it can be an imposition to make an additional visit. If three doses have been shown, on proper evaluation, to be effective in the circumstances prevailing, then this should be an advantage in delivery of a hepatitis B vaccine.

5. Use of Workers Appropriate for the Task

Hepatitis B vaccines are safe, and adverse events so few, that nurses are the logical operators for delivery of vaccine. A team of two nurses can, in some settings (e.g., vaccinating in schools), immunize up to 10,000 children per month at very low cost. It is not appropriate that doctors be employed for such public health work if the cost of this would delay implementation of a program.

6. Integration of Hepatitis B Vaccination into the Expanded Programme on Immunization (EPI)

Such an integration is logical not only in those areas where workers are required to make arduous or infrequent trips into remote areas, but in all countries where efficiency is desired.

III. EVALUATION

Every immunization program should be subject to proper evaluation of the process and the outcome, especially where costs are high or the delivery is demanding of resources.

A. Process Evaluation

Planning should be thorough and not unduly hurried. Authorities should attempt a formal assessment of the process of delivering the vaccine. For mass vaccination it is advisable to attempt the following, at as little cost as possible:

1. Identification of high-risk ethnic groups and compliance by each group for each dose.
2. Check on the suitability of venues, including the convenience of times and dates of clinics, and cost-effectiveness, where appropriate. All these matters can have an impact on the overall success of a program.
3. Check that adequate means of communication exists at a community level, so that babies (and children) can be brought in.
4. Check that the funding allocated is reaching controllers at the front line and that it is enough to see the task completed.
5. Ensure that the staffing is appropriate in numbers, knowledge, and skill.
6. Ensure that supplies are adequate and that vaccine is appropriately stored (hepatitis B vaccine should not be discarded lightly, for example, because it may have been unrefrigerated overnight).
7. If possible, arrangements should be made to vaccinate absentees at a later date, bearing in mind the great flexibilities in scheduling possible with hepatitis B vaccines. For example, dose 2 may be given from about 2 weeks to 3 months after dose 1 if circumstances demand this. Some support for this may be found in Figure 3, which presents anti-HBs prevalence and levels in

child vaccinees one year after the third dose of 2 μg MSD plasma-derived vaccine. It may be seen that there is no significant difference in anti-HBs persistent between children given vaccine over a 2-month period (0,1,2) or a 6-month period (0,1,6).

8. The national coordinator should be keenly aware of the progress of the program and should report promptly to the controlling officer or government if difficulties arise or targets are not met.

Process evaluation will require modification if, for example, only babies are to be vaccinated, or if vaccine is given in doctors' offices.

B. Outcome Evaluation

This should also be planned well in advance of the commencement of vaccinations and should include, wherever possible:

1. Preprogram hepatitis B seroprevalence studies in appropriate age groups, e.g., 12–18 months, 4–5 years, 10–12 years, young mothers.
2. Following vaccination, properly designed, preferably random selection of suitable subjects from different areas or different operators. For example, the New Zealand outcome evaluation involved sampling of an average of 27 children aged 4–5 years from 39 different locations throughout the country.
3. Outcome in terms of disease reduction when compared with historical controls, e.g., babies of HBeAg carrier mothers, or rates of incidence of infection in similar age groups in the recent past.

In the New Zealand evaluation, postvaccination sera were tested for anti-HBc and HBsAg to identify children with a history of past or current infection and for anti-HBs to check for seroconversion. These tests were done by EIA, which is suitably sensitive and practicable even for less sophisticated laboratories. Also, 100 randomly selected sera were assayed by radioimmunoassay so as to determine the GMT of anti-HBs.

C. Model Hepatitis B Immunization Projects and Programs

A number of countries have introduced hepatitis B vaccination programs or have set up trial projects, often in difficult areas, as a prelude to the introduction of a long-term control program. We report on three of these.

1. Indonesia. Integration of Hepatitis B Immunization into the EPI in Lombok.

The Indonesian Ministry of Health, in association with the International Task Force on Hepatitis B, set up a large field project for one fifth of the communities on the island of Lombok in 1987. A principal aim was to integrate hepatitis B immunization into the EPI schedule in a manner that would improve delivery of both, and a requirement was that the process should be sustainable in Lombok and replicable in other parts of Indonesia. Vaccine supply was put to tender, and a sealed bid from Korea Green Cross of 95 cents per pediatric dose was obtained.

Prior HBV serum prevalence studies confirmed the endemicity of the virus. A cluster survey of EPI coverage was conducted for comparison with coverage during the project. Community education was intensive and staff training was thorough, contributing to the high compliance reported. A major benefit of the program was that uptake of other EPI vaccines was dramatically improved, even in nonproject villages served by the same vaccinators.

The coverage rate for hepatitis B vaccine dose 3 (HB3) in the core villages was 61%, short of the 65% target. However, HB1 was delivered to 98% of newborn, and HB2 to 79%, a remarkable achievement in the conditions prevailing.

Despite the major reduction, the cost of HB vaccine remains an impediment to nationwide implementation of a vaccination program. Local production of vaccine is being considered as an option to overcome this.

Outcome evaluation, in terms of seroconversion and protective efficacy, has yet to be reported but will be of great interest in view of the variation in immunogenicity of hepatitis B vaccines.

2.   The Gambia Hepatitis Intervention Study (GHIS)

The government of The Gambia, The International Agency for Research on Cancer (IARC), and the Medical Research Council Laboratories (MRCL) in The Gambia are jointly responsible for the conduct of this major study, which is funded by the Ministry of Foreign Affairs of Italy. Plasma-derived hepatitis B vaccine donated by Merck Sharp & Dohme was used at the commencement of the study and was to be replaced by rDNA vaccine when supplies of the plasma vaccine were exhausted. Hepatitis B vaccine was introduced into the EPI in the first study zone in July 1986 and national coverage was achieved in 1990.

The timetable for implementation of the program was adhered to, and compliance for the vaccinations (by dose) was remarkably good for the study group reported, with 97% of children receiving dose 1, 95% dose 2, and 91% dose 3. Delivery of dose 4, at 77%, was impressive.

An outcome evaluation in 764 children, tested one year after vaccination, showed that 94% of children had detectable vaccine-induced immunity and an additional 4% had natural immunity, with 0.5% being HBsAg positive. A large proportion of immune children (>80%) had levels of anti-HBs exceeding 100 mIU/ml.

The GHIS team is conducting a number of ancillary studies in conjunction with their hepatitis B vaccination program, including studies on immune response in the presence of HBV-positive family contacts, the genetic contribution to the immune response (in twins), cost-effectiveness of hepatitis B vaccination, and a number of studies on other vaccine-preventable diseases. In addition, the natural history of HBV infection is being studied. A number of papers have resulted (34–37), and others will follow.

The GHIS produces an annual report, which contains valuable information on organization, conduct, and evaluation of such programs, and is recommended even for those countries that already have hepatitis B vaccination programs in operation.

3. New Zealand

This relatively wealthy country is unique in that the indigenous Maori, who make up 11% of the population of 3.3 million, have very high HBV seroprevalence rates, as have immigrant Pacific Islanders. In many communities HBsAg positivity exceeds 10% in Maori teenagers, and HBV has spread to Europeans, resulting in rates of infection as high as 50% in 7-year-old children in some communities.

Following successful trials of reduced doses of MSD plasma–derived vaccine, all children up to 13 years old in the eastern Bay of Plenty were offered community-funded vaccination using 2-μg doses of MSD plasma–derived vaccine at 0,1,2 months in hyperendemic areas and 0,1,6 months in endemic areas, beginning in late 1984. This regimen has proved efficacious, with elimination of clinical infections in vaccinated children.

The New Zealand Department of Health now funds universal vaccination of all newborns and routine blood testing of all pregnant women to identify those whose babies will have HBIG as well as vaccine. In 1988 free immunization was extended to all preschool (0–4 years old) children, and in 1990 a further extension to children up to the age of 15 years was approved.

The latter extension has been criticized for two reasons:

1. It is difficult to justify expensive state-funded vaccination of teenagers, who have a low risk of becoming carriers if infected.
2. Vaccination of Maori and Pacific Islander teenagers, without prior, relatively inexpensive blood tests, is covering up the problem of the many carriers in these groups. Proponents of prevaccination screening are prevailing, and the focus is now on identification and management of hepatitis B carriers, who have most to fear from HBV and who are the source of most infections.

REFERENCES

1. C-J. Chen, Y. C. Chang, S-F. Tsai, A. S. Chang, T-M. Lin, S-N. Lu, W-Y. Chang, Y-F. Liaw, Epidemiological studies of multiple risk factors in hepatocellular carcinoma in Taiwan, *Viral Hepatitis and Liver Disease*, Alan R. Liss, Inc., pp. 723–725 (1988).
2. M-H. Chang, H-S. Chen, H-C. Hsu, M-Z. Wu, H-Y. Hsu, C-Y. Lee, Childhood hepatocellular carcinoma in Taiwan: The prominent role of perinatally transmitted

hepatitis B virus infection, *Viral Hepatitis and Liver Disease*, Alan R. Liss, Inc., pp. 726–727 (1988).

3. M. C. Whittle, K. McLauchlan, A. K. Bradley, A. B. Adjukiewitz, C. R. Howard, et al., *Lancet* 1203–1206 (1983).

4. T. Kuberski, G. Le Gonidee, I. D. Gust, M. Dimitrikakis, D. Cantaloube, et al., Hepatitis B virus infections in Melanesians and Polynesians in New Caledonia. *Am. J. Epidemiol.*, 114:355–361 (1981).

5. I. D. Gust, N. I. Lehmann, M. Dimitrikakis, A seroepidemiological study of infection with hepatitis A virus and hepatitis B virus in five Pacific islands, *Am. J. Epidemiol.*, 110:237–242 (1979).

6. P. Maupas, A. Goudeau, P. Coursaget, J-P. Chion, J. Drucker, et al., Hepatitis B virus infection and primary hepatocellular carcinoma: epidemiological, clinical and virological studies in Senegal, *Viruses in Naturally Occurring Carriers* (M. Essex et al., eds.), Cold Spring Harbor Laboratories, Cold Spring Harbor, NY, pp. 401–421 (1980).

7. R. P. Beasley, L-Y. Hwang, C-C. Lin, M-L. Leu, C. E. Stevens, et al., Incidence of hepatitis B virus infections in preschool children in Taiwan, *J. Infect. Dis.*, *146*: 198–204 (1982).

8. E. K. Yeoh, W. K. Chang, J. P. W. Kwam, Epidemiology of viral hepatitis B infection in Hong Kong, *Viral Hepatitis B Infection* (S. K. Lam et al., eds.), World Sci. Publ. Corp., Singapore, p. 33 (1984).

9. J. F. Botha, M. J. J. Ritchie, G. M. Dusheiko, H. W. K. Mouton, M. C. Kew, Hepatitis B virus carrier state in black children in Ovamboland: role of perinatal and horizontal infections, *Lancet* 1210–1212 (1984).

10. C. J. Tibbs, Hepatitis B, tropical ulcers, and immunization strategy in Kiribati, *Br. Med. J.*, *294*: 537–540 (1987).

11. F. Barin, J. Perrin, J. Chotard, F. Denis, R. N'Doye, et al., Cross-sectional and longitudinal epidemiology of hepatitis B in Senegal, *Prog. Med. Virol.*, *27*: 148–162 (1981).

12. A. Milne, G. K. Allwood, C. D. Moyes, N. E. Pearce, C. R. Lucas, Prevalence of hepatitis B infection in a multiracial New Zealand community, *N.Z. Med. J.*, *98*: 529–532 (1985).

13. P. Coursaget, B. Yvonnet, J. Chotard, P. Vincelot, M. Sarr, et al., Age and sex-related study of hepatitis B virus chronic carrier state in infants from an endemic area, *J. Med. Virol.*, *22*: 1–5 (1987).

14. C. E. Stevens, R. A. Neurath, R. P. Beasley, W. Szmuness, HBsAg and antiHBe detection by RIA: correlation with vertical transmission of hepatitis B virus in Taiwan, *J. Med. Virol.*, *3*: 237–241 (1979).

15. A. W. Dimisceglie, M. C. Kew, G. M. Dusheiko, E. L. Berger, E. Song, et. al., Prevalence of hepatitis B infection among black children in Soweto, *Br. Med. J.*, *292*: 1440–1442 (1986).

16. K. Zhao, Epidemiology of hepatitis B in China, *Viral Hepatitis B Infection* (S. K. Lam et al., eds.), World Sci. Publ. Corp., Singapore, p. 23 (1984).

17. A. Milne, Viral hepatitis in the eastern Bay of Plenty, *N.Z. Med. J.*, *92*: 85–87 (1980).

18. R. P. Beasley, G. C-Y. Lee, C. H. Roan, L-Y. Hwang, C-C. Lam, et al.,

Prevention of perinatally transmitted hepatitis B virus infections with hepatitis B immuno globulin and hepatitis B vaccine, *Lancet, 2*: 1099–1102 (1983).

19. Y. Poovorawan, S. Sampavat, W. Pongpumlert, S. Chumdermpadetsuk, P. Sentra-kul, et al., Comparison of a recombinant DNA hepatitis B vaccine alone or in combination with hepatitis B immuno globulin for the prevention of perinatal acquisition of hepatitis B carriage, *Vaccine, 8*: S56–S59 (1990).

20. P. Coursaget, B. Yvonnet, E. Rolyveld, A. Brizard, C. Bourdil, et al., Simultaneous injection of hepatitis B vaccine with BCG, diptheria and tetanus toxoids, pertussis and polio vaccines, *Progress in Hepatitis B Immunization* (P. Coursaget, M. J. Tong, eds.), John Libbey Eurotext, 194, pp. 319–324 (1990).

21. Y. Chengde et al., Observations on immune response and reactions to simultaneous administration of hepatitis B vaccine with other routine vaccines in children, *Chinese J. Epidemiol., 10*: 210–214 (1989).

22. A. Milne, C. D. Moyes, Response to hepatitis B vaccine in New Zealand children: Using low doses in two month versus six month schedule, *Viral Hepatitis and Liver Disease* (A. J. Zuckerman, ed.), Alan Liss, New York, pp. 977–979 (1988).

23. P. Coursaget, B. Yvonnet, J. Chotard, M. Sarr, A. Samb, et al., Long-term efficacy of hepatitis B vaccine in infants from an endemic area, *Progress in Hepatitis B Immunization* (P. Coursaget, M. J. Tong, eds.), John Libbey Eurotext, 194, pp. 287–300 (1990).

24. C. D. Moyes, A. Milne, J. Waldon, Very low dose hepatitis B vaccination in the newborn: anamnestic response to booster at 4 years, *J. Med. Virol., 30*: 216–218 (1990).

25. A. Milne, J. Waldon, S. Hadler, C. D. Moyes, S. Krugman, C. R. Lucas, N. E. Pearce, 5 year efficacy and booster studies in children who received reduced doses of plasma derived hepatitis B vaccine. *NZ Med J* (Aug 1992) in press.

26. A Goudeau, F. Dubois, M-C. Dubois, C. Long, M-C. Maxert, Immunogenicity of low dose (1.25 and 3 mcg) hepatitis B vaccine, *Lancet, 2*: 1091–1092 (1984).

27. C. Scaravelli, E. Bianchi, V. Biraghi, G. Mariani, G. C. Calligori, Efficacy of minimal doses of an American hepatitis B vaccine in neonates, *Clin. Ther., 6*: 680–683 (1985).

28. A. Milne, G. K. Allwood, N. E. Pearce, C. R. Lucas, S. Krugman, Low dose hepatitis B vaccination in children, *N.Z. Med. J., 99*: 47–49 (1986).

29. A. Milne, T. A. Brawner, P. C. Dumbill, I. Kawachi, N. E. Pearce, Comparison of immunogenicity of reduced doses if two recombinant DNA hepatitis B vaccines in New Zealand children, *J. Med. Virol, 27*: 264–267 (1989).

30. A. Milne, C. D. Moyes, J. Waldon, N. E. Pearce, S. Krugman, Mass vaccination against hepatitis B in preschool children: Immunogenicity after 3 reduced doses, *N.Z. Med. J., 102*: 429–430 (1989).

31. N. E. Pearce, A. Milne, C. D. Moyes, Hepatitis B virus: The importance of age of infection, *N.Z. Med. J., 101*: 788–790 (1988).

32. C. D. Moyes, A. Milne, M. Dimitrikakis, P. N. Goldwater, N. E. Pearce, Very low dose hepatitis B vaccination in neonates: an economic option for control in endemic areas, *Lancet*, (Jan. 5): 29–31 (1987).

33. A. Milne, J. Waldon, C. D. Moyes, N. E. Pearce, Hepatitis B vaccine boosters: Further studies in children, *N.Z. Med. J., 103*: 539–541 (1990).

34.   The Gambia Hepatitis Study Group, The Gambia hepatitis intervention study, *Cancer Res.*, *47*: 5782–5787 (1987).

35.   The Gambia Hepatitis Study Group, Hepatitis B vaccine in the expanded programme of immunization: The Gambian experience, *Lancet*, *1*: 1057–1060 (1989).

36.   W. R. Gilks, A. J. Hall, N. E. Day, Timing of booster doses of hepatitis B vaccine, *Lancet*, *2*: 1273–1274 (1989).

37.   J. Chotard, A. J. Hall, H. M. Inskip, et al., The Gambia hepatitis intervention study: Preliminary results of the two year follow up, *Progress in Hepatitis B Immunization*, John Libbey Paris, Colloque Inserm., 194, pp. 501–508 (1990).

15

Prevention of Hepatitis B Virus Infection Among Health-Care Workers

Eric E. Mast and
Miriam J. Alter

Centers for Disease Control,
Atlanta, Georgia

I. INTRODUCTION

Hepatitis B virus (HBV) infection is a well-recognized occupational risk for health-care workers. The risk of infection has been demonstrated to be primarily related to the degree of contact with blood in the workplace. In serological studies conducted in the United States during the 1970s, health-care workers were demonstrated to have a prevalence of HBV infection up to 10 times higher compared to the general population. Because of the high risk of hepatitis B among health-care workers, routine preexposure vaccination of health-care workers against hepatitis B and the use of universal precautions to prevent exposure to blood and other potentially infectious body fluids have been recommended since the early 1980s. Regulations recently issued by the Occupational Safety and Health Administration (OSHA) should increase compliance with these recommendations and further decrease the risk of HBV transmission in the workplace.

II. MODES OF HBV TRANSMISSION IN THE HEALTH-CARE SETTING

Blood contains the highest HBV titers of all body fluids and is the most important vehicle of transmission in the health-care setting. Hepatitis B surface antigen (HBsAg) has been detected in a wide variety of other body fluids including breast milk, bile, cerebrospinal fluid, feces, nasopharyngeal washings, saliva, semen, sweat, and synovial fluid (1). However, the concentration of HBsAg in body fluids can be 100- to 1000-fold higher than the concentration of infectious HBV particles. Therefore, most body fluids are not efficient vehicles of transmission because they contain low quantities of infectious HBV, despite the presence of HBsAg. The principle modes of HBV transmission in the health-care setting are (a) direct percutaneous inoculation of blood or body fluids containing HBV via needlestick or other injuries from sharp instruments, (b) direct inoculation of blood or body fluids containing HBV onto mucous membranes, cutaneous scratches, abrasions, burns, or other lesions, and (c) indirect inoculation of HBV from environmental surfaces contaminated with blood or body fluids onto mucous membranes, cutaneous scratches, abrasions, burns, or other lesions.

A.   HBV Transmission from Needlesticks and Other Sharp Instrument Injuries

Injuries from needles containing HBV-infected blood are one of the most efficient means of HBV transmission in the health-care setting. The average volume of blood inoculated during a needlestick injury with a 22-gauge needle is approximately 1 μl (2), a sufficient quantity to contain up to 100 infectious doses of HBV (3). In studies of health-care workers who sustained injuries from needlesticks contaminated with blood from HBsAg-positive persons (and who received normal titer immune serum globulin), 6–14% developed clinical hepatitis and 27–45% developed serological evidence of HBV infection (4, 5). The risk of developing clinical hepatitis from a needle contaminated with hepatitis B *e* antigen (HBeAg)–positive blood was 22–31%, and serological evidence of HBV infection developed in 37–62%. By comparison, the risk of developing clinical hepatitis from a needle contaminated with HBeAg-negative blood was 1–6% and a serological response to HBV developed in 23–37%.

In studies conducted during the late 1970s and early 1980s, the reported frequency of needlestick and other sharp instrument injuries in hospitals ranged from 7.5 to 16 per 100 employees per year (6–10). However, the reported injury rates in earlier studies may have substantially underestimated actual injury rates occurring in the health-care setting. In one study, a threefold increased injury rate was reported after greatly increased efforts to reduce injuries because of the risk of human immunodeficiency virus (HIV) infection (11). Regardless of the time period of the study, higher injury rates were reported among nursing, housekeeping, and laboratory personnel compared to rates reported among physicians, students, and x-ray technicians. Moreover, injuries were reported to occur most commonly during disposal of used needles, administration of parenteral injections, drawing blood, recapping needles after use, and handling trash with uncapped needles.

B. HBV Transmission from Other Direct Blood or Body Fluid Exposures

Although overt percutaneous injuries are one of the most efficient modes of HBV transmission, these exposures probably account for only a minority of HBV infections among health-care workers. In several investigations of nosocomial hepatitis B outbreaks, most infected health-care workers could not recall an overt percutaneous injury (12–14). Similarly, in case series of health-care workers with acute hepatitis B, only a small proportion could recall a specific percutaneous injury (<10%); however, 29–38% could recall caring for a HBsAg-positive patient within 6 months prior to onset of illness (15–17). Direct blood or body fluid exposures that may result in HBV infections can include inoculation of HBV into cutaneous scratches, abrasions, burns, or other lesions or inoculation of HBV on to mucosal surfaces such as by mouth pipetting or accidental splashes in the eyes.

Other possible types of direct blood or body fluid exposures have been determined to be unlikely modes of HBV transmission. Although airborne transmission of HBV has been suggested (18, 19), aerosolized HBsAg or blood could not be detected in experimental studies conducted in environments where such transmission would be expected to occur, including dialysis centers, laboratories, and dental offices (20, 21). Therefore, the respiratory tract is an unlikely route of HBV transmission. HBV transmission by way of the gastrointestinal tract is also unlikely to occur. HBV infection has occurred after oral administration of serum containing HBV in experimental studies in children (22), but studies in animals suggest that the site of infection after oral inoculation of HBV is either through the oral mucosa or through mucosal lesions (23).

C. HBV Transmission from Environmental Surfaces

HBV has been shown to survive in dried blood at room temperature on environmental surfaces for a least one week (24). Since HBV is stable on environmental surfaces, indirect inoculation of HBV onto mucous membranes, cutaneous scratches, abrasions, burns, or other lesions can occur via inanimate objects. In an investigation in a hemodialysis unit, HBsAg was detected on 25 (13%) of 195 surfaces, including needle clippers and choppers, gloved hands, and dialysis machine carts (25). In a similar investigation in a clinical laboratory area, 26 (34%) of 76 environmental surfaces sampled were positive for HBsAg including the outer surface of blood and serum specimen containers, pipetting devices, marking devices (ballpoint pens, felt markers), and machine surfaces (26). Many of the HBsAg-positive specimens collected in both of these investigations were from areas where no visible blood was noted. The titer of HBV in blood can be so high that blood can be diluted to an extent that it cannot be seen and still contain 10^4–10^5 infectious particles (27).

The potential for HBV transmission through contact with environmental surfaces has been demonstrated in investigations of HBV outbreaks among patients and staff of hemodialysis units (28–30). Contact with HBV-contaminated blood from the surface of dialysis machines and instruments and transfer of HBV on the hands of medical personnel to patients was suspected to be the primary mode of transmission in these outbreaks. Most reported outbreaks of hepatitis B in dialysis units occurred before HBsAg-positive patients were routinely isolated from susceptible patients and before other routine infection control practices were initiated during the late 1970s. With the extensive use of these infection control procedures in the United States, the annual incidence of HBV infection among staff in dialysis centers decreased more than 25-fold from 2.6% during 1976 to 0.1% during 1989 (31, 32). A similar decline was also demonstrated among dialysis patients during this time period.

III. SEROPREVALENCE OF HBV INFECTION AMONG HOSPITALIZED PATIENTS

The risk of HBV infection among health-care workers is directly related to the prevalence of hepatitis B carriers in the patient population. In seroprevalence studies of patients consecutively admitted to hospitals in the United States, 0.9–1.5% were found to be HBsAg-positive (33–35). In one such study, a substantially higher precentage of hospitalized patients was found to be HBsAg-positive compared to first-time volunteer blood donors from the same geographic area (34). The prevalence of hepatitis B carriers among patients has been found to vary by geographic location and by the degree of specialization of the hospital; the highest prevalence was found in urban, tertiary care hospitals (36–38). Only a small fraction (<20%) of hepatitis B carriers admitted to hospitals had a history of liver disease (34, 35). This finding provides the rationale for using universal precautions to prevent exposure to blood or body fluids in hospitals and for vaccination of all health-care workers who have exposure to blood, since health-care workers may treat five HBsAg-positive persons for each one they recognize.

IV. SEROPREVALENCE OF HBV INFECTION AMONG HEALTH-CARE WORKERS

In serological studies conducted during the 1970s, 3–35% of health-care workers were found to have evidence of HBV infection (36, 39–44); by comparison, about 4% of first-time blood donors in the United States had serological markers of HBV infection (42). Estimates of the annual risk of HBV infection among selected health-care worker groups range from 0.5 to 6% in various studies (43, 45, 46).

The prevalence of HBV infection has been found to vary considerably among persons in the same profession including dentists (4–30%) (39, 42, 44, 47–50), physicians (9–35%) (36, 39–42, 47, 51, 52), nurses (3–32%) (37, 39–41, 47, 53), and laboratory personnel (3–26%) (39, 41, 46, 47, 53). Prevalence estimates have also been found to vary by hospital work area (36, 40, 43, 53). This variation appears to be related to differences in the frequency of blood contact (33, 37, 40, 41, 43, 46, 53). The frequency of patient contact has not been associated with the prevalence of HBV infection when health-care workers did not also have contact with blood (33, 40, 41, 43). There also appears to be an increased risk of infection associated with a longer duration of time in medical practice (36, 39, 41, 43, 46, 47) and for persons recently entering medical practice (36, 43, 47). The latter finding may be the result of an increased frequency of incidents leading to exposure to blood, either because of inexperience in performing procedures or because of the nature of training programs for health-care workers.

Although health-care workers continue to have a substantial risk of acquiring HBV infection, there is evidence that this risk is declining. In a Centers for Disease Control (CDC) study conducted in four sentinel counties in the United States, the proportion of acute heptititis B cases accounted for by health-care employment decreased 75% between 1981 and 1988, presumably as a result of hepatitis B vaccination (54). In some studies, however, a declining incidence of HBV infection was noted prior to the availability of hepatitis B vaccine. In Minnesota, annual rates of hepatitis B among health-care workers declined more than fivefold, from 101 to 8 cases per 100,000 persons, between 1974 and 1983 (38). A similar decline was also noted among health-care workers in Sweden between 1969 and 1983 (55). Despite these declines, an estimated 6500–9500 acute HBV infections occurred among health-care workers in the United States during 1990 (CDC, unpublished data).

V. STRATEGIES FOR CONTROL OF HBV TRANSMISSION IN THE HEALTH-CARE SETTING

A. Use of Hepatitis B Vaccine

Vaccination of health-care workers who are regularly exposed to blood is the most effective means of preventing HBV infection in the health-care setting. In two studies of hepatitis B vaccine efficacy and immunogenicity among health-care workers, seroconversion rates of 96–97% were demonstrated, and no severe adverse reactions occurred (56, 57). The most frequent side effect was a sore arm at the injection site, which was reported by 17–26% of vaccine recipients and by

15–24% of placebo recipients. In one of these studies the point estimate of vaccine efficacy was 92% (57); in the other the number of infections was small, but a trend towards efficacy in preventing HBV infections was observed (56).

In a survey of hospitals in the United States conducted during 1990 by OSHA, 91% of hospitals had hepatitis B vaccination programs for their employees; of these, 64% paid for the cost of vaccination for employees involved in direct patient care and laboratory work (high-risk employees) (OSHA, personal communication). Responses to this survey indicated that an estimated 46% of these high-risk employees had received hepatitis B vaccine. In a survey of dentists conducted in 1990, the estimated percentage of dentists who had received hepatitis B vaccine was 56% (American Dental Association, personal communication), an increase from 17% in 1983 and 36% in 1985 (58). Since there is a substantial risk of HBV infection for persons recently entering medical practice, vaccination of students in schools of medicine, dentistry, nursing, medical technology, and other fields is especially important. In a survey of medical schools in the United States conducted during 1988, 71% of schools offered hepatitis B vaccination to students at some time during their training, and 19% required hepatitis B vaccination (59). In a similar survey conducted during 1989, hepatitis B vaccine was offered to students in 81% of laboratory schools and in 23% of nursing schools (CDC, unpublished data).

Several problems have been encountered when implementing hepatitis B vaccination programs in the health-care setting. In many hospitals, there has been poor acceptance of hepatitis B vaccine by employees despite the availability of vaccine free of charge. Concern about the safety and efficacy of hepatitis B vaccine and lack of perceived risk were the major reasons cited for not being vaccinated in studies of vaccine acceptance among hospital employees (60–63). Low seroconversion rates (50–80%) after vaccination have also been reported among hospital employees (64–67). Factors that may be associated with lower antibody response to hepatitis B vaccine include freezing the vaccine prior to administration (68), older age at vaccination (69), use of the intradermal rather than the intramuscular route for vaccination (70), and genetic factors (71). Administration of hepatitis B vaccine in the buttock rather than in the deltoid muscle has also been associated with a lower antibody response (64, 65, 72). For this reason, vaccine administration in the buttock is contraindicated; persons who fail to develop an adequate antibody response ($\geq$10 mIU/ml) after inadvertently receiving vaccine in the buttock should be revaccinated with one or more additional doses (70). Revaccination should also be considered for persons who fail to develop an adequate antibody response after receiving a primary vaccine series administered in the deltoid muscle. An adequate antibody response has been reported to occur in 15–25% of such persons after one additional vaccine dose and in 30–50% of persons after three additional doses (73).

The long-term efficacy of hepatitis B vaccine and the need for vaccine booster doses have not been fully determined. In long-term studies of healthy adults, immunologic memory has been demonstrated to remain intact for at least 9 years following vaccination. Up to 50% of adults who initially respond to vaccination may have low or undetectable antibody levels (<10 mIU/ml) within 7 years after vaccination; the risk of antibody loss has been found to be inversely related to the peak anti-HBs level after vaccination (74, 75). However, despite declining antibody levels, no episodes of clinical illness have been reported and chronic HBV infection has only rarely been reported among persons who initially responded to vaccination. (75, 76). Therefore, for persons with normal immune status, booster doses are not currently recommended within 9 years after vaccination (70). The need for vaccine booster doses after longer intervals will need to be assessed with further studies.

In some health-care settings, there may be a need for either prevaccination serological testing to screen for susceptibility to HBV infection or postvaccination testing to determine serological response to vaccination. The decision to screen health-care workers for susceptibility to HBV infection prior to vaccination is based primarily on cost considerations (i.e., the cost of vaccinating all persons in the target group, regardless of their immune status, compared to the cost of serological testing plus vaccination of susceptible individuals) (70). Prevaccination testing is usually not cost-effective for groups with a low expected prevalence of HBV serological markers (≤20%), such as health-care professionals in training or during their early career years. If a decision is made to do prevaccination serological testing, only one antibody test is generally needed (anti-HBs or anti-HBc) (70). For groups expected to have hepatitis B carrier rates of <2%, such as health-care workers, neither test has a particular advantage. Testing for serological response to vaccination should be considered for persons whose subsequent management depends on knowing their immune status, such as dialysis patients and staff, and for persons who may have needlestick exposures necessitating postexposure prophylaxis (70). When necessary, postvaccination serological testing for anti-HBs should be done between 1 and 6 months after completion of the hepatitis B vaccine series; routine serologic testing after longer intervals is not recommended.

B. Use of Infection Control Practices

A substantial proportion of hepatitis B morbidity and mortality occurring in the health-care setting can be prevented by vaccinating health-care workers against hepatitis B. However, some health-care workers will not develop an adequate antibody response to hepatitis B vaccine. Therefore, other infection control practices are needed to prevent transmission of HBV in the health-care setting. The most important of these infection control practices is the use of "universal precautions" (77). Universal precautions emphasize that all patients should be assumed to be infectious for HBV and other bloodborne pathogens and that precautions should be taken to prevent exposure to all blood and blood-derived body fluids.

A variety of barrier precautions can be used when appropriate to prevent exposures to blood and blood-derived body fluids including use of gloves, gowns, masks, and protective eyewear. Measures that can be taken to prevent needlestick and other sharp instrument injuries include avoidance of recapping needles before disposal, use of impervious containers for the disposal of needles, use of self-sheathing needles for blood drawing and intravenous lines, use of gloves that are puncture resistant, and use of laser cutting devises as substitutes for scalpels. Measures to prevent mucous membrane exposure to HBV include avoidance of practices such as mouth pipetting, eating and smoking in the work area. Environmental control measures are also important, including appropriate use of hand washing (78) and rigorous maintenance of a work environment that is free of blood contamination (27, 79).

Routine screening of patients for serological evidence of HBV infection is recommended only in dialysis units; those who are found to be HBsAg positive should be isolated (80, 81). Use of postexposure prophylaxis with hepatitis B immune globulin (HBIG) is about 75% effective in preventing HBV infection when initiated within 1 week of exposure (4, 5, 82), and detailed algorithims for postexposure prophylaxis with HBIG and/or hepatitis B vaccine have been recommended (70). However, use of postexposure prophylaxis will prevent only a fraction of occupationally acquired hepatitis B cases, since only a small proportion of health-care workers with acute HBV infection report a discrete exposure incident.

D. OSHA Regulations

In 1986, various unions representing health-care workers petitioned OSHA to take action to reduce the risk to health-care workers from exposure to certain infectious agents, including HBV. In response to these requests, OSHA developed regulations to protect workers from occupational exposures to bloodborne hazards (83). These regulations became law in December 1991 and require all employers to provide the following: (a) hepatitis B vaccine free of charge to employees who have occupational exposure to blood or other potentially infectious materials; (b) personal protective clothing and equipment when there is a potential for exposure to blood or blood-derived body fluids including gloves, gowns, fluid-proof aprons, face shields, and eye protection when necessary to prevent mucous membrane exposure; (c) engineering and work-practice controls including facilities for hand washing, provisions for immediate disposal of needles after use without recapping, and prohibition of eating, drinking, or smoking in areas where there is a potential for occupational exposure; (d) appropriate housekeeping procedures, including cleaning and disinfection of equipment and environmental surfaces after contact with blood or other potentially infectious material, and appropriate disposal of infectious waste and laundry; (e) medical follow-up of exposure incidents, including use of HBIG, when appropriate; and (f) training of health-care workers regarding the measures they can take to prevent exposure to HBV in the workplace.

VI. CONCLUSION

The incidence of occupationally-acquired HBV infections has declined substantially in the United States through the use of hepatitis B vaccine and other infection-control practices. However, an estimated 6500–9500 acute HBV infections still occur annually among health-care workers. As a result of these infections, 300–950 (5–10%) health-care workers may develop chronic HBV infection, and of these, 100–150 (25%) will be expected to die of cirrhosis and 25–40 (4%) will be expected to die of primary hepatocellular carcinoma at some time in the future. The morbidity and mortality associated with occupationally acquired hepatitis B can be virtually eliminated if all health-care workers rigorously adhere to universal precautions and if all susceptible health-care workers are vaccinated against hepatitis B.

REFERENCES

1. W. W. Bond, N. J. Petersen, M. S. Favero, Viral hepatitis B: Aspects of environmental control, *Health. Lab. Sci.* 14:235–252 (1977).
2. V. M. Napoli, J. E. McGowan, How much blood is in a needlestick? *J. Infect. Dis.*, 155:828 (1987).
3. T. Shikata, K. Karasawa, K., Abe, T. Uzawa, et al., Hepatitis B e antigen and infectivity of hepatitis B virus, *J. Infect. Dis.*, 136:571–576 (1977).
4. G. F. Grady, V. A. Lee, A. M. Prince, G. L. Gitnick, et al., Hepatitis B immune globulin for accidental exposures among medical personnel: Final report of a multicenter controlled trial, *J. Infect. Dis.*, 138:625–638 (1978).
5. L. B. Seeff, E. C. Wright, H. J. Zimmerman, H. J. Alter, et al., Type B hepatitis after needlestick exposure: Prevention with hepatitis B immune globulin. Final report of the Veterans Administration Cooperative Study, *Ann. Intern. Med.*, 88:285–293 (1978).
6. J. T. Jacobson, J. P. Burke, M. T. Conti, Injuries of hospital employees from needles and sharp objects, *Infect. Control*, 4:100–102 (1983).
7. F. L. Ruben, C. W. Norden, K. Rockwell, E. Kruska, Epidemiology of accidental needle-puncture wounds in hospital workers, *Am. J. Med. Sci.*, 286:26–30 (1983).
8. R. D. McCormick, D. G. Maki, Epidemiology of needle-stick injuries in hospital personnel, *Am. J. Med.*, 70:928–932 (1981).
9. S. E. Dandoy, B. L. Kirkman-Liff, F. M. Krakowski, Hepatitis B exposure incidents in community hospitals, *Am. J. Public Health*, 74:804–807 (1984).

10. J. S. Reed, A. C. Anderson, G. R. Hodges, Needlestick and puncture wounds: Definition of the problem, *Am. J. Infect. Control*, 8:101–106 (1980).

11. R. D. McCormick, M. Meisch, F. Ircinik, D. G. Maki, Epidemiology of hospital sharps injuries: A 14-year perspective in the pre-AIDS and AIDS eras, (Abstract) presented at the 30th Interscience Conference on Antimicrobial Agents and Chemotherapy, Atlanta, October 21–24, 1990 (1990).

12. J. A. Bryan, H. E. Carr, M. B. Gregg, An outbreak of non-parenterally transmitted hepatitis B, *JAMA*, 223:279–283 (1973).

13. C. P. Pattison, K. M. Boyer, J. E. Maynard, P. C. Kelly, Epidemic hepatitis in a clinical laboratory: possible association with computer card handling, *JAMA*, 230:854–856 (1974).

14. J. L. Rosenberg, D. P. Jones, L. R. Lipitz, J. B. Kirsner, Viral hepatitis: An occupational hazard to surgeons, *JAMA*, 223:395–400 (1973).

15. A. K. R. Chaudhuri, E. A. C. Follett, Hepatitis B virus infection in medical and health care personnel, *Br. Med. J.*, 284:1408 (1982).

16. M. E. Callender, Y. S. White, R. Williams, Hepatitis B virus infection in medical and health care personnel, *Br. Med. J.*, 284:324–326 (1982).

17. Public Health Laboratory Service, Acute hepatitis B, *Br. Med. J.*, 3:603 (1975).

18. J. D. Almeida, G. D. Chisholm, A. E. Kulatilake, A. B. McGregor, et al., Possible airborne spread of serum hepatitis virus within a hemodialysis unit, *Lancet*, 2:849–850 (1971).

19. R. A. Garibaldi, F. E. Hatch, A. L. Bisno, M. H. Hatch, M. B. Gregg, Non-parental serum hepatitis: Report of an outbreak, *JAMA*, 220:963–966 (1972).

20. N. J. Petersen, An assessment of the airborne route in hepatitis B transmission, *Ann. N.Y. Acad. Sci.*, 353:157–166 (1980).

21. N. J. Petersen, W. W. Bond, M. S. Favero, Air sampling for hepatitis B surface antigen in a dental operatory, *JADA*, 99:465–467 (1979).

22. S. Krugman, J. P. Giles, J. Hammond, Infectious hepatitis: Evidence for two distinctive clinical, epidemiological, and immunological types of infection, *JAMA*, 200:365–373 (1967).

23. D. P. Francis, M. S. Favero, J. E. Maynard, Transmission of hepatitis B virus, *Semin. Liver Disease*, 1:27–32 (1981).

24. W. W. Bond, M. S. Favero, N. J. Petersen, C. R. Gravelle, J. W. Ebert, J. E. Maynard, Survival of hepatitis B virus after drying and storage for one week, *Lancet*, 1:550–551 (1981).

25. M. S. Favero, J. E. Maynard, N. J. Petersen, K. M. Boyer, et al., Hepatitis-B antigen on environmental surfaces, *Lancet*, 2:1455 (1973).

26. J. L. Lauer, N. A. VanDrunen, J. W. Washburn, H. H. Balfour, Transmission of hepatitis B virus in clinical laboratory areas, *J. Infect. Dis.*, 140:513–516 (1979).

27. M. S. Favero, Control measures for preventing hepatitis transmission in hospitals, *Hepatitis A* (R. J. Gerety, Ed.), Academic Press, Inc., Orlando, FL, pp. 163–184 (1984).

28. C. H. Hennekens, Hemodialysis-associated hepatitis: An outbreak among hospital personnel, *JAMA*, 225:407–408 (1973).

29. R. A. Garibaldi, J. N. Forrest, J. A. Bryan, B. F. Hanson, W. E. Dismukes, Hemodialysis-associated hepatitis, *JAMA*, 225:384–389 (1973).

30. D. R. Snydman, J. A. Bryan, E. J. Macon, M. B. Gregg, Hemodialysis-associated hepatitis: Report on an epidemic with further evidence on mechanisms of transmission, *Am. J. Epidemiol.*, 104:563–570 (1976).

31. M. J. Alter, M. S. Favero, J. E. Maynard, Impact of infection control strategies on the incidence of dialysis-associated hepatitis in the United States, *J. Infect. Dis.*, 153:1149–1151 (1986).

32. M. J. Alter, M. S. Favero, L. A. Moyer, L. A. Bland, National surveillance of dialysis-associated diseases in the United States, *A.S.A.I.O. Trans.*, 37:97–109 (1991).

33. J. E. Maynard, Nosocomial viral hepatitis, *Am. J. Med.*, 70:439–444 (1981).

34. J. P. Mahoney, A. V. Richman, P. O. Teague, Admission screening for hepatitis B surface antigen in a university hospital, *South Med. J.*, 71:624–628 (1978).

35. C. C. Linnemann, M. E. Hegg, N. Ramundo, G. M. Schiff, Screening hospital patients for hepatitis B surface antigen, *Am. J. Clin. Pathol.*, 67:257–259 (1977).

36. A. E. Denes, J. L. Smith, J. E. Maynard, I. L. Doto, K. R. Berquist, A. J. Funkel, Hepatitis B infection in physicians: Results of a nationwide seroepidemiologic survey, *JAMA*, 239:210–212 (1978).

37. J. R. Harris, R. F. Finger, J. M. Kobayashi, S. C. Hadler, et al., The low risk of hepatitis B in rural hospitals: Results of a seroepidemiologic study, *JAMA*, 252:3270–3272 (1984).

38. M. T. Osterholm, S. M. Garayalde, Clinical viral hepatitis B among Minnesota hospital personnel: Results of a ten-year statewide survey, *JAMA*, 254:3207–3212 (1985).

39. H. E. Segal, C. H. Llewellyn, G. Irwin, W. H. Bancroft, G. P. Boe, D. J. Balaban, Hepatitis B antigen and antibody in the U.S. Army: Prevalence in health care personnel, *Am. J. Public Health*, 66:667–671 (1976).

40. C. P. Pattison, J. E. Maynard, D. R. Berquist, H. M. Webster, Epidemiology of hepatitis B in hospital personnel, *Am. J. Epidemiol.*, 101:59–64 (1975).

41. J. L. Dienstag, D. M. Ryan, Occupational exposure to hepatitis B virus in hospital personnel: Infection or immunization? *Am. J. Epidemiol.*, 115:26–29 (1982).

42. J. L. Smith, J. E. Maynard, K. R. Berquist, I. L. Doto, H. M. Webster, M. J. Sheller, Comparative risk of hepatitis B among physicians and dentists, *J. Infect. Dis.*, 133:705–706 (1978).

43. S. C. Hadler, I. L. Doto, J. E. Maynard, J. Smith, et al., Occupational risk of hepatitis B infection in hospital workers, *Infect. Control*, 6:24–31 (1985).

44. F. B. Hollinger, J. W. Grander, F. R. Nickel, M. S. Suarez, Hepatitis B prevalence within a dental student population, *JADA*, 94:521–527 (1977).

45. J. F. Jovanovich, L. D. Sarovolatz, L. M. Arking, The risk of hepatitis B among select employee groups in an urban hospital, *JAMA*, 250:1893–1894 (1983).

46. B. I. Hirshowitz, C. A. Dasher, F. J. Whitt, G. W. Cole, Hepatitis B antigen and antibody and tests of liver function: A prospective study of 310 hospital laboratory workers, *Am. J. Clin. Pathol.*, 73:63–68 (1980).

47. D. R. Snydman, A. Munoz, B. G. Werner, B. F. Polk, et al., A multivariate analysis of risk factors for hepatitis B virus infection among hospital employees screened for vaccination, *Am. J. Epidemiol.*, 120:684–693 (1984).

48. J. W. Mosley, V. M. Edwards, G. Casey, A. G. Redecker, E. White, Hepatitis B virus infection in dentists, *N. Engl. J. Med.*, 293:729–734 (1975).

49. R. B. Weil, D. O. Lyman, R. J. Jackson, B. Bernstein, A hepatitis serosurvey of New York dentists, *N.Y. State Dent. J.*, 43:587–590 (1977).

50. Council on Dental Therapeutics, Type B (serum) hepatitis and dental practice, *JADA*, 92:153–159 (1976).

51. S. Krugman, H. Friedman, C. Lattimer, Hepatitis A and B: Serologic survey of various population groups, *Am. J. Med. Sci.*, 275:249–255 (1978).

52. W. Szmuness, Large-scale efficacy trials of hepatitis B vaccines in the USA: Baseline data and protocols, *J. Med. Virol.*, 4:327–340 (1979).

53. B. S. Levy, J. C. Harris, J. L. Smith, J. W. Washburn, et al., Hepatitis B in ward and clinical laboratory employees of a general hospital, *Am. J. Epidemiol.*, 106:330–335 (1977).

54. M. J. Alter, S. C. Hadler, H. S. Margolis, W. J. Alexander, et al., The changing epidemiology of hepatitis B in the United States: Need for alternative vaccination strategies, *JAMA*, 263:1218–1222 (1990).

55. B. Christenson, Acute infections with hepatitis B virus in medical personnel during a 15-year follow-up, *Am. J. Epidemiol.*, 122:411–417 (1985).

56. J. L. Dienstag, B. G. Werner, B. F. Polk, D. R. Snydman, et al., Hepatitis B vaccine in health care personnel: Safety, immunogenicity, and indicators of efficacy, *Ann. Intern. Med.*, 101:34–40 (1984).

57. W. Szmuness, C. E. Stevens, E. J. Harley, E. A. Zang, et al., Hepatitis B vaccine in medical staff of hemodialysis units: Efficacy and subtype cross-protection, *N. Engl. J. Med.*, 307:1481–1486 (1982).

58. C. Siew, S. E. Gruninger, E. W. Mitchell, K. H. Burrell, Survey of hepatitis B exposure and vaccination in volunteer dentists, *JADA*, 114:457–459 (1987).

59. G. A. Poland, K. L. Nichol, Medical schools and immunization policies: Missed opportunities for disease prevention, *Ann. Intern. Med.*, 113:628–631 (1990).

60. K. B. Crossley, D. N. Gerding, R. A. Petzel, Acceptance of hepatitis B vaccine by hospital personnel, *Infect. Control*, 6:147–149 (1985).

61. D. L. Palmer, R. King, Attitude toward hepatitis vaccination among high-risk hospital employees, *J. Infect. Dis.*, 147:1120–1121 (1983).

62. H. C. Bodenheimer, J. P. Fulton, P. D. Kramer, Acceptance of hepatitis B vaccine among hospital workers, *Am. J. Public Health*, 76:252–255 (1986).

63. J. P. Fulton, H. C. Bodenheimer, P. D. Kramer, Acceptance of hepatitis B vaccine among hospital workers: a follow-up, *Am. J. Public Health*, 76:1339–1340 (1986).

64. F. E. Shaw, H. A. Guess, J. M. Roets, F. E. Mohr, et al., Effect of anataomic injection site, age and smoking on the immune response to hepatitis B vaccination, *Vaccine*, 7:425–430 (1989).

65. P. J. Pead, A. A. Saeed, W. G. Hewitt, R. N. Brownfield, Low immune responses to hepatitis B vaccination among healthy subjects, *Lancet*, 1:1152 (1985).

66. D. M. Schaaf, M. Lender, P. Snedeker, L. A. Graham, Hepatitis B vaccine in a hospital, *Ann. Intern. Med.*, 101:720–721 (1984).

67. A. C. Strickler, P. C. Kibsey, H. Vellend, Seroconversion rates with hepatitis B vaccine, *Ann. Intern. Med.*, 101:564 (1984).

68. A. A. McLean, R. Shaw, Hepatitis B virus vaccine, *Ann. Intern. Med.*, 97:451 (1982).

69. A. A. McLean, E. B. Buynak, B. J., Kuter, M. R. Hilleman, D. J. West, Clinical experience with hepatitis B vaccine, *Hepatitis B: The Virus, the Disease, and the Vaccine* (I. Millman, T. K. Eisenstein, B. S. Blumberg, Eds.), Plenum Press, New York, pp. 149–159 (1984).

70. Centers for Disease Control, Hepatitis B Virus: A comprehensive strategy for eliminating transmission in the United States through universal childhood vaccination. Recommendations of the Immunization Practices Advisory Committee (ACIP), *MMWR*, 40:1–25 (1991).

71. D. E. Craven, Z. L. Awdeh, L. M. Kunches, E. J. Yunis, et al., Nonresponsiveness to hepatitis B vaccine in health care workers: Results of revaccination and genetic typings, *Ann. Intern. Med.*, 105:356–360 (1986).

72. Centers for Disease Control, Suboptimal response to hepatitis B vaccine given by injection into the buttock, *MMWR*, 34:105–108, 113 (1985).

73. S. C. Hadler, D. P. Francis, J. E. Maynard, S. E. Thompson, et al., Long term immunogenicity and efficacy of hepatitis B vaccine in homosexual men, *N. Engl. J. Med.*, 315:209–214 (1986).

74. S. C. Hadler, Are booster doses of hepatitis B vaccine necessary? *Ann. Intern. Med.*, 108:457–458 (1988).

75. S. C. Hadler, P. Coleman, P. O'Malley, F. N. Judson, N. Altman, Evaluation of long term protection by hepatitis B vaccine in homosexual men followed for 7 to 9 years. Viral Hepatitis and Liver Disease (F. B. Hollinger, S. M. Lemon, H. S. Margolis, Eds.). Williams & Wilkins, Baltimore, MD, pp. 766–768 (1991).

76. R. B. Wainwright, B. J. McMahon, L. R. Bulkow, A. J. Parkinson, et al., Duration of immunogenicity and efficacy of hepatitis vaccine in a Yupik Eskimo population–preliminary results of an 8-year study. In: Viral Hepatitis and Liver Disease (F. B. Hollinger, S. M. Lemon, H. S. Margolis, Eds.). Williams & Wilkins, Baltimore, MD, pp. 762–766 (1991).

77. Centers for Disease Control, Update: Universal precautions for prevention of transmission of human immunodeficiency virus, hepatitis B virus, and other blood-borne pathogens in health-care settings, *MMWR*, 37:377–382, 387–388 (1988).

78. J. S. Garner, M. S. Favero, Guideline for handwashing and hospital environmental control, 1985. Atlanta: Public Health Service, Centers for Disease Control, 1985. HHS publication no. 99-1117 (1985).

79. M. S. Favero, Sterilization, disinfection, and antisepsis in the hospital, *Manual of Clinical Microbiology*, 4th ed., American Society for Microbiology, Washington, DC, pp. 129–137 (1985).

80. G. R. Najem, D. B. Louria, I. S. Thind, M. A. Lavenhar, et al., Control of hepatitis B infection: The role of surveillance and an isolation hemodialysis center, *JAMA*, 245:153–157 (1981).

81. M. S. Favero, M. J. Alter, L. A. Bland, Dialysis-associated infections and their control, *Hospital Infections* (J. V. Bennett, P. S. Brachman, Eds.), Little, Brown and Co., Boston, MA, pp. 375–403 (1992).

82. A. M. Prince, W. Szmuness, M. K. Mann, G. N. Vyas, et al., Hepatitis B "immune" globulin: Effectiveness in prevention of dialysis-associated hepatitis, *N. Engl. J. Med.*, 293:1063–1067 (1975).

83. Occupational Safety and Health Administration, Occupational exposure to blood-borne pathogens; final rule, *Fed. Reg.*, 56:64005–64182 (1991).

16

Global Control of Hepatitis B Through Universal Infant Immunization

Mark A. Kane

World Health Organization,
Geneva, Switzerland

I. INTRODUCTION

When safe, immunogenic, and effective hepatitis B (HB) vaccines became available in the early 1980s, expert groups met to decide on the proper strategy for their use. Most of these groups decided that proper control strategy in areas of high and intermediate HBV endemicity was the universal immunization of infants as part of the Expanded Programme on Immunization (EPI), and that the recommended control strategy in areas of low endemicity was the immunization of high-risk groups (1, 2).

There is now considerable evidence to suggest that high-risk group immunization, although medically indicated for many individuals, will not lead to control of HBV infection on a population basis, and that universal immunization of infants is the only strategy that will lead to control of HBV infection in all regions of the world (3–5).

Approximately 50 countries have begun to routinely immunize all infants with hepatitis B vaccine either nationwide or in selected provinces. The barrier to more widespread use of this vaccine is financial: there are no technical impediments to its use. An analysis of the economic situation with respect to this vaccine provides important lessons about the introduction of future vaccines into public health use. This chapter will discuss the issue of universal immunization with HB vaccine within the context of the public health, economic, and political realities of the global immunization effort.

309

II. WHERE DO VACCINES COME FROM?

The public, scientists, and physicians in developed countries often have little idea how vaccines are obtained and delivered to most of the world's children. Approximately 80% of the children in the world now receive primary immunization with six "universal" antigens (DTP, polio vaccine, BCG, and measles vaccine) (6). These vaccines are usually administered to them under a national immunization program: these programs, as well as certain regional and international programs, are linked together in a network called the Expanded Programme on Immunization (EPI), which is headquartered at the World Health Organization (WHO) in Geneva, Switzerland.

The EPI is the most successful public health program in the world, reaching more people than the postal service. At its inception in 1974 it was estimated that less than 5% of the world's children were receiving primary immunizations. For most children, the vaccines that they receive through the EPI may be the only immunizations they will ever receive.

Approximately 50% of the vaccines used worldwide is purchased by the United Nations Children's Fund (UNICEF) and supplied to countries for their EPI programs (T. Hill, personal communication). Countries with relatively more resources purchase vaccines directly from commercial manufacturers or manufacture vaccines themselves in public sector or semi-public sector institutes. UNICEF is able to obtain vaccine at very low prices: the cost of the vaccine needed to fully immunize a child (one BCG, three polio, three DTP, one measles) is approximately $0.65 per child (7).

Vaccine represents only a small portion (less than 10%) of the cost to fully immunize a child, which averages about $13–20 (J. Clements, personal communication). Immunizers' salaries, vaccine storage, the cold chain, sterilizers, transportation, training, surveillances, and other costs are greater than those of the vaccine. Most of those costs are borne by the country or by bilateral or multilateral donors.

UNICEF relies on donor contributions to purchase vaccines. It currently spends approximately $85 million for vaccine purchases, and this is expected to increase to $100 million over the next few years (J. Sherry, personal communication). If UNICEF were to begin to purchase HB vaccine at current prices ($1.00 per dose) for 100 million children, it would cost 300 million dollars, more than three times their current vaccine expenditure. Of course, HB vaccine price would fall dramatically if tenders were issued for tens or hundreds of millions of doses. Even assuming that HB vaccine price fell to $0.25 per dose, the vaccine would cost $75,000,000. UNICEF and its donors are at present unwilling to make this commitment.

Vaccine manufacturers have a multilevel pricing structure for their products, selling smaller volumes of vaccine in developed countries for relatively high prices, and larger volumes to developing countries at lower prices. The manufacturers claim that they must sell at high prices in developed countries to recover the huge costs of research and development, to make a profit, and to be able to make the product available to the developing world. Currently, the developing world price of $1–2 per dose is too high for UNICEF. The manufacturers claim that they cannot lower the price substantially unless they get large guaranteed orders, and UNICEF claims it cannot give large guaranteed orders until the price is lower. Efforts are being made to break out of this unproductive cycle.

Approximately 50 countries with more resources in areas of high and intermediate endemicity in Asia, the Middle East, and the Pacific Basin are using HB vaccine as a routine infant immunogen (8). Those with the most resources have already initiated national programs, and those with fewer resources (Thailand, Indonesia, Philippines) have begun programs in selected provinces with the intent of moving to universal immunization over the next few years. China produces approximately 10 million doses per year of HB vaccine, but charges parents for the vaccine, limiting its use among the poor, especially in rural areas.

The fact that donors, to date, have not funded the purchase of HB vaccine means that the poorest children in the world, most of whom are at highest risk of HBV infection, do not receive HB vaccine. Only one country in sub-Saharan Africa, The Gambia, routinely gives HB vaccine to all infants (9). A number of African countries with excellent EPI coverage are ready to use HB vaccine but cannot find donor funding.

HB immunization is cost-effective in both developing and developed countries. An excellent study of the cost-effectiveness of adding HB vaccine to the EPI in Gambia found that the cost per carrier prevented was in the range of $30–40 at a vaccine cost of $1 per dose. The undiscounted cost per death averted was approximately $150–$200 ($1000–1400 discounted) (10). This result compared favorably with the cost-effectiveness of other EPI antigens, the cost per carrier averted being higher than that for preventing a case of measles or pertussis, but lower than the cost of preventing a case of neonatal tetanus, polio, or diphtheria (11, 12).

Numerous studies of the cost-effectiveness of immunizing health-care personnel (13) and infants of carrier mothers (14) have been published in developed countries, but few studies have looked at the cost-effectiveness of universal infant immunization in areas of low endemicity. One such study, commissioned by the CDC Hepatitis Branch, found the strategy not only cost-effective, but actually cost saving (P. Coleman, personal communication). More studies of this type in developed countries are urgently needed.

III. GLOBAL EPIDEMIOLOGY OF HBV INFECTION

The basic argument for the use of HB vaccine as a universal childhood immunogen derives from the epidemiology and natural history of HBV infection (see Chapter 7). Most people are infected with HBV during childhood, and childhood infection is especially likely to lead to the chronic carrier state and serious sequellae of HBV infection. Approximately 2000 million individuals worldwide have serological evidence of prior HBV infection (15), and approximately 300 million individuals are chronically infected carriers of this virus (16). It has been estimated that approximately 25% of these carriers will die from the chronic sequellae of this infection, primarily liver cirrhosis and primary hepatocellular carcinoma (PHC) (17).

The epidemiology of HBV infection varies geographically from being an almost universal infection in childhood to being an infection of adults in certain high-risk groups defined by lifestyle or occupation. Hepatitis researchers, for conceptual purposes, have divided the world into zones of high, intermediate, and low endemicity.

Most countries in Africa, the Middle East, Asia east of the Indian subcontinent, the Pacific Basin, the Amazon Basin, and the Arctic Rim have 50–90% of the population seropositive for at least one marker of HBV infection, with 5–15% of the population being chronically infected carriers positive for hepatitis B surface antigen (HBsAg). In these areas of the world, referred to as regions of high endemicity, most people in the population are infected during childhood either by transmission from child to child or from an infected mother to her newborn (perinatal transmission.)

Perinatal transmission is a highly efficient mode of transmission from mothers who are positive for both HBsAg and hepatitis B e antigen (HBeAg). Infants born to such mothers have an approximately 70–90% risk of being infected and becoming a chronic carrier (18). The role of HBeAg itself may be only as a marker denoting active viral replication and high titers of circulating infectious HBV. High levels of circulating HBV DNA also correlate with perinatal transmission, but the test for DNA is more difficult and expensive than that for HBeAg.

Approximately 40% of HBV carrier women of childbearing age in Asia are HBeAg-positive, and thus perinatal transmission plays an important role in generating the carrier pool in Asian countries (19). If 10% of women are HBsAg positive and 40% of them are HBeAg-positive, then 4% of children are born to such mothers. Assuming that the carrier state develops in 70% of such children, 2.8% of the population are carriers generated by perinatal transmission. If 12% of the population are carriers, then 23% of the carriers are generated by perinatal transmission. In Africa, approximately 10% of mothers are HBsAg-positive, but only about 13% are HBeAg-positive (20, 21). Using the same calculations as above, 1.3% of infants are born to such HBeAg-positive carrier mothers, and perinatal transmission accounts for about 8% of chronic carriers in Africa.

In all areas of high endemicity, child-to-child transmission is more common and generates more carriers than perinatal transmission. This point is often misunderstood and leads to the misconception that if HB vaccine cannot be given at birth to prevent perinatal transmission, it is not worth using. In fact, even in areas with high levels of perinatal transmission, most infection and most carriers can be prevented even if HB vaccine is first used several months after birth.

The relative importance of the various described modes of transmission of HBV in childhood are not well understood. Child-to-child transmission in residential settings occurs in both developed and developing countries, so siblings living closely together or young clients in crowded orphanages or institutions for the retarded readily infect one another (22–24). Some investigators feel that skin lesions such as impetigo, scabies, cuts, scrapes, and scratched insect bites play a major role by providing a route for virus to exit the body of carriers and enter the body of susceptibles as they play together and sleep in the same bed. Certainly, sharing household articles such as toothbrushes and razors, traditional medical procedures (25), circumcision, scarification, and use of reused unsterile medical and dental equipment is responsible for various amounts of HBV transmission in different societies. Arthropod transmission has been discussed for decades, but there is no good evidence that it is an important mode of transmission.

HBV infection during childhood is especially likely to lead to the chronic carrier state. The immunological reasons for this are not well understood, but it is clear that the younger the age at infection, the more likely it is that the carrier state will develop (26). Development of the carrier state at a younger age allows sufficient time for chronic active hepatitis, cirrhosis, and PHC to develop. PHC is the number one or two leading cause of cancer death in males in most sub-Saharan African countries and in many countries in Asia and the Pacific Basin (27).

IV. HB VACCINES

HB vaccines have characteristics that make them easy to integrate into primary infant immunization programs. Vaccines derived from either plasma or recombinant technology may be used in EPI programs. HB vaccines are safe, with an exceptionally low rate of serious or unacceptable side effects and are immunogenic in up to 97% of infants. The efficacy in preventing clinical HB infection and the carrier state exceeds 90% in many field trials (see Chapter 10). HB vaccines are effective from birth, and passively transferred maternal antibodies, or those derived from hepatitis B immune globulin (HBIG), do not interfere with the immune response to this vaccine (see also Chapter 12).

HB vaccines do not interfere with the immune response to BCG, inactivated or live attenuated polio vaccines, DTP, measles, or yellow fever vaccines. Conversely, these other EPI antigens do not interfere with the antibody response to HB vaccine (28). HB vaccines are flexible enough to be effective in any existing EPI schedule without additional visits. Although the EPI has a recommended schedule, in practice, most countries have immunization schedules that vary from it.

HB vaccines are among the most stable vaccines at temperatures above freezing and may be stable for months at room temperature, a characteristic that may make it possible to use it beyond the cold chain in the future. Currently, however, it is recommended that the vaccine be transported and stored at 4–8°C, like DTP. HB vaccine is alum adjuvanted, and thus cannot be frozen (29).

In the future, HB vaccine may be combined with DTP, a combination that will have enormous advantages with respect to shipping, storage, number of injections given at a visit, number of syringes used, training of immunizers, and cost. Several manufacturers are currently working on this formulation. Because DTP cannot be given at birth, monovalent HB vaccine will still need to be used when a dose at birth is desired. Combined HB vaccine with BCG, which may be given at birth, may be developed in the future.

Currently three doses of HB vaccine are recommended to ensure a good immunological response (30). Vaccines given in one dose would have obvious advantages, since the cost of a visit to a health-care provider for immunization may be much greater than the cost of the vaccine, and the dropout rate for repeated visits is quite substantial in many developing countries (and in settings such as prisons, drug treatment centers, and clinics for sexually transmitted diseases [STD]). The WHO Programme for Vaccine Development is developing polymer-coated, slow-release antigens, which may make one-shot vaccines feasible in the near future. This technology is first being developed for tetanus toxoid, and work on polymer-coated HBsAg has begun.

The duration of immunity conferred by HB vaccine is not yet known. It is clear that virtually all responders to this vaccine are protected against clinical HB infection and the development of the carrier state for the length of time we have studied this vaccine (31) (see also Chapter 10). It is also clear that the protection against clinical disease and the carrier state lasts longer than detectable anti-HBs antibodies, calling into question the complex schemes for antibody testing and booster doses proposed by some investigators. It appears that the strong anamnestic response seen after exposure to the virus in vaccinated individuals coupled with the long incubation period of HBV infection makes booster doses unnecessary at this time. Continued follow-up of vaccinated populations will tell us how long protection lasts, and whether booster doses will be necessary in the future.

Strategies sometimes recommended for use of HB vaccine in health-care workers, including prevaccination antibody testing, postvaccination testing, and booster doses, have little or no place in universal immunization programs (in fact, they probably prevent little or no disease in the health-care setting, but serve to reassure personnel and may have medico-legal functions). In most cases, HB vaccine will be given to all infants with no antibody testing. Small subgroups of the population may be tested for anti-HBs to monitor the potency of the vaccine and to assess vaccine coverage, and special studies adding anti-HBc and HBsAg testing may be done to monitor long-term efficacy of the vaccine program.

V. MATERNAL HBsAg SCREENING AND THE TIMING OF THE FIRST DOSE OF VACCINE

Countries embarking on universal immunization programs for control of HBV infection must clearly understand the issues involved in maternal HBsAg screening and the relative importance of the timing of the first dose of vaccine. Newborns of HBsAg- and HBeAg-positive mothers are at high risk of perinatal transmission, and almost 90% will develop the chronic carrier state if infected. Before the advent of HB vaccine it was shown that HBIG had an efficacy of 75% in preventing these newborns from developing the carrier state (33), although the protection provided was of short duration, and many of the infants were infected during the second year of life, probably from their mother or infectious siblings at home. With the advent of HB vaccine it was shown that one dose of HBIG plus a course of HB vaccine could increase the efficacy of treatment to 85–95%, and the protection was of long duration (34, 35). A number of developed countries recommended maternal HBsAg screening of all pregnant women, or of pregnant women belonging to high-risk groups. The strategy of high-risk group screening proved to be ineffective in the United States, and current recommendations state that all pregnant women in the United States should be screened (36).

The use of HBIG and HB vaccine in newborns of carrier mothers, although efficacious, has several problems associated with it. HBIG is quite expensive and not available in many developing countries. In order to use this strategy, it is necessary to screen pregnant women with HBsAg to identify infectious mothers. This testing may be costly, but more importantly depends on the availability of laboratories that run this test and an organized system of prenatal care, which are often not available in developing countries. In fact, many mothers deliver at home with minimal or no prenatal care.

Fortunately, studies have shown that HB vaccine alone, without HBIG, is approximately 75% effective in preventing the carrier state from developing in infants of HBsAg- and HBeAg-positive mothers if the first dose is given near birth (37). Some studies have reported efficacies approaching 90% for HB vaccine alone (38; K. M. Tin, personal communicaton). If HB vaccine is given to all newborns, the cost-effectiveness (cost per additional carrier prevented) of adding expensive prenatal HBsAg screening and HBIG is such that this addition is quite questionable. Many developed countries who have started maternal HBsAg screening may continue to do so, but developing countries should carefully examine the ramifications of this practice, and not automatically follow the policy of other countries with different epidemiological, socioeconomic, and medicolegal situations.

The timing of the first HBV vaccine dose may depend on the realities of vaccine delivery in a given country. When births occur in hospitals or clinics where vaccines are routinely given, HB vaccination at birth may not be difficult. However, home births are usually not attended by persons trained to give immunizations, and immunization under these conditions may be difficult. For immunization to occur, vaccinators must either visit the home or mothers must bring their newborns to an immunization clinic. A system of rapid birth notification and home visits may be difficult and expensive to develop, as this is not the usual immunization routine. Although this may be feasible in densely populated areas, people in remote rural areas, on islands, and in areas difficult to access because of poor roads may be difficult to reach. A demonstration project in Lombok, Indonesia, has been successful in developing a system of early birth notification and home visits (39).

It may also be difficult for mothers to bring their newborns to immunization clinics soon after birth. There may be cultural restrictions about taking the infant out of the home for periods up to several months, and it may be difficult or extremely inconvenient for a mother to travel to a distant immunization clinic. In some countries, rural areas are served by outreach vaccination teams that may visit only a few times a year. One suggested approach is to train local birth attendants in the use of a single-dose HB vaccine apparatus that is kept outside of the cold chain by the birth attendant.

Countries should begin HB immunization by doing the best that they can and giving HB vaccine at the first contact between the child and the immunization teams. As previously discussed, most HBV infection occurs well after the perinatal period and can be prevented by immunization started even at 3 months of age. If perinatal transmission is important and resources are available, special efforts like training birth attendants to give vaccine or early birth notification and home visits for home births may be developed.

VI. BEYOND INFANT IMMUNIZATION

Primary infant immunization with HB vaccine as part of the EPI should be the first step and cornerstone of HBV control. When routine infant immunization is well established and additional resources are available, priorities must be established. Some countries have elected to immunize older cohorts of children, for example, all children under 10 years of age. Other countries, especially in areas of lower endemicity where infection occurs primarily during adulthood, adolescent immunization at the age of 12 or 13 is recommended in addition to infant immunization (Italy) (40). The Spanish state of Catalonia is planning adolescent immunization before they introduce infant immunization. Other countries will choose to use additional resources by immunizing adult high-risk groups such as health-care workers, STD patients, drug users, or prostitutes.

VII. STRATEGY IN COUNTRIES OF LOWER ENDEMICITY

Most developed countries in areas of low endemicity have as their policy to control heptatitis B recommendations to immunize members of groups at high risk of HBV infection. Data from many countries supports the notion that this strategy has failed to control HB infection on a population basis. Certainly, high-risk group immunization is good medical practice, in that it protects high-risk individuals, but it will not eliminate the transmission of HBV infection in the population.

The reasons for the failure of this strategy fall into two categories. First are the practical issues that make implementation difficult or impossible, and second are issues based on the epidemiology of HBV infection that makes the strategy questionable even if great effort and resources are devoted to pursuing it.

Approximately 85–90% of vaccine used in developed countries has gone to health-care personnel, a group that represents less than 5% of reported cases of HBV infection in the United States. Health-care personnel are easy to access, funding for their vaccine is usually provided by employers, and pharmaceutical companies have spent huge sums promoting the immunization of this group. The other high-risk groups are not so easy to reach; members of the groups may have little motivation to seek immunization and funding has generally not been available to immunize them.

The largest single group of reported hepatitis B cases do not admit belonging to any defined high-risk group, and vaccine obviously cannot be targeted to them. The second largest group are people who become infected through sexual transmission. Homosexually active males were recognized as a high-risk group before vaccine became available, but very few municipalities have attempted to vaccinate them. In any case, because of behavior changes secondary to the AIDS epidemic, homosexually active men represent a much smaller proportion of reported cases than they did during the early 1980s. The proportion of cases due to heterosexual transmission is now greater than that due to homosexual transmission. The heterosexually active population is too large a group to reach through selective immunization. Subsets of this population, such as STD patients or persons with multiple partners, have been discussed as target groups for selective immunization, but no programs have been devised to effectively reach them with vaccine or to determine what the impact might be on the overall incidence of HBV infection (41).

Drug users who share needles are an important high-risk group, but reaching them with vaccine is extremely difficult. One attempt during a large HBV and hepatitis delta virus (HDV) epidemic with more than a dozen deaths, utilizing free vaccine, neighborhood clinics, and anonymous recording, found little interest in participation, and over 85% of those tested were already immune or infected. Drug users accessed in prisons or drug treatment programs were also usually immune and rarely returned for the second or third dose unless they were still confined.

Although the prevalence of carriers in European and North American countries may be low in the general population, important subpopulations exist in most countries. In the United States, blacks have an anti-HBs prevalence of approximately 40% by the age of 60 (11), and many Asians born in Asia have a carrier prevalence of over 10%. In European countries, Gypsy populations, North Africans, Africans, and Asians may represent significant subpopulations. Some Eastern European countries (Bulgaria, Albania, Romania, parts of the former U.S.S.R.) have HBV carrier rates in the range of 5–10% in the general population (15).

It is becoming clear to many hepatitis experts and public health officials that the only way to control HBV infection on a population basis in countries with low prevalence is to immunize the population before they begin behaviors, lifestyles, or occupations that put them at risk for HBV infection. Infant immunization is easiest since a well-developed system to administer vaccines to infants is already in operation This strategy will prevent childhood infection in populations where this occurs, but it will take more than 20 years to have a major impact on the incidence of acute HBV infection in populations where adult infection is the predominant pattern.

Immunization of all adolescents will have a more rapid impact on disease rates and can be stopped or reduced to one booster dose (if necessary) after the infant cohorts reach adolescence. Many countries, including the United States, have no existing health programs to deliver vaccines to adolescence, so adoption of this strategy would necessitate building a new delivery structure, a difficult and expensive proposition. There is now increasing interest in reaching adolescents for health interventions such as measles vaccine boosters, cardiovascular screening, and STD, pregnancy, and drug counseling. Adolescent immunization may be more feasible in the near future. Adolescent immunization is much less of a problem for many European countries, which have effective government-run school health programs, and Italy and parts of Spain began adolescent hepatitis B immunization in 1992.

In November 1991, the Immunization Practices Advisory Committee (ACIP) of the U.S. Public Health Service issued a statement entitled "Hepatitis B Virus: A Comprehensive Strategy for Eliminating Transmission in the United States Through Universal Childhood Vaccination" (32). In this document the ACIP recommends routine immunization of all infants in the United States, as well as extended recommendations for immunization of persons in high-risk groups, including adolescents at risk because of drug use, sexual behavior, or because they live in communities where teenage pregnancies, STDs, and injecting drug use is common. Approximately 50% of children receive their primary immunizations in public clinics, paid for by the federal government. Congress will need to allocate sufficient funds through immunization grants to the states if the vaccine is to be made available. Although the government will obtain a reasonable vaccine price through competitive bidding, it remains to be seen what the vaccine will cost parents who go to private pediatricians and how that price will influence compliance with these recommendations.

VIII. CONCLUSION

The EPI has now recommended universal infant immunization with HB vaccine for all countries as the only strategy that will lead to long-term control of HBV infection. The Working Group on Viral Hepatitis of the European Regional Office of WHO, the Immunization Practices Advisory Committee of the U.S. Centers for Disease Control, the Red Book Committee of the American Academy of Pediatrics, and the governments of Italy and New Zealand have now called for universal infant immunization in areas classified as low endemicity. These recommendations recognize that HB immunization of high-risk groups, although medically indicated, will not control HB infection on a population basis.

Universal infant immunization for areas of intermediate and high endemicity has been recommended for many years, and almost 50 countries have begun such programs nationwide or in selected provinces. However, HB vaccine is still considerably more expensive than other EPI vaccines, and many countries cannot afford to buy it. Because UNICEF and other donors have not yet begun to provide HB vaccine to the poorest countries, HB immunization in those areas has, in general, not begun.

Universal infant HB immunization is cost-effective, and HB vaccine has characteristics that make it ideal for introduction into EPI programmes. Development of a safe and effective vaccine against hepatitis B was one of the major medical advances of this century, and we must work to ensure that it is made available to all of the world's children.

REFERENCES

1. Centers for Disease Control. Protection against viral hepatitis: Recommendations of the Immunization Practices Advisory Committee (ACIP). MMWR 1990;39(no. RR-2):1–26.
2. Progress in the control of viral hepatitis: Memorandum from a WHO meeting. Bull. WHO 1988,66:443.
3. Kane MA, Alter MJ, Hadler SC, Margolis HS. Hepatitis B infection in the United States: Recent trends and future strategies for control. Am J Med 1989;87(suppl 3A):11s–13s.
4. Bernier RH, Kane MA, Nathanson N, Francis DP. The vaccine: Priorities for the use of hepatitis B vaccine. In: Millman I, Eisenstein TK, Blumberg BS (eds.).

Hepatitis B: The Virus, the Disease, and the Vaccine. New York and London: Plenum Press, 1984:175–187.

5. Alter MJ, Hadler SC, Margolis HS, et al. The changing epidemiology of hepatitis B in the United States. Need for alternative vaccine strategies. JAMA 1990; 263:1218–1222.

6. WHO, Report of the Global Advisory Group of the Expanded Programme on Immunization. WHO Wkly Epidem Rec 1991; No. 3:9–12.

7. T. Hill, personal communication.

8. WHO Expanded Programme on Immunization. Hepatitis B vaccine: Attacking a pandemic. Update, Nov. 1989.

9. Hall AJ. The Gambian hepatitis B control programme. In: Hollinger FB, Lemon SM, Margolis HS (eds.). Viral Hepatitis and Liver Disease: Proceedings of the 1990 International Symposium on Viral Hepatitis and Liver Disease. Williams & Wilkins, Baltimore, 1990.

10. Robertson RL, Hall AJ, Crivelli PE, et al. Cost effectiveness analyses of the Expanded Program on Immunization (EPI) and of the addition of hepatitis B virus vaccination to the EPI of The Gambia, (in press).

11. McQuillan GM, Townsend TR, Fields HA, et al. The seroepidemiology of hepatitis B infection in the United States, 1976–1980. Am J Med 1989; 87(3A):55

12. Robertson RL, et al. Cost effectiveness of immunization in the Gambia. J Trop Med Hyg 1985; 88:343–351.

13. Mulley AG, et al. Indications for use of hepatitis B vaccine, based on cost-effectiveness analysis. N Engl J Med 1982; 307(11):644–652.

14. Arevalo JA, Washington AE. Cost-effectiveness of prenatal screening and immunization for hepatitis B virus. JAMA 1988; 259(3):365–369.

15. WHO, Division of Communicable Diseases and European Regional Office. Unpublished data. 1991.

16. Maynard JE, Kane MA, Hadler SC. Global control of hepatitis B through vaccination: role of hepatitis B vaccine in the Expanded Programme on Immunization. Rev Infect Dis 1989; 11(s3):s574–578.

17. Beasley RP, Hwang L-Y. Epidemiology of hepatocellular carcinoma, in Vyas GN, Dienstag JL, Hoofnagle JH (eds), Viral Hepatitis and Liver Disease. Orlando, FL, Grune and Stratton, 1984; 209–224.

18. Beasley RP, et al. The 'e' antigen and vertical transmission of hepatitis B surface antigen. Am J Epidemiol 1977; 105:94–98.

19. Stevens CE, et al. Vertical transmission of hepatitis B antigen in Taiwan. N Engl J Med 1975; 292:771–774.

20. Prince AM, et al. Epidemiology of hepatitis B infection in Liberian infants. Infect Immun 1981; 32:675–680.

21. Kiire CF, et al. Hepatitis B infection in subSaharan Africa. Vaccine 1990; 8 (Suppl.):s107–112.

22. Franks AL, Berg, CJ, Kane MA, Browne BB, Sikes RK, Elsea WR, Burton AH. Hepatitis B virus infection in U.S. born children of Southeast Asian refugees. N Engl J Med 1989; 321:1301–1305.

23. Hershow RC, Hadler SC, Kane MA, Adoption of children from countries with endemic hepatitis B: Transmission risk and medical issues. Pediatr Infect Dis J 1987; 6:431–437.

24. Bernier RH, Sampliner R, Gerety R, et al. Hepatitis B infection in households of chronic carriers of hepatitis B surface antigen. Am J Epidemiol 1982; 116:199–211.

25. Kent GP, Brondum J, Keenlyside RA, et al. A large outbreak of acupuncture associated hepatitis B. Am J Epidemiol 1988; 127:591–598.

26. McMahon BJ, Alward WLM, Hall DB, et al. Acute hepatitis B virus infection: Relation of age to the clinical expression of disease and subsequent development of the carrier state. J Infect Dis 1985; 151:599.

27. Parkin DM (ed.). Cancer occurrence in developing countries. IARC Scientific Publications No. 75, Lyon, 1986.

28. Coursaget P, et al. Simultaneous injection of hepatitis B vaccine with BCG, diphtheria and tetanus toxoids, pertussis and polio vaccines. Progress in Hepatitis B Immunization, P. Coursaget, M. J. Tong, eds. Colloque INSERM/John Libbey Eurotext Ltd., 1990, 194:319–324.

29. Kane MA, Clements CJ, Hu DJ. The global control of hepatitis B. In: Douglas RG and Hilleman MR (eds.). Assessment and Management of Risks Associated with Hyperlipidemia, Osteoporosis, and Hepatitis B: Effectiveness of Intervention. Hanley and Belfus, Inc., Philadelphia, 1991:247–263.

30. Hilleman MR. The vaccine solution to the problem of human hepatitis B and its sequellae. In: Douglas RG and Hilleman MR (eds.). Assessment and Management of Risks Associated with Hyperlipidemia, Osteoporosis, and Hepatitis B: Effectiveness of Intervention. Hanley and Belfus, Inc., Philadelphia, 1991:191–207.

31. Hadler SC, Francis DP, Maynard JE. Long term immunogenicity and efficacy of hepatitis B vaccine in homosexual men. N Engl J Med 1986; 315:209.

32. Centers for Disease Control. Hepatitis B virus: a comprehensive strategy for eliminating transmission in the United States through universal childhood vaccination: Recommendations of the Immunization Practices Advisory Committee (ACIP). MMWR 1991; 40(no. RR-13).

33. Beasley RP, Hwang L-Y, Stevens CE, et al. Efficacy of hepatitis B immune globulin for preventing perinatal transmission of the hepatitis B virus carrier state: Final report of a randomized double-blind placebo-controlled study. Hepatology 1983; 3:135–141.

34. Beasley RP, Hwang LY, Lee GC, et al. Prevention of perinatally transmitted hepatitis B virus infection with hepatitis B immune globulin and hepatitis B vaccine. Lancet 1983; 2:1099–1102.

35. Stevens CE, Taylor PE, Tong MJ et al. Yeast recombinant hepatitis B vaccine: Efficacy with hepatitis B immune globulin in prevention of perinatal hepatitis b virus transmission. JAMA 1987; 257:2612–2616.

36. Centers for Disease Control. Hepatitis B virus: A comprehensive strategy for eliminating transmission in the United States through universal childhood vaccination: recommendations of the Immunization Practices Advisory Committee (ACIP). MMWR 1991:40 (No. RR-13):1–25.

37. Smego, RA, Halsey NA, The case for routine hepatitis B immunization in infancy for populations at increased risk. Pediatr Infect Dis J 1987; 6:11–19.

38. Poovorawan Y, Sanpavat S, Pongpunlert W, et al. Comparison of a recombinant DNA hepatitis B vaccine alone or in combination with hepatitis B immune globulin

for the prevention of perinatal acquisition of hepatitis B carriage. Vaccine 1990; 8 (Suppl.);s56–s59.

39. International Task Force on Hepatitis B Immunization: Report on Lombok, Indonesia Demonstration Project, 1991.

40. WHO, Report of the European Working Group on Viral Hepatitis, 1991.

41. Alter MJ, Hadler SC, Margolis HS, et al. The changing epidemiology of hepatitis B in the United States. Need for alternative vaccine strategies. JAMA 1990; 263:1218–22.

17

Needs Unfulfilled by Current Hepatitis B Vaccines

Patricia L. Hibberd, Robert H. Rubin, and Jules L. Dienstag

*Harvard Medical School and
Massachusetts General Hospital, Boston, Massachusetts*

In 1982, a safe and effective plasma-derived hepatitis B virus (HBV) vaccine was introduced. Although it should have been a major breakthrough in the control of hepatitis B (1–4), the vaccine met with limited acceptance because of the concurrent awareness of the unprecedented epidemic of human immunodeficiency virus (HIV) infection and the unfounded fears regarding vaccine safety (5–14). In 1987, a second-generation hepatitis B vaccine was introduced. This new vaccine is derived from recombinant yeast expressing hepatitis B surface antigen (HBsAg, the product of the S gene of HBV), and its availability has relieved the persistent, unfounded fears about the source and safety of the original plasma-derived vaccine (5). Two commercially available preparations of the recombinant yeast-derived vaccine are now available (15). All three vaccines are safe, immunogenic, and effective in the prevention of hepatitis B. Hepatitis B vaccination is recommended for patients who are at high or moderate risk of acquiring hepatitis B infection.

Three concerns regarding the prevention of hepatitis B remain. First, the annual incidence rate of hepatitis B is at best stable through the 1980s (16) despite widespread availability of the vaccine, suggesting that current strategies for vaccination are inadequate. Second, the duration of protection is unclear, and the need for and timing of booster doses is uncertain (17–21). The third concern is the growing population who fail to acquire protective levels of antibody following vaccination (13, 22–41). This population consists of both immunocompromised and immunocompetent individuals. In this chapter, we address these three problems and discuss possible strategies that may offer solutions.

I. FAILURE OF HEPATITIS B IMMUNIZATION POLICY

The incidence of hepatitis B in the United States continued to increase in the early 1980s (42) and remained relatively stable at approximately 13 cases per 100,000 population in the late 1980s (16). There are several important reasons for the lack of an impact of hepatitis B vaccines on the transmission of hepatitis B.

The first problem is that fewer than 10% of the estimated 22 million persons considered at high risk of acquiring hepatitis B infection have actually been vaccinated (43, 44). In other countries, intensive vaccination strategies have demonstrated a reduction in the incidence of hepatitis B infection (45, 46); unfortunately, in the United States, high-risk patients are difficult to reach with current immunization policies. The second problem is that during the 1980s, the epidemiology of hepatitis B infection has been changing (16). The proportion of cases accounted for by homosexual males and health-care workers has decreased by 62 and 75%, respectively. It is likely that availability of hepatitis B vaccine is responsible for the decrease in hepatitis B among health-care workers, but modification of high-risk sexual behavior is the more likely explanation for the reduction in hepatitis B in homosexual men. The proportion of cases accounted for by parenteral drug use has increased by 80%, while cases attributed to heterosexual behavior have increased by 38%. In addition, 30–40% of cases of hepatitis B have occurred in patients with no known risk factor for exposure to hepatitis B (16).

An analogous situation, showing that selective screening is an ineffective method of preventing hepatitis B infection, was the initial recommendations to screen only those pregnant women in high-risk groups for evidence of hepatitis B exposure. Approximately 50% of HBsAg-positive pregnant women were missed, all of whom were capable of transmitting hepatitis B infection to their offspring (47). The result of this observation has been the recent recommendation that all pregnant women be screened for HBsAg to identify all infants that need to be vaccinated at birth (48).

Clearly, immunization of high-risk patients such as intravenous drug users and no-risk patients is difficult to achieve with current policies and has led to the increasingly frequent cry for either expanded or universal vaccination programs, as recommended recently by the Centers for Disease Control (16) (see also Chapter 16). The major obstacle to the initiation of this program is its currently prohibitive cost. Advances in techology resulting in cheaper vaccine production, marketplace competition, purchase of large quantities of vaccine by government contract, changes in the route and schedule of vaccination or use of decreased doses (49) may alleviate some of these cost issues in the near future. The timing of vaccine administration in a universal vaccine program is not yet defined. The simplest approach would be to administer hepatitis B vaccine on a schedule similar to the routine childhood immunizations; however, vaccination early in life may be inadequate to protect against infection during adolescence or early adulthood, when most infections occur. It is possible that preadolescent booster doses would be necessary following a primary series. This proposed booster may be logistically feasible if attached to school attendance and may be combined with a future recommendation for a measles, mumps, and rubella reimmunization.

II. DURATION OF PROTECTION BY HEPATITIS B VACCINE

The duration of protection by the vaccine has been the subject of intense debate in the recent years. Decline in antibody after vaccination has been quantified for up to 7 years (17–21). Antibody levels decline most rapidly in the first 6 months following completion of primary immunization, and more slowly afterwards (19). Regardless of this decline, current data suggest that protection persists at least as long as measurable antibody to HBsAg is detectable in the circulation: 5 years after vaccination, about 90% of patients retain detectable antibody, and approximately 80% have antibody levels that are considered protective (i.e., >10 mIU/ml) (17,50–51).

Even loss of detectable antibody after vaccination does not necessarily correlate with loss of protection, as is demonstrated by the following three observations. First, B cells obtained from vaccine responders with no anti-HBs or a level less than 10 mIU/ml after 7 years in vitro have evidence of intact immunological memory (52). Second, booster vaccination 7 years after primary vaccination produces an anamnestic increase in anti-HBs titer, suggesting that exposure to natural infection would stimulate the same immune response (53). Third, patients whose anti-HBs level has become undetectable after primary immunization who are subsequently exposed to natural hepatitis B develop an immediate, boosterlike anamnestic increase in anti-HBs titer to levels adequate to protect against infection (51).

The maximal level of anti-HBs after completion of the three-part vaccination schedule is predictive of the persistence of antibody (50,54,55). The rate of decline of antibody is similar among all vaccinees and is independent of initial antibody titer. In a large cohort of vaccinated homosexual males, 7% of those whose peak postvaccination anti-HBs level was at least 100 serum radioimmunoassay units (SRU) had no detectable antibody after 5 years (50). In this same population, 54% of patients whose peak titer was below 50 SRU had lost detectable antibody within 5 years.

Long-term protection against hepatitis B has been best studied in homosexual males, in Alaskan natives, and in health-care workers (17, 21, 50) (see also Chapter 12). In one cohort of homosexual males, evidence of HBV infection developed in a small proportion, long after vaccination, that was detected by the de novo appearance of antibody to hepatitis B core antigen (anti-HBc). All but one case was subclinical; the clinical case occurred in one patient in whom detectable HBsAg antigenemia and transient aminotransferase elevation developed. As mentioned above, the risk of subclinical seroconversion was inversely related to the peak anti-HBs level achieved after primary immunization. This cohort of patients was evaluated in the early 1980s, before many homosexual men were avoiding high-risk sexual behavior, and may represent a worst-case scenario with continued high-level exposure to HBV infection. In contrast, in a cohort of vaccinated health-care workers, no cases of clinical or subclinical infection were encountered (17). Even in the cited cohort of homosexual men, clinical illness and HBsAg antigenemia were rarely observed; protection from clinical illness, detectable antigenemia, and chronic infection was the rule (56).

Based on the apparent long-term protection provided by vaccination and the absence of data suggesting that booster immunization has an advantage over natural reexposure, there are no formal recommendations for booster vaccinations except for hemodialysis patients (43, 57) (see below). As mentioned above, if universal vaccination is implemented, future studies may provide answers to the unsolved questions of duration of protection and the need for and timing of booster doses.

A recently recognized related problem is the emergence of "escape mutants" of HBV resulting from evolutionary pressures. Clinical or subclinical infection with hepatitis B after vaccination may be attributable not only to vaccine nonresponsiveness or to loss of protection over time, but also to disease caused by a HBV mutant that may elude protection provided by anti-HBs. For example, in HBsAg-positive liver transplant recipients, suppression of detectable HBsAg can be achieved initially with a high-potency human-mouse hybrid monoclonal anti-HBs. Over several months of therapy, however, HBsAg that is no longer recognized by the monoclonal antibody may become detectable. The emerging variants have been shown to differ from the original HBV isolate by a single amino acid in the highly conserved hydrophobic antigenic domain of the HBsAg/*a* determinant, indicating that even this minimal difference between the two strains is sufficient to interfere with the efficacy of the protective antibody (58).

These escape mutants are not just theoretical concerns following vaccination. In a group of immunized contacts of hepatitis B carriers, including infants born to HBsAg-positive mothers, all of whom developed protective anti-HBs after vaccination, a breakthrough infection developed in one infant (59). The genome of the breakthrough mutant had the identical point mutation in the *a* determinant of HBsAg, as was observed in the transplant recipients described above. The clinical implications and importance of these recent observations in terms of lack of vaccine efficacy or limited duration of protection is unknown.

III. NONRESPONSIVENESS AND HYPORESPONSIVENESS TO THE HEPATITIS B VACCINE

Nonresponsiveness is defined as the failure to acquire detectable levels of anti-HBs after vaccination. Hyporesponsiveness is defined as the failure to acquire protective levels of anti-HBs following vaccination (i.e., at least 10 mIU/ml). Both have been observed in the immunocompetent and immunocompromised patient.

A. Immunocompetent Patients

Between 2.5 and 5% of immunocompetent patients fail to acquire anti-HBs following the routine three administrations of hepatitis B vaccine (1, 14). In these nonresponders, a second course of vaccine injections induces an antibody response in 40% of cases; however, the response tends to be weak and limited in duration. By comparison, in hyporesponders, revaccination is successful in inducing an immune response in most patients, and the immune response is more likely to be adequate and sustained (60).

In addition, among immunocompetent patients, one of the major determinants of response to hepatitis B vaccine is age of the patient at the time of vaccination (22–24). Adult response is inversely related to age, decreasing from more than 95% in young adults to between 50 and 70% in patients over the age of 60 (22, 23). Other factors such as sex, weight, smoking, and presence of other chronic diseases (e.g., diabetes and alcoholic liver disease) have not been associated consistently with decreased responsiveness to the vaccine (23,61,62). Extrinsic factors such as freezing of the vaccine during transport, site of administration (the deltoid being superior to the buttock), and altered timing of vaccine administration have all been associated with decreased immune response to the vaccine (24, 61).

Investigations of immunological nonresponsiveness to HBsAg in mice have demonstrated that antibody production to this antigen is an inherited genetic trait (63,64). In humans, the presence of an immune response gene accounting for anti-HBs production is supported by the identification of a higher than expected frequency of specific extended haplotypes among nonresponders to the hepatitis B vaccine. Specifically, HLA B8, SC01, DR3 and B44, DR7, FC31 have been found in increased frequency in nonresponders and hyporesponders who failed to improve their responsiveness even after a second complete course of hepatitis B vaccine (60). In a follow-up study, patients known to be homozygous or heterozygous at one of these extended haplotypes were vaccinated; heterozygotes responded normally, homozygotes did not. This finding supports the hypothesis that a dominant immune response gene in the MHC is required for a humoral response to HBsAg and that patients who lack this gene cannot mount an adequate anti-HBs response (65). Other nonresponder genotypes have also been described (66,67).

In the murine model, strategies to overcome genetically determined nonresponsiveness to HBsAg have been developed and include alterations in the route of immunization, dose, and the vaccine antigen (68,69). For example, in the murine system, immune responsiveness to HBsAg, the product of the S gene, and responsiveness to the products of Pre-S regions of the hepatitis B genome are linked to different histocompatibility loci. If data from the murine system can be extrapolated to humans, nonresponsiveness may be overcome by use of vaccines containing Pre-S proteins (see also Chapter 20). To date, vaccination of susceptible chimpanzees with a synthetic Pre-S2 polypeptide has been shown to provide protection against challenge with HBV (70). A stable vaccine incorporating the Pre-S2 and S regions has been developed and is currently being tested in normal immunocompetent patients and in patients who have had a limited response to the currently available vaccines (71). Preliminary data in healthy adults show that levels of anti-HBs induced by the new Pre-S2 plus S vaccine are comparable to levels induced by commercially available recombinant vaccine (72).

B.   HIV-Infected Patients

It is well recognized that patients infected with HIV have a variety of defects in immune function that lead to their increased risk of life-threatening infection. In addition to the severe depression in cell-mediated immunity caused by infection and depletion of CD4+ lymphocytes and dysfunction of monocytes and macrophages, these patients also have a severe defect in B-lymphocyte dysfunction. These abnormalities result in decreased responsiveness to many vaccines (73) including heptatitis B. On the other hand, poor responsiveness in this population is not invariable; there is a continuum of immune compromise and vaccine responsiveness. Therefore, in order to accomplish effective protection against hepatitis B in these patients whose high-risk behaviors for HIV infection place them at risk of acquiring hepatitis B infection, vaccination of susceptibles must be initiated as early as possible in the course of HIV infection.

In two small studies of HIV-infected homosexual men, hepatitis B vaccination resulted in seroconversion rates of 53 and 56%, respectively (25, 29). Loss of vaccine-acquired or naturally acquired anti-HBs has also been reported in HIV-positive patients with hemophilia (30). Evidence is also mounting that HIV-positive patients lack both humoral and cellular immune response to HBV and are at increased risk of becoming chronically infected with hepatitis B virus (74, 75). Thus, protection against hepatitis B infection is of critical importance in these patients. It can be achieved in part by elimination of high-risk behavior, but active immunization is also important. Unfortunately, efficacy of the vaccine is limited in this setting. As with other immunosuppressed patients, novel strategies to improve vaccine response are necessary.

C. Oncology Patients

Oncology patients are heterogeneous with respect to their risk for infection in general, but those that have multiple exposure to blood products are at increased risk of acquiring hepatitis B. The risk of hepatitis B infection derives not only from primary infection but also from reactivation of infection associated with intensive chemotherapy (76–81). Unfortunately, as with other immunosuppressed patients, the efficacy of hepatitis B vaccine is limited, varying from under 10% in patients who do not survive malignancy to 70% in survivors (31). Although the response rate is variable and protection after vaccination is not assured during intensive chemotherapy, vaccination is currently recommended for these high-risk patients.

D. Patients with Renal Failure

A wide range of defects in white cell and immune function can be demonstrated in patients with uremia. Although these defects increase the risk of many infections, chronically hemodialyzed patients are at risk of acquiring hepatitis B because of their frequent exposure to blood products (although this risk may decrease as the transfusion requirement is reduced in patients receiving erythropoietin). Unfortunately, vaccine efficacy in this group of patients varies between 44 and 74% (27, 28, 32–38), although administration of extra doses may increase response rates to as high as 86% (39). These results are the best that can be achieved even with double the usual dose of vaccine. More disturbing, despite a 50% rate of seroconversion during one placebo-controlled trial, the incidence of hepatitis B was 6.4% in the vaccinated group and 5.4% in the placebo-treated group. At least 4 of these 67 patients had initially seroconverted, although anti-HBs levels were low or undetectable before detection of HBsAg. The vaccination status of the remaining patients is not clearly specified, but it is possible that in patients on hemodialysis, induced anti-HBs, at least at low titers, cannot be relied upon to protect against hepatitis B infection (28). Higher response rates have been reported with other hepatitis B vaccines not licensed in the United States, i.e., those produced by the Pasteur Institute (13) and the Netherlands Red Cross (40). Still, neither the initial response to hepatitis B vaccine nor the level and duration of responses in hemodialysis patients is entirely satisfactory. The response rate does appear to depend on the degree of uremia at the time of vaccine administration, and therefore vaccination should be considered when chronic progressive renal failure is present but prior to endstage renal disease. Future strategies to improve vaccine efficacy may include concurrent administration of hepatitis B vaccine and immunoadjuvants. Preliminary data in hemodialysis patients show benefit from a combination of hepatitis B vaccine and either interleukin-2 (82) or gamma interferon (83) (see below).

E. Transplant Recipients

Hepatitis B is not an uncommon infection among transplant recipients because of frequent exposure to blood products, prior to transplantation or peri-operatively. Once acquired, hepatitis B infection persists indefinitely in these immunosuppressed patients (84), and occasionally the exogenous immunosuppression necessary to prevent allograft rejection may actually reactivate latent infection (85–87). There is also a risk of progressive liver disease and hepatocellular carcinoma in these patients (88, 89). Again, the seroconversion rate following vaccination is low, varying between 18 and 32%, even when vaccine is administered to patients on stable, maintenance-level immunosuppression (34, 41). Even in those patients who seroconvert, the rate of antibody decline is more rapid than is seen in the normal patient population (34). The message is clear: hepatitis B immunization should occur prior to transplantation and initiation of immunosuppression whenever possible (73).

IV. FUTURE CONSIDERATIONS

Two common themes run through the preceding discussion. Timely delivery of vaccine is inadequate for both immunocompetent and immunocompromised populations and available vaccines are insufficient in both high-risk immunocompromised patients and in immunocompetent genetic nonresponders. Inadequacy of delivery can be overcome by implementation of a universal vaccination program commencing in childhood, enhanced perhaps by booster vaccination prior to adolescence and at the earliest sign of evolving immunocompromising illness. Although financial constraints remain a major obstacle, anticipated reductions in cost will facilitate the implementation of this policy.

Development of new vaccines may provide immunogens to overcome genetic nonresponsiveness to HBsAg (see Chapter 20). Pre-S vaccines are one example. Others include vaccine-adjuvant combinations and vaccines containing hepatitis B core proteins (90, 91). In the murine system, immunization with core proteins provides T-cell help for the humoral immune response to HBsAg and can overcome HBsAg nonresponsiveness (92). In immunocompromised persons, however, a specific genetic defect is unlikely to explain vaccine nonresponsiveness (a report of genetic nonresponsiveness in dialysis patients notwithstanding (93)). Instead, global immunosuppression is the predominant factor. An important and promising new direction for this group of patients is the use of immunomodulators in conjunction with existing vaccines to induce improved immune response. There is already some evidence for an enhanced benefit from hepatitis B immunization in hemodialysis patients when vaccination is combined with immunomodulators such as interleukin-2 and gamma interferon (82, 83).

We continue to urge that extensive evaluation of novel vaccines, alternative vaccination strategies, and immunomodulator or adjuvant combinations be conducted (94). These approaches appear to represent the most promising and rational strategies for resolving the needs unfulfilled by currently available hepatitis B vaccines.

REFERENCES

1. W. Szmuness, C. E. Stevens, E. J. Harley, et al. Hepatitis B vaccine: Demonstration of efficacy in a controlled clinical trial in a high risk population in the United States. *N Engl J Med 303:* 833–841 (1980).

2. S. Krugman, The newly licensed hepatitis B vaccine. Characteristics and indications for use. *JAMA 247:* 2012–2015 (1982).

3. Centers for Disease Control, Recommendations of the Immunization Practices Advisory Committee (ACIP): inactivated hepatitis B virus vaccine. *MMWR 31:* 317–322 327–328 (1982).

4. A. G. Mulley, M. D. Silverstein, J. L. Dienstag. Indications for use of hepatitis B vaccine, based on cost-effectiveness analysis. *N Engl J Med 307:* 644–652 (1982).

5. E. M. Scolnick, A. A. McLean, D. J. West, et al. Clinical evaluation in healthy adults of a hepatitis B vaccine made by recombinant DNA. *JAMA 251:* 2812–2815 (1984).

6. S. Krugman, J. P. Giles, J. Hammond. Hepatitis virus: Effect of heat on infectivity and antigenicity of the MS-1 and MS-2 strains. *J Infect Dis 122:* 432–436 (1970).

7. S. Krugman, J. P. Giles, J. Hammond, Viral hepatitis type B (MS-2 strain). *JAMA 217:* 41–45 (1971).

8. P. Maupas, A. Goudeau, P. Coursaget, et al. Immunisation against hepatitis B in man. *Lancet 1:* 1367–1370 (1976).

9. P. Maupas, J.-P. Chiron, F. Barin, et al. Efficacy of hepatitis B vaccine in prevention of early HBsAg carrier state in children: Controlled trial in an endemic area Senegal. *Lancet 1:* 289–292 (1981).

10. W. Szmuness, C. E. Stevens, E. A. Zhang, et al. A controlled clinical trial of the efficacy of the hepatitis B vaccine (Heptavax B): A final report. *Hepatology 1:* 377–385 (1981).

11. W. Szmuness, C. E. Stevens, E. J. Harley, et al. Hepatitis B vaccine in medical staff of hemodialysis units: Efficacy and subtype cross-protection. *N Engl J Med 307:* 1481–1486 (1982).

12. J. Crosnier, P. Jungers, A.-M. Courouce, et al. Randomized placebo-controlled trial of hepatitis B surface antigen vaccine in French haemodialysis units, I: Medical staff. *Lancet 1:* 455–459 (1981).

13. J. Crosnier, P. Jungers, A.-M. Courouce, et al. Randomized placebo-controlled trial of hepatitis B surface antigen, II: Haemodialysis patients. *Lancet 1:* 797–800 (1981).

14. J. L. Dienstag, B. G. Werner, B. F. Polk, et al. Hepatitis B vaccine in health care

personnel: Safety, immunogenicity, and indicators of efficacy. *Ann Intern Med 101:* 34–40 (1984)

15. J. Petre, F. Van Wijnedaele, B. de Neys, et al. Development of a hepatitis B vaccine from transformed yeast cell. *Postgrad Med J 63* (Suppl 2): 73–81 (1987).

16. Centers for Disease Control Hepatitis B Virus: A comprehensive strategy for eliminating transmission in the United States through universal childhood vaccination: recommendation of the Immunization Practices Advisory Committee (ACIP). *MMWR 40* (no. RR-13) (1991).

17. A. Gibas, E. Watkins, J. L. Dienstag. Long-term persistence of protective antibody after hepatitis B vaccination of healthy adults. *Viral Hepatitis and Liver Disease* (A. J. Zuckermann, ed.), Alan R. Liss, New York, pp. 998–1001 (1988).

18. S. C. Hadler, M. A. Monzon, D. R. Lugo, et al. Effect of timing of hepatitis B vaccine doses on response to vaccine in Yucpa Indians. *Vaccine 7:* 106 (1989).

19. W. Jilg, M. Schmidt, F. Deinhardt. Persistence of specific antibodies after hepatitis B vaccination. *J. Hepatol 6:* 201 (1988).

20. P. R. Taylor, C. E. Stevens. Persistence of antibody to hepatitis B surface antigen after vaccination with hepatitis B vaccine. *Viral Hepatitis and Liver Disease* (A. J. Zuckermann, ed.), Alan R. Liss, New York, p. 995 (1988).

21. R. B. Wainwright, B. J. McMahon, L. R. Bulkow, et al. Duration of immunogenicity and efficacy of hepatitis B vaccine in a Yupik Eskimo population. *JAMA 261:* 2362 (1989).

22. F. Denis, M. Mounier, L. Hessel, et al. Hepatitis B vaccination in the elderly. *J. Infect Dis 149:* 1019 (1984).

23. W. L. Heyward, T. R. Bender, B. J. McMahon, et al. The control of hepatitis B virus infection with vaccine in Yupik Eskimos. *Am J Epidemiol 121:* 914 (1985).

24. A. A. McLean, M. R. Hilleman, W. J. McAleer, et al. Summary of worldwide experience with HB-Vax (R) (B,MSD). *J Infect Dis 7* (Suppl): 95 (1983).

25. A. C. Collier, L. Corey, V. L. Murphy, et al. Antibody to human immunodeficiency virus and suboptimal response to hepatitis B vaccination. *Ann Intern Med 109:* 101–105 (1988).

26. S. C. Hadler. Hepatitis B prevention and human immunodeficiency virus infection. *Ann Intern Med 109:* 92 (1988).

27. B. Seaworth, J. Drucker, J. Starling, et al. Hepatitis B vaccine in patients with chronic renal failure before dialysis. *J Infect Dis 157:* 332–337 (19880.

28. C. E. Stevens, H. J. Alter, P. E. Taylor, et al. Hepatitis B vaccine in patients receiving hemodialysis—immunogenicity and efficacy. *N Engl J Med 311:* 496–501 (1984)

29. C. A. Carne, I. V. D. Weller, J. Waite, et al. Impaired responsiveness of homosexual me with HIV antibodies to plasma derived hepatitis B vaccine. *Br Med J 294:* 866–868 (1987).

30. J. H. Drake, R. T. Parmley, H. A. Britton. Loss of hepatitis B antibody in human immunodeficiency virus-positive hemophilia patients. *Pediatr Infect Dis 6:* 1051–1054 (1987).

31. A. B. Weitberg, S. A. Weitzman, E. Watkins, et al. Immunogenicity of hepatitis B vaccine in oncology patients receiving chemotherapy. *J Clin Oncol 3:* 718–722 (1985).

32. G. R. Aronoff, D. R. Maxwell, B. E. Batteiger, et al. Hepatitis B virus vaccine: A randomized trial of a reduced dose regimen in hemodialysis patients. *Am Soc Kidney Dis 6:* 170–172 (1985).

33. M. Bruguera, M. Cremades, A. Mayor, et al. Immunogenicity of a recombinant hepatitis B vaccine in haemodialysis patients. *Post Grad Med J 63* (Suppl 2): 155–158 (1987).

34. P. J. Grob, U. Binswanger, K. Zaruba, et al. Immunogenicity of a hepatitis B subunit vaccine in hemodialysis and in renal transplant recipients. *Antiviral Res 3:* 43–52 (1983).

35. H. Kohler, W. Arnold, G. Renschin, et al. Active hepatitis B vaccination of dialysis patients and medical staff. *Kidney Int 25:* 124–128 (1984).

36. M. T. Pasico, W. R. Bartholomew, T. R. Beam, et al. Long term evaluation of the hepatitis B vaccine (heptavax-B) in hemodialysis patients. *Am J Kidney Dis 11:* 326–331 (1988).

37. F. G. Regenstein, R. P. Perrillo, C. Bodicky, et al. Clinical and immunological features of chronic dialysis patients who fail to respond to hepatitis B vaccine. *Vaccine 3:* 27–30 (1985).

38. R. W. Steketee, M. E. Ziarnik, J. P. Davis. Seroresponse to hepatitis B vaccine in patients and staff of renal dialysis centers, Wisconsin. *Am J Epidemiol 127:* 772–782 (1988).

39. J. A. Van Geelen, S. W. Schlam, E. M. de Visser, et al. Immune response to heptatitis B vaccine in hemodialysis patients. *Nephron 45:* 216–218 (1987).

40. J. Desmyter, J. Colaert, G. de Groote, et al. Efficacy of hear inactivated hepatitis B vaccine in haemodialysis patients and staff. *Lancet 2:* 1323–1327 (1983).

41. I. M. Jacobson, G. Jaffers, J. L. Dienstag, et al. Immunogenicity of hepatitis B vaccine in renal transplant recipients. *Transplantation 39:* 393–395 (1985).

42. Centers for Disease Control. Annual summary 1984: Reported mobidity and mortality in the United States. *MMWR 33:* 125 (1986).

43. Centers for Disease Control. Update on hepatitis B prevention: Recommendations of the Immunization Practices Advisory Committee. *Ann Intern Med 107:* 353–357 (1987).

44. W. W. Williams, M. A. Hickson, M. A. Kane, et al. Immunization policies and vaccine coverage among young adults: The risk for missed opportunities. *Ann Intern Med 108:* 616–625 (1988).

45. P. J. Grob, M. Rickenbach, R. Stefen, et al. Hepatitis B vaccination campaign in a low endemicity area. *Eur J Public Health 4:* 408–411 (1985).

46. H.-M. Hsu, D.-S. Chen, C.-H. Chuang, et al. Efficacy of a mass hepatitis B vaccination program in Taiwan: Studies on 3464 infants of hepatitis B surface antigen-carrier mothers. *JAMA 260:* 2231–2235 (1988).

47. M. M. Jonas, E. R. Schiff, M. J. O'Sullivan, et al. Failure of Centers for Disease Control criteria to identify hepatitis B infection in a large municipal obstetrical population. *Ann Intern Med 107:* 335–337 (1987).

48. Centers for Disease Control. Prevention of perinatal transmission of hepatitis B virus: Prenatal screening of all pregnant women for hepatitis B surface antigen. *MMWR 37:* 341–346,351 (1988).

49. J. P. Bryan, M. Sjogren, M. Iqbal, et al. Comparative trial of low-dose, intradermal, recombinant- and plasma-derived hepatitis B vaccines. *J Infect Dis 162:* 789–793.

50. S. C. Hadler, D. P. Francis, J. E. Maynard, et al. Long-term immunogenicity and efficacy of hepatitis B vaccine in homosexual men. *N Engl J. Med 315:* 209–214 (1986).

51. C. E. Stevens, P. E. Taylor, M. J. Tong, et al. Hepatitis B vaccine: An overview. *Viral Hepatitis and Liver Disease* (G. N. Vyas, J. L. Dienstag, J. H. Hoofnagle, eds.), Grune & Stratton, Orlando, FL, pp. 275–291 (1984).

52. J. van Hattum, T. Maikoe, J. Poel, et al. Persistance of immune memory in responders to hepatitis B vaccination who subsequently lost anti-HBs titer (abstract). *Hepatology 12:* 885 (1990).

53. S. Krugman, M. Davidson, Hepatitis B vaccine: Prospects for duration of immunity. *Yale J Biol Med 60:* 333–338 (1987).

54. W. Jilg, M. Schmidt, F. Deinhardt. Hepatitis B vaccination: How long does protection last? (letter) *Lancet 2:* 458 (1984).

55. M. T. Pasko, T. R. Beam. Persistence of anti-HBs among health care personnel immunized with hepatitis B vaccine. *Am J Public Health 80:* 590–593 (1990).

56. Hepatitis B Expert Panel. Immunization against hepatitis B. *Lancet 2:* 875 (1988).

57. Centers for Disease Control. Protection against viral hepatitis: Recommendations of the Immunization Practices Advisory Committee (ACIP). *MMWR 39:* 1–26 (1990).

58. G. McMahon, L. A. McCarthy, D. Dottavio, et al. Surface antigen and polymerase gene variation in hepatitis B virus isolates from a monoclonal antibody treated liver transplant patient. *Viral Hepatitis and Liver Disease.* (F. B. Hollinger, S. M. Lemon, H. S. Margolis, eds.), Williams & Wilkins, Baltimore, in press.

59. W. F. Carman, A. R. Zanetti, P. Karayiannis, et al. Vaccine-induced escape mutant of hepatitis B virus. *Lancet 336:* 325–329 (1990).

60. D. E. Craven, Z. L. Awdeh, L. M. Kunches, et al. Nonresponsiveness to hepatitis B vaccine in health care workers: Results of revaccination and genetic typings. *Ann Intern Med 105:* 356–360 (1986).

61. F. E. Shaw, H. A. Guess, J. M. Roets, et al. The affect of anatomic injection site, age, and smoking on the immune response to hepatitis B vaccination. *Vaccine 7:* 425 (1989).

62. D. J. Weber, W. A. Rutala, G. P. Samsa, et al. Obesity as a predictor of poor antibody response to hepatitis B plasma vaccine. *JAMA 254:* 3187 (1985).

63. D. R. Milich, F. V. Chisari. Genetic regulation of the immune response to hepatitis B surface antigen (HBsAg). I. H-2 restriction of the murine humoral response to the a and d determinants of HBsAg. *J Immunol 129:* 320–325 (1982).

64. D. R. Milich, G. G. Leroux-Roels, F. V. Chrisari. Genetic regulation of the immune response to hepatitis B surface antigen (HBsAg). II. Qualitative characteristics of the humoral immune response to the a, d, and y determinants of HBsAg. *J Immunol 130:* 1395–1400 (1983).

65. C. A. Alper, M. S. Kruskall, D. Marcus-Bagley, et al. Genetic Prediction of nonresponse to hepatitis B vaccine. *N Engl J Med 321:* 708–712 (1989).

66. M. E. Walker, W. Szmuness, C. E. Stevens, et al. Genetics of anti-HBs responsive-

ness. I. HLA-DR7 and non-responsiveness to hepatitis vaccination (abstract). *Transfusion 21:* 601 (1981).

67. H. Waranabe, S. Matsushita, N. Kamikawaji, et al. Immune suppression gene on HLA-Bw54-DR4-DRw53 haplotype controls nonresponsiveness in human to hepatitis B surface antigen via CD8+ suppressor T cells. *Hum Immunol 22:* 9–17 (1988).

68. D. R. Milich, G. B. Thornton, A. R. Neurath, et al. Enhanced immunogenicity of the pre-S region of hepatitis B surface antigen. *Science 228:* 1195–1199 (1985).

69. D. R. Milich, M. K. McNamara, A. McLachlan, et al. Distinct H 2-linked regulation of T-cell responses to the pre-S and S regions of the same hepatitis B surface antigen polypeptide allows circumvention of non-responsiveness to the S region. *Proc Natl Acad Sci USA 82:* 8168–8172 (1985).

70. Y. Itoh, E. Takai, H. Ohnuma, et al. A synthetic peptide vaccine involving the product of the pre-S(2) region of hepatitis B virus DNA: Protective efficacy in chimpanzees. *Proc Natl Acad Sci USA 83:* 9174–9178 (1986).

71. R. W. Ellis, P. J. Kniskern, A. Hagopian, et al. Preparation and testing of recombinant-derived hepatitis B vaccine consisting of pre-S2 + S polypeptides. *Viral Hepatitis and Liver Disease.* (A. J. Zukermann, ed.), Alan R. Liss, New York, pp. 1079–1086 (1988).

72. E. Miskovsky, K. Gershman, M. L. Clements, et al. Comparative safety and immunogenicity of yeast recombinant hepatitis B vaccines containing S and pre-S2+S antigens. *Vaccine 9:* 346–350 (1991).

73. P. L. Hibberd, R. H. Rubin. Approach to immunization in the immunosuppressed host. *Infect Dis Clin North Am 4:* 123–142 (1990).

74. S. C. Hadler, F. Judson, D. Echenberg, et al. Effect of prior human immunodeficiency virus on outcome of hepatitis B virus infection. *J Med Virol 21:* 87A (1987).

75. P. E. Taylor, C. E. Stevens, R. de Cordobas, et al. Hepatitis B virus and human immunodeficiency virus: Possible interactions. *Viral Hepatitis and Liver Disease* (A. J. Zuckerman, ed.), Alan R. Liss, New York, pp. 198–200 (1988).

76. J. H. Hoofnagle, G. M. Dusheiko, D. F. Schafer, et al. Reactivation of chronic hepatitis B virus infection by cancer chemotherapy. *Ann Intern Med 96:* 447–449 (1982).

77. C. J. Lightdale, H. Ikram, C. Pinsky, Primary hepatocellular carcinoma with hepatitis B antigenemia-effects of chemotherapy. *Cancer 46:* 1117–1122 (1980).

78. A. N. Schulman, N. D. Fagan, C. M. Ling, et al. Repeated type B hepatitis infections-Ten cases studied prospectively. *Gastroenterology 72:* 1182 (1977).

79. A. Locasciulli, M. Santamaria, G. Masera, et al. Hepatitis B virus makers in children with acute leukemia-the effect of chemotherapy. *J Med Virol 15:* 29–33 (1985).

80. J. R. Wands, C. M. Chura, F. J. Roll, et al. Serial studies of hepatitis-associated antigen and antibody in patients receiving antitumor chemotherapy for myeloproliferative and lymphoproliferative disorders. *Gastroenterology 68:* 105–112 (1975).

81. J. R. Wands, J. A. Walker, T. T. Davis, et al. Hepatitis B in an oncology unit. *N Engl J Med 291:* 1371–1375 (1974).

82. P. J. Grob, H. I. Joller-Jemelka, U. Bingswanger et al. Interferon as an adjuvant for

hepatitis vaccination in non- and low- responder populations. *Eur J Clin Microbiol 3:* 195–198 (1984).

83. S. C. Mueur, H. Dumann, K. H. Bushenfelde zum Meyer, et al. Low dose interleukin-2 induces systemic immune responses against HBsAg in immunodeficient non-responders to hepatitis B vaccination. *Lancet 1:* 15–17 (1989).

84. G. P. Coughlin, A. G. Van Deth, A. P. S. Disney, et al. Liver dysfunction and the e antigen in HBsAg carriers with chronic renal failure. *Gut 21:* 118–122 (1980).

85. G. Dusheiko, E. Song, S. Bowyer, et al. Natural history of hepatitis B virus infection in renal transplant recipients—a fifteen year follow-up. *Hepatology 3:* 330–336.

86. J. Nagington, Y. E. Cossart, B. J. Cohen. Reactivation of hepatitis B after transplantation operations. *Lancet 1:* 558–560 (1977).

87. E. Villa, A. Theodossi, B. Portmann, et al. Reaction of hepatitis B virus infection in two patients—immunofluorescence studies of liver tissue. *Gastroenterology 80:* 1048–1053 (1981).

88. P. S. Parfrey, R. D. C. Forbes, T. A. Hutchinson, et al. The clinical and pathological course of hepatitis B liver disease in renal transplant recipients. *Transplantation 37:* 461–466 (1984).

89. G. P. J. Schroler, R. Weill, I. Penn, et al. Hepatocellular carcinoma associated with chronic hepatitis B virus infection after kidney transplantation. *Lancet 2:* 381–382 (1982).

90. E. Tabor, R. J. Gerety. Possible role of immune responses to HBcAg in protection against hepatitis B infections. *Lancet 1:* 72 (1984).

91. K. Murray, S. A. Bruce, P. Wingfield, et al. Protective immunization against hepatitis B with an internal antigen of the virus. *J Med Virol 23:* 101–107 (1987).

92. D. R. Milich, A. McLachlan, G. B. Thornton, J. L. Hughes. Antibody production to the nucleocapsid and envelope of the hepatitis B virus primed by a single synthetic T cell site. *Nature 329;* 547–549 (1987).

93. S. Pol, C. Legendre, B. Mattlinger, et al. Genetic basis of nonresponse to hepatitis B vaccine in hemodialyzed patients. *J Hepatol 11:* 385–387 (1990).

94. P. L. Hibberd, R. H. Rubin. Immunization strategies for the immunocompromised host: The need for immunoadjuvants. *Ann Intern Med 110:* 955–956 (1989).

18

Variant Hepatitis B and D Viruses

Tim J. Harrison and Arie J. Zuckerman

The Royal Free Hospital School of Medicine,
University of London,
London, United Kingdom

I. INTRODUCTION

It is now more than a decade since the genetic organization of hepatitis B virus (HBV) was elucidated following the molecular cloning and nucleotide sequencing of the 3.2-kilobase viral genome. As the sequences of a number of independent clones representing various subtypes of the virus became available, it was clear that a number of features were highly conserved, most particularly four large open reading frames (ORFs). Other features, such as the 11-base pair, directly repeated motifs involved in the replication of the genome, enhancers, promoters, and signals for the termination of transcription are also largely conserved among the sequences that have been reported to date.

Two of the ORFs encode structural proteins and will be considered in detail in this chapter. The first encodes the nucleocapsid protein, hepatitis B core antigen (HBcAg), and a nonstructural protein, hepatitis B e antigen (HBeAg), which is secreted by the infected hepatocytes. This ORF contains two in-phase methionine codons, which may initiate translation of the messenger RNA. Translation from the downstream codon yields the structural protein, HBcAg. The region upstream of this codon, the so-called precore region, encodes a protein domain which resembles a secretory signal, and translation from the first initiation codon yields a protein which, following proteolytic removal of the carboxyl-terminal domain, is secreted as HBeAg with cleavage of the signal sequence. Recently, there have been a number of reports of virus isolates with variant precore regions, many of which contain in-phase termination codons. These are discussed below.

The second ORF encodes the envelope proteins of the virus, hepatitis B surface antigen (HBsAg). There are three in-phase translational start signals, which yield the large, middle, and major forms of the surface protein. The major protein has been used in natural (plasma-derived) and recombinant (yeast-derived) form as first- and second-generation hepatitis B vaccines, and the emergence of variants that may escape neutralization by vaccine-induced antibody is of particular concern.

Hepatitis delta virus (HDV) is a satellite of HBV, which requires a coat of HBsAg for its transmission. Currently, no specific anti-delta vaccine is available, though a successful response to immunization with hepatitis B vaccine should also protect against HDV. Carriers of HBsAg who are currently HDV-negative are at risk of superinfection by HDV and cannot be protected in this fashion. The HDV genome encodes a protein, hepatitis delta antigen (HDAg), which forms the nucleocapsid of the virus and may be a suitable target for the development of a specific anti-delta vaccine. Variation in the sequence of this protein is therefore of great interest.

II. METHODOLOGY

The small size of the HBV genome (approximately 3200 nucleotides) along with (in most cases) a unique site for the restriction endonuclease *Eco*RI facilitated its cloning into plasmid vectors. Improved methods for the sequencing of DNA based on chemical modification and cleavage (1) or the incorporation of chain-terminating dideoxynucleotides (2) enabled the nucleotide sequence of such clones to be determined rapidly (3–5). By comparing the translation of their nucleotide sequence to protein sequence data available for the amino-terminal 19 residues and carboxyl-terminal three residues of HBsAg, Valenzuela et al. (3) were able to locate the region of the genome encoding the major form of the surface protein. Pasek et al. (5) were able to obtain expression of another region of the genome in *E. coli* and so were able to locate the sequences encoding HBcAg. Complete nucleotide sequences of other isolates of HBV have been reported since these early studies (e.g., 6–9).

Nucleotide sequence analysis of HBV isolates has been facilitated by the development of the polymerase chain reaction (PCR) (10). Briefly, oligonucleotides that are complementary to sites on either strand of the viral genome several hundred base pairs apart are constructed and used to prime synthesis of DNA in repeated rounds of denaturation, annealing, and polymerization using a thermostable DNA polymerase. The logarithmic increase in progeny molecules may result in an amplification of target sequences in the order of 10^6-fold. Two approaches are commonly used for sequence analysis of the product. In the first, the product is subcloned into a suitable vector (such as the bacteriophage M13) and a number of templates sequenced. This method has the disadvantage that minor populations of molecules may be missed in cases where sequence heterogeneity is present. In the second method, the product is used directly as template in a sequencing reaction without subcloning, and sequence heterogeneity may be recognized when the reaction product is analyzed by gel electrophoresis. It should be noted that there is no guarantee that nucleotide sequences obtained by these methods, particularly when only a segment of the genome is amplified by PCR, are derived from viable HBV genomes.

Analysis of the HDV genomes was greatly complicated by the fact that it is a circular RNA molecule (11). Complementary DNA was originally synthesized by self-priming using a nick in the RNA (11), by priming RNA polyadenylated in vitro using an oligo(dT)-linked plasmid, or by random priming of native RNA (12), or by priming with oligonucleotides synthesized on the basis of data from RNA sequencing (13). The current availability of the entire HDV sequence means that selected regions of the genome may be amplified by PCR following reverse transcription of the RNA using the antigenomic oligonucleotide as a primer.

III. VARIATION IN THE HEPATITIS B CORE GENE

Transcription of the core open reading frame is controlled by a promoter situated immediately upstream. The resultant family of transcripts have heterogeneous 5' ends, and the shortest are destined to become "pregenomes" and to serve as templates for the synthesis of progeny genomic DNA. Other transcripts that lack the precore initiation codon are translated from the second in-phase methionine codon to the end of the core open reading frame yielding the nucleocapsid protein (p21), HBcAg. The amino acid sequences of this protein were compared for a number of HBV sequences of various subtypes by Neurath and Kent (14), who found it to be highly conserved. The carboxyl terminus of the protein is arginine rich, and this highly basic domain is believed to interact with the pregenomic RNA in the formation of precores during replication in the hepatocyte and with the genome itself in virions.

The longest of this family of transcripts contain the precore initiation codon and are translated from that codon to produce a protein (p25) that is processed to yield the 15.5-kD HBeAg. The precore region comprises some 29 residues at the amino terminus of the protein, and the first 19 from a signal sequence that directs it to the endoplasmic reticulum (15, 16) where they are cleaved off by a signal peptidase. The protein is later secreted through the endoplasmic reticulum and Golgi apparatus following further proteolysis at the carboxyl terminus (17, 18). A highly conserved aspartyl protease–like domain is located near to the amino terminus of the core protein, and it has been postulated that this may be responsible for the latter cleavage events (19). However, site-directed mutagenesis aimed at the inactivation of this protease does not interfere with the normal processing of HBeAg (20, 21), and it appears likely that a cellular enzyme is responsible for cleavage of the carboxyl-terminal domain.

HBeAg secreted by infected hepatocytes may be detected in serum as a soluble antigen and may be regarded as a marker of infectivity. Clearance of virus-infected hepatocytes from the liver and cessation of viral replication is usually accompanied by seroconversion to anti-HBe. When DNA-DNA hybridization replaced the less sensitive assay for the endogenous DNA polymerase as a method for the direct serological detection of HBV, it became clear that some patients with anti-HBe were seropositive for virus. Lieberman et al. (22) found that 13 of 24 HBsAg carriers from Greece who were HBeAg negative and anti-HBe positive were seropositive for HBV DNA, sometimes at relatively high levels. Similar findings were reported by Hadziyannis et al. (23), who found evidence of continued viral replication in 14 of 18 HBsAg-positive and anti-HBe-positive patients with liver disease. A similar study in Israel also provided evidence of HBV replication in the absence of serum HBeAg, with 10 of 153 HBsAg-positive, HBeAg-negative patients seropositive for HBV DNA (24). In this study, it was clear that HBV DNA positivity in the absence of HBeAg was more common in patients with acute or chronic liver disease (4/20) than in HBsAg carriers without hepatitis (4/111). In our own studies of a healthy (blood donor) population of HBsAg carriers in the United Kingdom, only five of 173 HBsAg-positive, HBeAg-negative donors were seropositive for HBV DNA, in all cases at very low levels (25). In contrast, four of 12 HBsAg- and anti-HBe-positive patients undergoing diagnostic liver biopsy were found to have evidence of HBV replication by Southern hybridization to liver DNA (26). Clearly, patients presenting with liver dysfunction are a selected population and are more likely to have HBV replication in the absence of HBeAg than the general population of HBsAg carriers. Nonetheless, there is evidence that this phenomenon may be more common in Greece and other Mediterranean regions than elsewhere, raising the possibility of involvement of a variant form(s) of HBV.

In 1988 we reported the nucleotide sequence of the genome of a strain of HBV cloned from the serum of a naturally infected chimpanzee (9). A surprising feature of this sequence is a point mutation in the penultimate codon of the precore region changing the tryptophan codon (TGG) to an amber termination codon (TAG). This finding was at odds with the apparent high levels of circulating HBeAg in the chimpanzee's serum (9), though it was known that, at least in the case of the related hepadnavirus, duck hepatitis B virus, an inactive precore region did not prevent active virus replication (27, 28).

The nucleotide sequence of the HBV precore region from a number of anti-HBe-positive Greek patients was investigated by Carman et al. (29) by direct sequencing of PCR-amplified serum HBV DNA. These workers found a mutation of the penultimate codon of the precore region to a termination codon, identical to that previously described by Vaudin et al. (9), in seven of eight anti-HBe-positive patients who were seropositive for HBV DNA by hybridization. In most cases there was a second mutation in the following codon, which may be related to regulation of initiation of translation of the 21-kD HBcAg (29). HBV DNA could also be amplified by PCR from the sera of five of seven patients who were anti-HBe positive but seronegative for HBV DNA by hybridization. In these cases, the patients appeared to be infected with a mixture of viruses with and without this termination codon. Interestingly, the stop codon was also present in virus from one patient who was HBeAg-positive.

Variant viruses were also found by amplification of serum HBV DNA from a further seven anti-HBe-positive patients, one of whom appeared to be coinfected with a wild-type virus (30). Again, the variation involved a G-to-A point mutation creating a termination codon accompanied by a second mutation adjacent to the HBcAg initiation codon and a variety of minor changes. Tong et al. (31) investigated the sequences of viruses from three anti-HBe-positive patients without PCR amplification and again found evidence of inactivation of the precore region. In most cases this was associated with a termination codon in the penultimate position, though in one isolate there was a single nucleotide insertion leading to a frameshift (31). It is clear that these variants are not confined to the Mediterranean region since Okamoto et al. (32) have observed the same nonsense mutation (without a second mutation in the adjacent codon) in patients from Japan and elsewhere along with more rare examples of defective precore regions caused by frameshifts or loss of the precore initiation codon. Mutations of the precore initiation codon have also been observed by Raimondo et al. (33) and Fiordialisi et al. (34) but, again, the latter workers found the nonsense mutation in the penultimate precore codon, with or without the associated adjacent mutation, to be much more common. The common occurrence of the mutation in the penultimate precore codon prompted Li et al. (35) to design specific oligonucleotide probes for its detection. Stringent hybridization of these probes to PCR-amplified DNA enabled the detection of the nonsense and/or the adjacent mutation(s) in a number of HBeAg-negative, DNA-positive sera.

It is clear from the above that HBeAg-negative patients with high levels of HBV replication and from various geographical areas may frequently be found to be infected by viruses with variant precore regions. Presumably, these viruses are able to replicate in the hepatocytes without secretion of HBeAg. The majority of patients who are infected with these variants are anti-HBe-positive, implying past infection with nondefective HBV. It is not clear whether these individuals were originally infected with a mixture of wild-type and mutant viruses or whether the variants arise throughout the course of natural infection. It is likely, however, that the process of seroconversion from HBeAg to anti-HBe positivity selects the variant viruses, and this may be related to the expression of HBeAg on the surface of hepatocytes infected by the wild-type virus (36).

Most of the studies described above involved patients with liver disease, and it is not clear that all carriers of HBsAg with viremia in the absence of HBeAg are infected with variant viruses. For example, in our own studies of United Kingdom blood donors, the rare cases of serum HBV DNA positivity in the absence of HBeAg appeared to have very low levels of circulating virus (25). Sequencing of PCR-amplified HBV DNA from these individuals reveals that the precore regions are intact (Dyal and Harrison, unpublished observations), and it is possible that the anti-HBe response is sufficient to titrate out the small amount of HBeAg produced by the infected hepatocytes. These individuals may be in the process of clearing HBV infection from the liver.

In many cases, precore variants have been described in patients with severe chronic liver disease who may have failed to respond to therapy with recombinant interferon (30), raising the question of whether they are more virulent than the wild-type virus. However, it is clear that such variants will come to the attention of clinicians and scientists when they are involved in causing morbidity while they may pass unnoticed in the asymptomatic HBsAg carrier population. To date there is no convincing evidence for increased virulence of these variants. It should also be noted that these viruses do not have variant surface antigen genes and should be protected against by the currently licensed hepatitis B vaccines.

Other, more complex rearrangements of the HBV core gene have been reported, but it is not clear that they represent viable virus sequences. Will et al. (37) found that an HBV genome with a defective precore region was noninfectious for chimpanzees, but there were other rearrangements of the DNA including a six-base-pair duplication at the end of the X gene. Another variant has been described with more elaborate rearrangements of the core ORF, which include an in-phase termination codon in the precore region, loss of the core initiation codon, and an in-frame insertion of 36 nucleotides with a new initiation codon resulting in a modification of the amino terminus of the core protein (38). The patient infected with this virus failed to make an anti-HBc response, but this may have been related to infection with the human immunodeficiency virus (HIV) (38). Rho et al. (39) have reported the complete nucleotide sequence of an HBV genome in which the termination codon of the X gene was mutated so that the ORF was fused with that of the core gene.

Reports of infections in Senegal characterized by low levels of HBsAg antigenaemia without detectable anti-HBc (40) led to speculation about a new strain of HBV (so-called HBV2). However, nucleotide sequence analysis reveals that the virus(es) involved are not significantly different from HBV, and the unusual serological patterns observed in these patients appear to be attributable to atypical immunological responsiveness on the part of the host rather than to a variant virus. Other examples of HBV infection associated with a complete failure of the immune system to respond to the virus (and which might be diagnosed as non-A, non-B hepatitis on the basis of serology) have been described (41). Again, HBV DNA may be detected by PCR, and subsequent nucleotide sequence analysis does not reveal any major divergence from the wild-type HBV sequence (41).

IV. VARIATION IN THE HEPATITIS B SURFACE GENE

The surface ORF has three in-phase initiation codons, which enable the production of the large (p39 and gp42), middle (gp33 and gp36), and major (p24 and gp27) forms of HBsAg. The pre-S1 region shows some variation between different isolates (14), particularly at the extreme amino terminus (see 9). The domain that binds to the receptor on the hepatocyte appears to reside in this region (42) and is rather more highly conserved. The pre-S2 region is relatively highly conserved but also shows regions of variability (14). The inclusion of the pre-S2 epitopes in future generations of hepatitis B vaccines is largely aimed at increasing the immunogenicity of the surface protein rather than inducing specific anti–pre-S2 antibodies so that variation in this region is not of great consequence.

The currently licensed hepatitis B vaccines contain the major surface protein, and an immune response to the immunodominant *a* epitope appears to induce protective immunity. This epitope, which covers amino acid residues 124–148, is common to all subtypes of the virus and appears to have a double loop conformation. Two minor epitopes responsible for the mutally exclusive subdeterminants *d* or *y* and *w* or *r* (reviewed in Ref. 43) appear to lie to either side of the *a* epitope (*d/y* at amino acid residue 122 and *w/r* at amino acid residue 160).

Studies on the immunogenicity and efficacy of two licensed hepatitis B plasma-derived vaccines, which met the WHO Requirements (HB-VAX produced by Merck Sharp & Dohme and HEVAC B produced by the Institut Pasteur) were carried out in Italy between 1982 and 1987 in infants born to HBsAg carriers and family contacts of carriers. The vaccines were given with and without hepatitis B immunoglobulin (HBIG). Of vaccinated subjects, 1590, mostly infants from two regions of southern Italy where the prevalence of HBsAg was greater than 5%, were followed up. Forty-four (2.8%) of the subjects became HBsAg-positive, 32 of whom had additional markers of replication of HBV, in the presence of specific surface antibody (anti-HBs). The preliminary findings were reported by Zanetti et al. (44). HBsAg was detected in the serum of children born to carrier mothers 14–27 months following completion of immunization with circulating anti-HBs titers ranging from 55 to

370 mIU/ml, and during the administration of booster doses of the vaccine 4–9 months after the first injection, with anti-HBs titers of 70–210 mIU/ml. Similar observations were made in children with family contact with hepatitis B during booster immunization 7–10 months after immunization, with antibody titers ranging from 12 to 2850 mIU/ml, and in adult family contacts 10–28 months after completion of a course of immunization in the presence of anti-HBs at a titer of 6 to more than 120 mIU/ml.

The circulating uncomplexed anti-HBs had a high titer of antibody to the group-specific *a* determinant. Analysis of the HBsAg with monoclonal antibodies showed that the circulating antigen did not carry the *a* determinant or that this determinant was masked. These findings suggested that the circulating viral antigen has an unusual epitopic conformation, which was not neutralized by anti-*a* antibody. Further studies revealed that HBsAg in these persons did not bear epitopes reactive with monoclonal RF-HBs-1 and 7 antibodies previously demonstrated within the *a* determinant of all types of HBV.

In the competitive inhibition format of the assay, both the HBsAg bearing the *a* epitope recognized by monoclonals RF-HBs-1, 7, or 18 and antibodies binding to these epitopes would have been detected. The failure of the serum to inhibit binding of these monoclonals to solid-phase antigen indicated that neither the epitopes nor antibodies binding to these epitopes were present in the patients' serum. In previous studies all HBsAg-positive specimens and the majority of anti-HBs-positive specimens from recovered patients or plasma of recombinant-vaccinated individuals have borne either the RF-HBs monoclonal-reactive epitopes or antibodies binding to these regions. The failure of the antigen to inhibit binding of these monclonal antibodies to solid-phase antigen from other sources suggested either that the epitope recognized by each of these antibodies is not present or that it is masked by antibodies. Failure to find free antibodies and the detection of free uncomplexed antigen by electron microscopy make the latter explanation unlikely. In addition, titration of a number of sera for specific anti-*a* antibody revealed titers of 150 mIU/ml together with free circulating antigen. In 32 out of the 44 immunized contacts of HBV carriers investigated, evidence of infection was confirmed by the presence of additional markers of viral replication. There was no evidence of concurrent infection with the HDV or with the HIV in any of these subjects.

In most cases there was only a transient appearance of HBsAg in the serum followed by anti-HBc and anti-HBe, and in several subjects HBsAg reappeared. However, in one child severe acute hepatitis B occurred followed by persistent elevation of alanine aminotransferase and establishment of the carrier state of HBsAg. The DNA encoding the major antigenic epitope of HBsAg from this child and his mother and from a number of control carriers of HBV were sequenced by Carman et al. (45). The virus from the child was found to have a different sequence from that of the virus infecting mother. A point mutation from guanosine to adenosine occurred at nucleotide position 587, numbered from the *Eco*R1 site of the HBV genome, resulting in an amino acid substitution from glycine to arginine at position 145 in the *a* determinant of HBsAg. This mutation was stable, since it was present in an isolate from the same child at the ages of 11 months and 5 years. The *a* determinant in this child and in some of the other subjects studied was partially lost, as shown by the failure of some monoclonal anti-*a* antibodies to bind to the circulating HBsAg. All cases tested had lost the *a* determinant as shown by polyclonal antibody subtyping assays. This might have been the result of high titers of anti-HBs masking the epitope.

The failure of monoclonal anti-*a* antibodies to neutralize the HBsAg implies that the changes in antigenicity may be specific to a single epitope. Carman et al. (45) found that the virus was intact in the rest of the coding region for the *a* determinant, and it seemed likely, therefore, that the region in which the mutation occurred is an important HBV epitope to which vaccine-induced neutralizing antibody binds and that the mutant virus can avoid this antibody. The mutant virus is able to replicate, and there is preliminary evidence that further spread of this escape mutant virus continues in Italy.

There is another recent report by McMahon et al. (46) of a patient with HBV-induced end-stage liver disease who received a liver transplant and was given monoclonal anti-HBs to prevent reinfection of the homograft. After treatment, HBV DNA became detectable again in the serum, and sequencing of the genome revealed an mutation identical to that described above in the immunized child.

There are thus two independent lines of evidence pointing to the susceptibility to mutation of this region of the viral envelope under "immune pressure." Long-term follow-up studies and surveillance are clearly required, and consideration may have to be given to the design of future hepatitis B vaccines to prevent the emergence of this escape virus mutant.

V. HEPATITIS DELTA VIRUS

Cloning and sequencing of the HDV genome revealed it to be a circular RNA molecule of around 1700 nucleotides with extensive sequence complementarity (11–13). There is considerable similarity to the viroids and virusoids of plants, and consensus sequences involved in the replication and processing of these agents appear to be highly conserved among HDV isolates. HDV encodes two species of HDAg (p24 and p27) which have both been shown to be derived from a single antigenomic open reading frame, originally designated ORF5 (47). In addition to its structural role in the HDV nucleocapsid, HDAg has been shown to be required for the replication of HDV RNA (48). It appears that the two species of HDAg are translated from heterogeneous HDV mRNA in which a single nucleotide change determines the presence or absence of an amber termination codon (yielding p24 and p27, respectively) (49, 50). Immunogenic epitopes of HDAg have been mapped using synthetic peptides, antipeptide antibodies, and human monoclonal antibodies (51) and by probing overlapping hexapeptides on pins using immune sera (52). These studies reveal a number of potential epitopes throughout the protein.

Recently, Chao et al. (53) reported the complete nucleotide sequence of an isolate of HDV obtained on Nauru Island in the Pacific which shows 14–17% divergence from other known HDV sequences. These authors identified three regions of the genome that are highly conserved: (a) the region around the autocatalytic cleavage site of genomic RNA, (b) the region around the auto-catalytic cleavege site of anti-genomic sense RNA, and (c) the region encoding the middle one-third domain of HDAg. This region is the RNA-binding domain of HDAg, which specifically interacts with HDV RNA (54). It remains to be determined whether the variable severity and transmissibility of HDV infection is related to sequence heterogeneity among different isolates.

REFERENCES

1. Maxam, A. M., and W. Gilbert. 1977. A new method for sequencing DNA. Proc. Natl. Acad. Sci. U.S.A. 74:560–564.
2. Sanger, F., S. Nicklen, and A. R. Coulson. 1977. DNA sequencing with chain-terminating inhibitors. Proc. Natl. Acad. Sci. U.S.A. 74:5463–5467.
3. Valenzuela, P., P. Gray, M. Quiroga, J. Zaldivar, H. M. Goodman, and W. J. Rutter. 1979. Nucleotide sequence of the gene coding for the major protein of hepatitis B virus surface antigen. Nature 280:815–819.
4. Galibert, F., E. Mandart, F. Fitoussi, P. Tiollais, and P. Charnay. 1979. Nucleotide sequence of the hepatitis B virus genome (subtype ayw) cloned in *E. coli*. Nature 281:646–650.
5. Pasek, M., T. Goto, W. Gilbert, B. Zink, H. Schaller, P. MacKay, G. Leadbetter, and K. Murray. 1979. Hepatitis B virus genes and their expression in *E. coli*. Nature 282:575–579.
6. Ono, Y., H. Onda, R. Sasada, K. Igarashi, Y. Sugino, and K. Nishioka. 1983. The complete nucleotide sequences of the cloned hepatitis B virus DNA; subtype adr and adw. Nucleic Acids Res. 11:1747–1757.
7. Kobayashi, M., and K. Koike. 1984. Complete nucleotide sequence of hepatitis B virus DNA of subtype adr and its conserved gene organization. Gene 30:227–232.
8. Okamoto, H., M. Imai, M. Shimozaki, Y. Hoshi, H. Iizuka, T. Gotanda, F. Tsuda, Y. Miyakawa, and M. Mayumi, 1986. Nucleotide sequence of a cloned hepatitis B virus genome, subtype ayr: comparison with genomes of the other three subtypes. J. Gen. Virol. 67:2305–2314.
9. Vaudin, M., A. J. Wolstenholme, K. N. Tsiquaye, A. J. Zuckerman, and T. J. Harrison, 1988. The complete nucleotide sequence of the genome of a hepatitis B virus isolated from a naturally infected chimpanzee. J. Gen. Virol. 69:1383–1389.
10. Saiki, R. K., S. Scharf, F. Faloona, K. B. Mullis, G. T. Horn, H. A. Erlich, and N.

Arnheim. 1985. Enzymatic amplification of beta-globin genomic sequences and restriction site analysis for diagnosis of sickle cell anemia. Science 230:1350–1354.

11. Kos, A., R. Dijkema, A. C. Arnberg, P. H. van der Meide, and H. Schellekens. 1986. The hepatitis delta (delta) virus possesses a circular RNA. Nature 323:558–560.

12. Wang, K. S., Q. L. Choo, A. J. Weiner, J. H. Ou, R. C. Najarian, R. M. Thayer, G. T. Mullenbach, K. J. Denniston, J. L. Gerin, and M. Houghton. 1986. Structure, sequence and expression of the hepatitis delta (delta) viral genome [published erratum appears in Nature 1987; 328(6129):456]. Nature 323:508–514.

13. Makino, S., M. F. Chang, C. K. Shieh, T. Kamahora, D. M. Vannier, S. Govindarajan, and M. M. Lai. 1987. Molecular cloning and sequencing of a human hepatitis delta (delta) virus RNA. Nature 329:343–346.

14. Neurath, A. R., and S. B. H. Kent. 1985. Antigenic structure of human hepatitis viruses. *Immunochemistry of Viruses. The Basis for Serodiagnosis and Vaccines* (Eds. M. H. V. Regenmortel and A. R. Neurath), Elsevier Science Publishers B.V., pp. 325–366.

15. Ou, J. H., O. Laub, and W. J. Rutter. 1986. Hepatitis B virus gene function: the precore region targets the core antigen to cellular membranes and causes the secretion of the e antigen. Proc. Natl. Acad. Sci. U.S.A. 83:1578–1582.

16. Roossinck, M. J., S. Jameel, S. H. Loukin, and A. Siddiqui. 1986. Expression of hepatitis B viral core region in mammalian cells. Mol. Cell Biol. 6:1393–1400.

17. Takahashi, K., A. Machida, G. Funatsu, M. Nomura, S. Usuda, S. Aoyagi, K. Tachibana, H. Miyamoto, M. Imai, T. Nakamura, Y. Miyakawa, and M. Mayumi. 1983. Immunochemical structure of hepatitis B e antigen in the serum. J. Immunol. 130:2903–2907.

18. Standring, D. N., J. H. Ou, F. R. Masiarz, and W. J. Rutter. 1988. A signal peptide encoded within the precore region of hepatitis B virus directs the secretion of a heterogeneous population of e antigens in Xenopus oocytes. Proc. Natl. Acad. Sci. U.S.A. 85:8405–8409.

19. Miller, R. H. 1987. Proteolytic self-cleavage of hepatitis B virus core protein may generate serum e antigen. Science 236:722–725.

20. Nassal, M., P. R. Galle, and H. Schaller. 1989. Proteaselike sequence in hepatitis B virus core antigen is not required for e antigen generation and may not be part of an aspartic acid-type protease. J. Virol. 63:2598–2604.

21. Jean-Jean, O., S. Salhi, D. Carlier, C. Elie, A. M. De Recondo, and J. M. Rossignol. 1989. Biosynthesis of hepatitis B virus e antigen: directed mutagenesis of the putative aspartyl protease site. J. Virol. 63:5497–5500.

22. Lieberman, H. M., D. R. LaBrecque, M. C. Kew, S. J. Hadziyannis, and D. A. Shafritz. 1983. Detection of hepatitis B virus DNA directly in human serum by a simplified molecular hybridization test: comparison to HBeAg/anti-HBe status in HBsAg carriers. Hepatology 3:285–291.

23. Hadziyannis,S. J., H. M. Lieberman, G. G. Karvountzis, and D. A. Shafritz. 1983. Analysis of liver disease, nuclear HBcAg, viral replication, and hepatitis B virus DNA in liver and serum of HBeAg vs. anti-HBe positive carriers of hepatitis B virus. Hepatology 3:656–662.

24. Tur-Kaspa, R., E. Keshet, M. Eliakim, and D. Shouval. 1984. Detection and

characterization of hepatitis B virus DNA in serum of HBe antigen-negative HBsAg carriers. J. Med. Virol. 14:17–26.

25. Harrison, T. J., V. Bal, E. G. Wheeler, T. J. Meacock, J. F. Harrison, and A. J. Zuckerman. 1985. Hepatitis B virus DNA and e antigen in serum from blood donors in the United Kingdom positive for hepatitis B surface antigen. Br. Med. J. Clin. Res. 290:663–664.

26. Harrison, T. J., M. G. Anderson, I. M. Murray-Lyon, and A. J. Zuckerman. 1986. Hepatitis B virus DNA in the hepatocyte. A series of 160 biopsies. J. Hepatol. 2:1–10.

27. Chang, C., G. Enders, R. Sprengel, N. Peters, H. E. Varmus, and D. Ganem. 1987. Expression of the precore region of an avian hepatitis B virus is not required for viral replication. J. Virol. 61:3322–3325.

28. Schlicht, H. J., J. Salfeld, and H. Schaller. 1987. The duck hepatitis B virus pre-C region encodes a signal sequence which is essential for synthesis and secretion of processed core proteins but not for virus formation. J. Virol. 61:3701–3709.

29. Carman, W. F., M. R. Jacyna, S. Hadziyannis, P. Karayiannis, M. J. McGarvey, A. Makris, and H. C. Thomas. 1989. Mutation preventing formation of hepatitis B e antigen in patients with chronic hepatitis B infection. Lancet 2:588–591.

30. Brunetto, M. R., M. Stemler, F. Bonino, F. Schodel, F. Oliveri, M. Rizzetto, G. Verme, and H. Will. 1990. A new hepatitis-B virus strain in patients with severe anti-HBe positive chronic hepatitis-B. J. Hepatol. 10:258–261.

31. Tong, S. P., J. S. Li, L. Vitvitski, and C. Trepo. 1990. Active hepatitis-B virus replication in the presence of anti-HBe is associated with viral variants containing an inactive pre-C region. Virology 176:596–603.

32. Okamoto, H., S. Yotsumoto, Y. Akahane, T. Yamanaka, Y. Miyazaki, Y. Sugai, F. Tsuda, T. Tanaka, Y. Miyakawa, and M. Mayumi. 1990. Hepatitis B viruses with precore region defects prevail in persistently infected hosts along with seroconversion to the antibody against e antigen. J. Virol. 64:1298–1303.

33. Raimondo, G., G. Rodino, V. Smedile, S. Brancatelli, D. Villari, G. Longo, and G. Squadrito. 1990. Hepatitis-B virus (HBV) markers and HBV-DNA in serum and liver tissue of patients with acute exacerbation of chronic type-B hepatitis. J. Hepatol. 10:271–273.

34. Fiordalisi G., E. Cariani, G. Mantero, A. Zanetti, E. Tanzi, M. Chiaramonte, and Primi D. 1990. High genomic variability in the pre-C region of hepatitis B virus in anti-HBe, HBV DNA-positive chronic hepatitis. J Med Virol 31:297–300.

35. Li, J., S. Tong, L. Vitvitski, F. Zoulim, and C. Trepo. 1990. Rapid detection and further characterization of infection with hepatitis B virus variants containing a stop codon in the distal pre-C region. J. Gen. Virol. 71:1993–1998.

36. Schlicht, H. J., and H. Schaller. 1989. The secretory core protein of human hepatitis B virus is expressed on the cell surface. J. Virol. 63:5399–5404.

37. Will H., C. Kuhn, R. Cattaneo and H. Schaller. 1982. Structure and function of the hepatitis B virus genome. In *Primary and Tertiary Structure of Nucleic Acids and Cancer Research,* vol. 12, pp. 237–247. Edited by M. Miwa, S. Nishimura, A. Rich, D. G. Soell and T. Sugimura. Tokyo: Japan Scientific Society Press.

38. Bhat, R. A., P. P. Ulrich, and G. N. Vyas. 1990. Molecular characterization of a new variant of hepatitis B virus in a persistently infected homosexual man. Hepatology 11:271–276.

39. Rho, H. M., K. Kim, S. W. Hyun, and Y. S. Kim. 1989. The nucleotide sequence and reading frames of a mutant hepatitis B virus subtype adr. Nucleic Acids Res. 17:2124–2124.

40. Coursaget, P., B. Yvonnet, C. Bourdil, M. N. Mevelec, P. Adamowicz, J. L. Barres, J. Chotard, R. N'Doye, I. Diop Mar, and J. P. Chiron. 1987. HBsAg positive reactivity in man not due to hepatitis B virus. Lancet 2:1354–1358.

41. Thiers, V., E. Nakajima, D. Kremsdorf, D. Mack, H. Schellekens, F. Driss, A. Goudeau, J. Wands, J. Sninsky, P. Tiollais, et al. 1988. Transmission of hepatitis B from hepatitis-B-seronegative subjects. Lancet 2:1273–1276.

42. Neurath, A. R., S. B. Kent, N. Strick, and K. Parker. 1986. Identification and chemical synthesis of a host cell receptor binding site on hepatitis B virus. Cell 46:429–436.

43. Zuckerman, A. J., and T. J. Harrison. 1990. Hepatitis B virus and hepatitis D virus. *Principles and Practice of Clinical Virology*, 2nd ed. (Eds. A. J. Zuckerman, J. E. Banatvala, and J. R. Pattison), John Wiley and Sons Ltd., pp. 153–172.

44. Zanetti, A. R., E. Tanzi, G. Manzillo, G. Maio, C. Sbreglia, N. Caporaso, H. Thomas, and A. J. Zuckerman. 1988. Hepatitis B variant in Europe [letter]. Lancet 2:1132–1133.

45. Carman, W. F., A. R. Zanetti, P. Karayiannis, J. Waters, G. Manzillo, E. Tanzi, A. J. Zuckerman, and H. C. Thomas. 1990. Vaccine-induced escape mutant of hepatitis B virus. Lancet 336:325–329.

46. McMahon, G., L. A. McCarthy, D. Dottavio, and L. Ostberg. Surface antigen and polymerase gene variation in hepatitis B virus isolates from a monoclonal antibody-treated liver transplant patient; in Hollinger F. B., S. M. Lemon, H. S. Margolis (eds): Viral Hepatitis and Liver Disease. Baltimore, Williams & Wilkins, 1991, pp. 219–221.

47. Weiner, A. J., Q. L. Choo, K. S. Wang, S. Govindarajan, A. G. Redeker, J. L. Gerin, and M. Houghton. 1988. A single antigenomic open reading frame of the hepatitis delta virus encodes the epitope(s) of both hepatitis delta antigen polypeptides p24 delta and p27 delta. J. Virol. 62:594–599.

48. Kuo, M. Y., M. Chao, and J. Taylor. 1989. Initiation of replication of the human hepatitis delta virus genome from cloned D. J. Virol. 63:1945–1950.

49. Luo, G. X., M. Chao, S. Y. Hsieh, C. Sureau, K. Nishikura, and J. Taylor. 1990. A specific base transition occurs on replication hepatitis delta virus RNA. J. Virol. 64:1021–1027.

50. Xia, Y. P., M. F. Chang, D. Wei, S. Govindarajan, and M. MC. Lai. 1990. Heterogeneity of hepatitis delta-antigen. Virology 178:331–336.

51. Bergmann, K. F., P. J. Cote, A. Moriarty, and J. L. Gerin. 1989. Hepatitis delta antigen. Antigenic structure and humoral immune response. J. Immunol. 143:3714–3721.

52. Wang, J. G., R. W. Jansen, E. A. Brown, and S. M. Lemon. 1990. Immunogenic domains of hepatitis delta virus antigen: peptide mapping of epitopes recognized by human and woodchuck antibodies. J. Virol. 64:1108–1116.

53. Chao, Y. C., M. F. Chang, I. Gust, and M. MC. Lai. 1990. Sequence conservation and divergence of hepatitis delta-virus RNA. Virology 178:384–392.

54. Lin, J. H., M. F. Chang, S. C. Baker, S. Govindarajan, and M. MC. Lai. 1990. Characterization of hepatitis delta-antigen-specific binding to hepatitis delta-virus RNA. J. Virol. 64:4051–4058.

19

Application of Synthetic Peptide Technology to Experimental HBV Vaccine Design

David R. Milich

The Scripps Research Institute, La Jolla, California

I. INTRODUCTION

Interest in the development of synthetic hepatitis B virus (HBV) vaccines began as soon as the viral genome was sequenced. Knowledge of the primary amino acid sequence of the structural proteins removed the first obstacle to the development of synthetic HBV immunogens, but a number of other factors remain to be considered. Our approach has been to utilize synthetic peptide reagents as probes to analyze basic aspects of the immune response to HBV proteins in a murine model system. This analysis may help us understand immune-mediated viral clearance mechanisms and provide the framework for the rational design of alternative HBV vaccines including the feasibility of a synthetic-based vaccine.

The original concept of a synthetic peptide vaccine was a B-cell epitope conjugated to an heterologous protein carrier such as tetanus toxoid. The phenomenon of carrier-induced suppression, the lack of well-defined carrier proteins suitable for human use, and the realization that priming a T-cell memory response relevant to the pathogen may be beneficial and possibly essential have altered this assumption. Only relatively recently has the desirability of including antigen-relevant T-cell recognition sites into the design of synthetic vaccines been considered. Therefore, definition of a synthetic vaccine will be expanded in this review to include composite peptides containing both T- and B-cell epitopes derived from the same HBV protein, composite peptides containing T- and B-cell epitopes from different HBV proteins, and peptide-protein chimeric subviral particles. The analysis of these various peptide immunogens has included the identification of relevant T- and B-cell recognition sites on the viral protein(s), linking the T- and B-cell components, immunogenicity tests in small animals, and ultimately protection trials in chimpanzees. Several of the experimental synthetic immunogens discussed in this chapter have progressed through chimpanzee protection trials successfully.

II. THE STRUCTURAL PROTEINS OF THE HBV

During HBV infection, at least four antigen-antibody systems are observed: (a) hepatitis B surface antigen (HBsAg) and its antibody (anti-HBs), (b) the preS antigens associated with HBsAg particles and their antibodies, (c) the particulate nucleocapsid antigen (HBcAg) and anti-HBc, and (d) an antigen structurally related to HBcAg, namely HBeAg and its antibody (anti-HBe). The specific serological marker of HBV infection is the HBsAg, which is present both in the intact virion and as free circulating filamentous and spherical 22-nm subviral particles. The HBsAg is composed of a major polypeptide, P24, and its glycosylated form, GP27. The HBsAg is a complex T-cell-dependent antigen possessing a common group-specific determinant, designated *a,* and two sets of subtype-specific determinants, *d/y* and *w/r.* Therefore, the four subtypes of HBsAg *(adw, ayw, adr,* and *ayr)* represent the major viral phenoptypes. Additional polypeptides of higher molecular weight (P39 and GP33) have recently been identified (1, 2).

The larger envelope polypeptides share the 226 amino acids of P24 (S region) at the carboxy terminus and possess additional residues at the amino terminus. The preS2 region consists of 55 residues amino-terminal to the S region (2), and the preS1 region consists of 119 residues amino-terminal to the preS2 region (1) (this region contains 108 or 119 amino acids depending on HBV subtype; numbering of amino acid residues in this chapter is based on 119 residues in the preS1 region). The relative proportions of P24 and GP33 are similar in the three morphological forms of HBsAg. However, the amount of P39 detected on intact virions, filaments, or spheres differs significantly in that P39 is associated preferentially with virions and filaments and only minimally with spheres (1) (Fig. 1). Herein HBsAg particle preparations are designated according to the highest molecular weight polypeptide present (i.e., HBsAg/P39, HBsAg/GP33, and HBsAg/P24).

The nucleocapsid of HBV is a 27-nm particle composed of multiple copies of a single polypeptide (P21), and the intact structure exhibits hepatitis B core antigenicity (HBcAg). A nonparticulate form of HBcAg designated HBeAg is secreted into the serum during HBV infection. Although HBcAg and HBeAg are serologically distinct, the primary amino acid sequences show significant identity [serum HBeAg (P15) lacks the C-terminal 34 residues of HBcAg (3) and possesses an additional 10 N-terminal residues (4)].

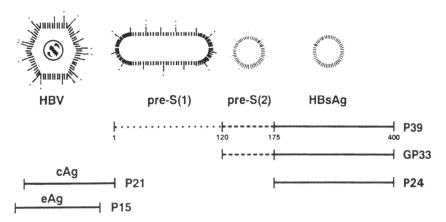

Figure 1 Representation of the antigen and polypeptide composition of envelope and nucleocapsid proteins of intact virons and spherical and filamentous subviral particles.

III. T-CELL VERSUS B-CELL ANTIGEN RECOGNITION

Prior to detailed analysis of the fine specificity of T- and B-cell recognition of the HBV structural proteins, a general discussion of mechanisms of T- and B-cell antigen recognition may be useful. In general, T-helper (Th) cells do not recognize native protein antigen, but only antigen that has been processed or physically altered (i.e., denatured, partially degraded, unfolded) and subsequently displayed in association with major histocompatibility complex (MHC)–encoded class II molecules (Ia) by the antigen-presenting cell (APC) (5). It has been suggested that intracellular processing represents events necessary to produce or select for that portion of the molecule or epitopes that have affinity for the Ia molecule and that the epitope associated with Ia molecules creates the determinant recognized by Th cells (6). The structural characteristics of the antigen required for its interaction with Ia have been the subject of numerous studies and is beyond the scope of this chapter. However, it should be noted that a T-cell determinant must possess at least two characteristics: the ability to interact with Ia molecules and the ability to interact with the T-cell receptor (TCR). Residues within the T-cell site involved in interaction with Ia have been termed *agretopic,* and residues involved in interaction with the TCR have been termed *epitopic* (7, 8). Agretopic and epitopic residues need not be segregated and are often interspersed within a 6- to 12-residue T-cell site. Examination of T-cell recognition in a number of protein systems has indicated that the T-cell response appears highly focused on a limited number of determinants (9–12). It has become apparent that the number of potential T-cell sites is not the limiting factor, but rather distinct sites are "selected" by each MHC haplotype, and even within a single haplotype immunodominant epitopes further focus the T-cell response (13). In the HBV system, the T-cell response to the HBcAg is focused on a general region; however, T cells of mice of five different MHC haplotypes predominantly recognize a distinct determinant within that region (12). Similarly, the fine specificity of the T-cell response to the preS2 region of the envelope of HBV is dependent on the MHC haplotype of the responding strain (14). Therefore, a protein antigen does not contain a preordained T-cell site or set of sites, but rather T-cell recognition sites will vary depending on the MHC of the immunized individual. Therefore, the constraints placed on T-cell recognition of antigen due to the dual recognition of antigen plus MHC molecules present theoretical problems to the design of T-cell components of a synthetic vaccine. This is quite different from B-cell recognition sites, which are relatively fixed on a protein antigen.

In terms of vaccine design, it is imperative that a synthetic T-cell determinant be capable of priming a memory T-cell response that can be recalled by a determinant on the pathogen. Sercarz and colleagues have categorized peptide T-cell determinants as immunodominant, subdominant, and cryptic dependent on the ability to recall a proliferative response from native protein-primed T-cells (13). In this regard, we have observed that very slight modifications in a peptide (i.e., minimal deletions or elongations), which do not effect peptide-specific T-cell activation, can dramatically affect the ability to generate a native protein-specific response (15). This phenomenon may reflect processing events within the native antigen that do not occur on a peptide antigen or vice versa (16). Therefore, great care must be taken in constructing synthetic T-cell sites, which are both immunogenic and relevant to the native protein.

In contrast to Th-cell recognition of antigen, B cells recognize their epitopes on native proteins in solution. Antibody-binding sites on proteins have long been categorized into two types, designated as sequential or continuous and conformational or discontinuous (17). Although it is acknowledged that most B-cell epitopes on protein antigens are of the conformational variety (18), a number of proteins possess (at least to some degree) sequential determinants dependent only on the linear amino acid sequence, which can be mimicked by techniques of peptide chemistry now in common use. Examples of such sequential epitopes are observed in a malaria circumsporozoite protein tandem repeat sequence (19), a number of epitopes within the preS regions of HBsAg/P39 and HBsAg/GP33 (20–22), a sequence within gp41 of the human immunodeficiency virus (HIV-1) (23), and a sequence within gp120 of HIV-1 (24, 25). These epitopes may be excellent candidates for synthetic vaccine design, whereas conformation-dependent epitopes are not, at least in the context of the present synthetic peptide technology. Unfortunately, B-cell epitopes of the S region of HBsAg (i.e., HBsAg/P24) and HBcAg appear to be of the conformational variety (26–28).

The classical approach to "searching" for B-cell recognition sites on a protein using synthetic peptides has been to synthesize a panel of candidate peptides, immunize, and test the antipeptide antisera for reactivity with the immunizing peptide and the native protein. Reciprocally, antibody to the native protein can be screened for reactivity on a panel of synthetic peptides. It was originally thought that antibodies reactive with native protein would only be produced if the fragment or peptide used for immunization closely reproduced the tertiary conformation of the protein. However, numerous studies showed that linear synthetic peptides corresponding to parts of a protein are able to elicit antibodies that react with the intact antigen (29–33). One can, at least operationally, define three categories of antipeptide antibodies: (a) an antipeptide that reacts with the immunizing peptide, but not with the native protein (i.e., peptide-specific), (b) an antipeptide that reacts with the immunizing peptide and with the native protein, but does not compete with antibodies produced by immunization with the native protein (i.e., peptide-unique), and (c) an antipeptide that reacts with the immunizing peptide and with native protein and that inhibits reactivity of antibodies elicited by immunization with the native protein (i.e., sequential determinant-specific). In other words, antibodies to a sequential determinant can be elicited by immunization with either a peptide or the native protein. In terms of synthetic vaccine design, only antipeptide antibodies capable of neutralizing infection are primarily of interest. Both peptide-unique and sequential determinant-specific antipeptide antibodies may be capable of neutralization, since both categories of antibodies bind native protein, whereas peptide-specific antibodies do not. The emphasis placed on using peptides that represent sequential determinants within the native protein is based on the desire to elicit antibody specificities that are elicited by the native protein during infection. However, it is possible that peptide-unique antibodies are also capable of possessing neutralizing function. For example, antibodies raised against residues 284–311 of the S region of HBsAg bind the immunizing peptide, bind native HBsAg, but do not compete with antinative monoclonal antibodies (unpublished observation); nevertheless, this peptide protected chimpanzees from infection with HBV (34). Therefore, in this case it appears that antipeptide antibodies that bound native HBsAg at "unique" sites other than those bound by antibodies to the native protein were capable of viral neutralization in vivo. The generality of this observation will require further studies in other viral systems and with other peptide antisera.

In summary, the challenge to the design of synthetic vaccines in terms of B-cell recognition is to overcome the conformational nature of many B-cell determinants by selecting only nonconformational epitopes or by learning to "structure" conformational peptides. The challenge in terms of T-cell recognition resides in the ability to provide a sufficient diversity of T-cell recognition sites to immunize an outbred population.

IV. IDENTIFICATION OF T- AND B-CELL SITES WITHIN HBV STRUCTURAL PROTEINS

A. Envelope Proteins

A prerequisite for the design of a synthetic HBV vaccine is the identification of relevant T- and B-cell recognition sites within the structural proteins. Although the antibody sites within the S region (resides 175–400) of HBsAg are primarily conformational (26–28), a number of investigators have predicted B-cell sites using synthetic peptides (Table 1) (see Ref. 35 for review). Although peptides derived from the entire S-region sequence have been synthesized, interest has focused on the major hydrophilic domain between residues 284 and 324 and on either side of the three cysteine residues (311–313). This region also contains numerous serological subtype substitutions (50). To address the issue of the requirement for intact disulfide bonds for HBsAg antigenicity, several investigators have prepared peptides with a cyclic structure by the formation of a disulfide bond between cysteines 298 and 311 (40, 41) or 313 and 321 (46). The cyclic versions were reported to react more efficiently with group-specific antisera (i.e., anti-*a*) (40, 46). These studies clearly reveal the importance of residues within the hydrophilic domain, but the inability of antipeptide sera (i.e., anti-284–311) to compete with antinative HBsAg monoclonal antibodies (unpublished observation) suggests that these linear and cyclic S-region peptides may not represent the entire epitope. Perhaps these peptides represent some part of greater conformational epitopes.

The problems in attempting to utilize peptides to mimic conformational B-cell determinants of HBsAg are not encountered with T-cell determinants since native conformation is not required for T-cell recognition of HBsAg (49). Accordingly, several T-cell recognition sites within the S region of HBsAg have been defined with synthetic peptides in humans and in mice (Table 1). The human and murine data indicate that the T-cell site recognized is dependent on the MHC haplotype of the responder. The S-region T-cell sites we have defined in mice are, in retrospect, relatively weak as compared to the T-cell sites identified within the preS region of HBsAg and within the HBcAg. This may reflect a relative decrease in the efficiency of T-cell recognition of the S region, which is consistent with studies using recombinant antigens (51, 54), or it may reflect improvement in technology in the more recent studies.

Numerous studies have been aimed at identifying T-cell and B-cell (antibody) recognition sites within the preS regions of HBsAg. These studies have been greatly facilitated by the fact that the preS regions of HBsAg contain continuous as opposed to discontinuous or topographical B-cell determinants (20, 22, 52, 53) unlike the S region (26–28). Denoting the amino terminus of the preS2 region as residue 120, synthetic peptides 120–145 (20) and 133–151 (55) were shown to bind human antibodies elicited by HBV infection or murine anti-preS2

Table 1 B- and T-Cell Recognition Sites Within the Envelope Proteins of HBsAg Defined with Synthetic Peptides

B-cell sites	Ref.	T-cell sites			Ref.
S region					
175–194	36	193–202	Th	DPw4	47
176–190	37	195–214	CTL	D^d	48
195–221	36	212–226	Th	A^q	49
222–239	38	269–283	Th	A^q	49
243–253	38	284–311	Th	$H-2^k$	49
269–283	37	314–328	Th	$H-2^k$	49
284–311[a]	34, 37				
291–311	39				
296–311	40, 41				
cyclic					
308–320	42				
309–329	43				
312–323	44, 45				
313–321	46				
cyclic					
330–359	36				
PreS2					
120–145[a]	20, 60	120–132	Th	$A^{q,s,k}$	63
126–140	57	120–134	Th, CTL	human	64
132–145	58	126–140	Th	human	57
133–151[a]	55, 61	148–174	Th	(see Fig. 2)	14, 17
137–143	56				
150–174	59				
PreS1					
1–21	53	12–21	Th	A^s	65
12–47[a]	66–68	21–28	CTL	A11	70
12–32	53	53–73	Th	A^s	65
16–27	65	94–117	Th	$H-2^{s,f,k,b}$	
27–35	69				
32–53	22				
41–53	65				
72–78[a]	69				
94–117[a]	22, 68				
94–105	65				
106–117	65				

[a]Peptides that have been shown to be protective in chimpanzee challenge experiments. Peptides derived from the hydrophilic domain of the S region of HBsAg are indicated by the box; Th, T-helper cell site; CTL, cytotoxic T-lymphocyte site.

antibodies elicited by immunization (52). Furthermore, these two synthetic peptides derived from the preS2 region sequence elicited antibodies cross-reactive with the native preS2 region (20, 52, 55). Antinative preS2 and anti-peptide antibodies were also cross-inhibitory in competitive inhibition assays (52). These studies indicate that the preS2 B-cell epitopes can be effectively represented by synthetic peptides. Further analysis using a combination of truncated synthetic peptides and monoclonal antibodies revealed that the murine antibody response to the preS2 region is predominantly focused on residues 133–143, and two distinct but overlapping epitopes were identified as 133–139 and 137–143 (56). Human HBV-infected sera also bind 133–143 and the constituent overlapping epitopes within this sequence (56) (see Table 1).

In terms of T-cell recognition, studies using a truncated preS2 polypeptide and a series of synthetic peptides illustrated that the C-terminal sequence (151–174) of the preS2 region is the dominant focus of T-cell recognition in multiple murine strains (14) and possibly in human vaccine recipients as well (T. Cupps and D. Milich, unpublished observation). Specifically, 17 distinct T-cell recognition sites were defined within the C-terminal half of the preS2 region (Fig. 2). The fine specificity of T-cell recognition of the preS2 region was dependent on the H-2 haplotype of the responding strain. T-cell recognition of all 17 sites was subtype specific, which is consistent with the fact that the C-terminal sequence is highly polymorphic between the d and y subtypes of the preS2 region (14). Additional studies have defined other T-cell sites within the preS2 region in humans as well as in mice (Table 1).

Several preS1-specific T-cell recognition sites have also been defined, which are relevant to the native HBsAg/P39. For example, the preS1 sequences 12–21, 57–67, and 94–117 can induce and elicit HBsAg/P39-specific T-cell activation in murine strains of the H-2^s haplotype (65). A number of preS1-specific antibody-binding sites have also been recently elucidated (Table 1). Identification of distinct T-cell and B-cell recognition sites within the preS region has allowed examination of the ability of a T-cell population specific for a single peptide to provide functional T-cell help for a series of B-cell specificities on HBsAg/P39. For this purpose, mice are primed with a synthetic T-cell determinant and challenged 4 weeks later with a suboptimal dose of HBsAg/P39 particles, and the fine specificities of the antibodies produced are measured. For example, priming with 12–21 elicited T-cell helper function resulting in in vivo antibody production to 12–32, 133–139, 137–143 in the preS region and group- and subtype-specific determinants in the S region. Similarly, priming with p94–117 elicited antibody production specific for p41–53, p94–105, 106–117, 133–139, and 137–143 in the preS region but did not prime antibody production to the S region determinants (65). Unprimed mice produced no antibody upon challenge. These results indicate that T cells primed to a single determinant are sufficient to provide functional help to multiple B-cell clones, which recognize unique epi-

HBsAg Pre-S(2) Region

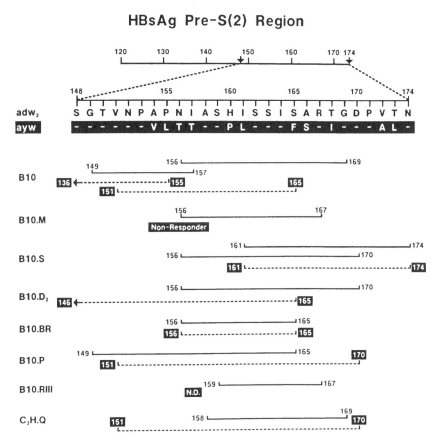

Figure 2 A summary of T-cell recognition sites within the *d* and *y* subtypes of the preS2 region identified among a panel of murine strains representing eight distinct H-2 haplotypes. The amino acid sequence of the p148–174 region of the *adw₂* subtype is shown, and the amino acid sequence of the *ayw* subtype is indicated by boxed letters. T-cell recognition sites relevant to the *adw₂* subtype sequence are indicated by solid lines, and sites relevant to the *ayw* subtype are indicated by dashed lines. The sites depicted do not necessarily represent the minimum size required to induce T-cell proliferation, but represent sequences capable of inducing T-cell proliferation at least 10-fold greater than background at a concentration of 10 μg/ml. The immunogens used to prime the T cells used to define these sites included HBsAg/GP33 *d* and *y*, p133–174 *d* and *y*, and p148–174 *d*. (From Ref. 14.)

topes on a complex HBsAg particle. This illustrates how T-cell recognition of sites within the preS regions can result in circumvention of nonresponse to the S region of HBsAg (22, 52, 54). It is noteworthy that 12–21 and p94–117 elicited antibody production to unique as well as common B-cell determinants. For example, p94–117 primed an anti-p41–53 response, whereas 12–21 did not. These data provide strong evidence that the fine specificity of the T-helper cell can influence the fine specificity of the antibody produced (65). These findings may have applications to the design of synthetic immunogens. For example, combinations of T- and B-cell sites can be preselected in order to elicit a desired antibody specificity.

B. Nucleocapsid Proteins

Examination of the fine specificity of T-cell recognition of HBcAg has shown that HBcAg-specific T cells from a variety of murine strains recognize multiple but distinct sites within the HBcAg/HBeAg sequence (12). T-cell recognition of HBcAg and HBeAg is highly cross-reactive both in the murine and human systems, which is consistent with the amino acid sequence identity between these two antigens (12, 71–74). T-cell recognition sites have been defined by 10- to 21-residue synthetic peptides. Although several strains recognize multiple T-cell sites, each strain recognizes a predominant T-cell determinant, and the fine specificity of this recognition process is dependent on the H-2 haplotype of the responding strain (Table 2). For example, T cells of H-2^s strains recognize 120–131 predominantly, H-2^b strains recognize 129–140, H-2^f strains recognize 100–110, H-2^q strains recognize a sequence within 100–120 distinct from H-2^f mice, and H-2^d mice recognize 85–96 predominantly (12, 75, 76). This murine model predicts that a human outbred population would exhibit similar complexity, and individuals may recognize distinct T-cell sites in the context of their HLA genotype. Indeed, recent studies indicate that human T cells recognize multiple sites within HBcAg/HBeAg that mostly overlap with the previously determined murine sites (77, 112) (Table 2). However, an apparent dominant T-cell site recognized by human HBcAg-specific T-cell clones has not been previously defined in the murine model (112). Although recognition of antibody-binding sites on HBV proteins appears conserved across many species, the diversity of Th-cell recognition sites within the murine species raises the question: Are Th-cell sites defined in the mouse relevant to human Th-cell recognition? We would argue that the definition of a Th-cell site in any species simply indicates that the sequence possesses the appropriate structural/chemical characteristics necessary to associate with MHC class II molecules. Whether a given MHC-binding sequence will function as a Th-cell site for a given individual of a particular species will, of course, depend on a number of additional factors such as MHC haplotype and TCR availability. However, the fact that MHC-encoded

Table 2 T-Cell Recognition Sites Within HBcAg/HBeAg Defined with Synthetic Peptides

		Ref.
Murine		
1–20	A^q	12
28–52	A^s	12
70–94	$H-2^d$	12
85–96	$H-2^d$	76
100–110	A^f	76
100–120	A^q	12
120–140	$H-2^{s,b,d}$	12
120–131	A^s	75
129–140	A^b	75
Human		
1–20		112
11–27(CTL)		115
50–69		112
72–90		77
90–99		77
108–122		77
117–131		112
126–146		77

class II molecules and the cellular mechanisms mediating T-cell recognition are well conserved across species makes the probability of overlaps in T-cell repertoires between species likely. In fact, a number of T-cell sites in the HBV system as well as in other systems have been identified that activate both murine and human T cells.

To determine the ability of synthetic T-cell sites to prime Th cells and facilitate anti-HBc production in vivo, the HBcAg-specific peptide 120–140 and amino-terminal (120–131) and carboxy-terminal (129–140) fragments were studied in the B10.S and B10 strains (75). Mice were primed with peptide and challenged with a suboptimal dose of HBcAg, and serum anti-HBc measured. In the B10.S strain, 120–140–primed and 120–131–primed mice produced IgG anti-HBc efficiently 7 days after the challenge, whereas 129–140–primed mice did not. Similarly, priming with 120–140 elicited anti-HBc in the B10 strain. In contrast to the B10.S strain, the carboxy-terminal 129–140 contained the active Th-cell site for B10 mice. These results are consistent with the T-cell proliferation results and indicate a concordance between T-cell proliferation and Th-cell fine specificities (75). Identification of HBcAg-specific T-cell recognition sites and characterization of their functional ability to elicit proliferation and to induce anti-HBc antibody in vivo have relevance to synthetic vaccine design and possibly to the use of peptide T-cell sites as immunotherapeutic agents in HBV chronic carriers.

Although several B-cell sites within HBcAg have been predicted [i.e., 107–118 (78) and 74–83 (79)], the dependence of HBcAg antigenicity on conformational integrity suggests that linear peptides may not be sufficient to completely mimic HBcAg B-cell epitopes. We have also noted the relative importance of the region bordering residue 80 in terms of antibody recognition of HBcAg. Our data indicate a contribution of residues 73–87 to anti-HBc binding, but similar to S-region peptides, this linear peptide does not appear to fully represent the entire native epitope (unpublished observation). We have been unable to confirm the importance of residues 107–118 in terms of antibody recognition of HBcAg using a similar peptide composed of residues 106–117. At least two HBeAg-specific epitopes designated HBe/α and HBe/β have been suggested (113). One group concluded that the HBe/β epitope is conformational residing around residue 140 plus an additional sequence at the N-terminus of HBeAg, and that HBe/α is linear and localized around residue 80 (79). More recently, another group has suggested that HBe/α is conformational and that HBe/β is linear and comprised of residues 128–133 (114). Our unpublished studies indicate that the "dominant" B-cell sites on HBeAg are primarily conformation dependent and are not faithfully mimicked by synthetic linear peptides. Antibody and T-cell sites have also been localized on nonstructural proteins of the HBV (see Ref. 80 for review).

V. SYNTHETIC PEPTIDES CAN PROTECT CHIMPANZEES AGAINST HBV INFECTION

The identification of B- and T-cell recognition sites within the structural proteins of HBV has provided the opportunity to determine the protective efficacy of immunization with peptide antigens. As previously discussed, immunization of chimpanzees with a synthetic peptide derived from the S region of HBsAg (residues 284–311) linked to KLH resulted in protection after HBV challenge (34). Immunization with a cyclic version of 284–311 resulted in complete protection in one chimp and an attenuated infection in another (81). These experiments identified a protective determinant within the S region and suggest that peptide-unique antibodies can neutralize infection in vivo.

Because preS-region B-cell epitopes appear to primarily represent sequential determinants in the native antigen (20, 52), it was anticipated that synthetic B-cell epitopes derived from preS sequences would be good candidates for eliciting protective antibodies. Indeed, three synthetic immunogens derived from the preS2 region—120–145-KLH (60), 133–151-KLH (61), and the entire 55–mer 120–174 (82)—have been shown to elicit protective antibodies in chimpanzees. These studies demonstrated that anti-preS2 antibodies in the absence of anti-S antibodies were sufficient to protect against HBV infection. Interestingly, in a second trial using free peptide unconjugated to a carrier protein 120–145 was also shown to be protective (68). Presumably, the presence of a T-cell determinant(s) within the amino terminus (i.e., 120–132) provided the Th-cell function necessary for anti-preS2 antibody production (63). It is notable that both outbred chimpanzees in this experiment responded to a single T-cell site, and similarly a majority of outbred baboons responded to unconjugated 120–145 (B. Thornton, personal communication). In this regard, in a previous study of HIV-1 vaccine recipients it was quite surprising that a high percentage of HIV-1 gp160-immune donors demonstrated a T-cell proliferative response to a single peptide (83). It is possible that the complexity of the human/primate MHC (i.e., number of loci and allelic polymorphism) and the fact that most humans are heterozygous in the MHC may actually increase the potential for any given peptide to interact with a MHC gene product. If true, this would have a profound effect on the design of synthetic vaccines, which is believed to be limited by the phenomenon of MHC-restricted T-cell recognition.

Recent studies have demonstrated that synthetic peptide sequences 12–47 (67, 68) and 94–117 (68) derived from the preS1 region of HBsAg are also protective in the chimpanzee challenge model. Note that both these pre-S1 synthetic immunogens possess both T- and B-cell epitopes (Table 1). Although the contribution of peptide-specific Th cells is difficult to interpret because the peptide immunogens were conjugated to KLH, 12–47–specific T-cell proliferative responses were observed in chimpanzees immunized with 12–47-KLH, and antibody titers were boosted upon injection of free peptide prior to infection with HBV (68).

VI. COMPOSITE SYNTHETIC IMMUNOGENS COMPRISED OF T- AND B-CELL RECOGNITION SITES

An ideal synthetic peptide vaccine will be composed of pathogen-specific T- and B-cell recognition sites. The use of heterologous protein carriers for B-cell epitopes would be problematic in human vaccine recipients and, more importantly, would not prime memory Th cells relevant to the pathogen should neutralizing antibody wane. For these reasons we have examined strategies to combine relevant T- and B-cell recognition sites into a single synthetic immunogen. The first example of a composite synthetic immunogen consisted of preS2 residues 120–145, which possesses a T-cell site on the amino-terminus (120–132) and two overlapping B-cell sites on the carboxyl-terminus (133–143)

(63). This unconjugated synthetic immunogen is very immunogenic in murine strains that can recognize the 120–132 T-cell sequence (i.e., H-2^{q,k,b}), but H-2^{d,f} strains are nonresponders and H-2^s strains are low responders (15). Importantly, the anti–133–143 antibody response is fully cross-reactive with the native preS2 region (63) (Table 3). However, a limitation of this synthetic immunogen is the fact that 120–132-specific Th cells are not cross-reactive with the native preS2 region (63). Therefore, the 120–132 T-cell site can serve to prime Th cell activity for anti-preS2 antibody production but would not provide long-term Th cell memory that would be recalled by exposure to HBV at a later date. Therefore, in a subsequent composite synthetic immunogen we chose the preS1 sequence 12–21 as the T-cell site because it represents a T-cell site within the native protein for H-2^{s,f}–bearing strains (65). The preS2 B-cell epitopes present within residues 133–151 were used in all studies because these B-cell sites are well characterized and anti–133–143 is protective (60, 61). Immunization with preS1 12–21–(133–151) resulted in efficient anti–133–143 antibody production, which was highly cross-reactive with preS2-containing native particles (i.e., HBsAg/GP33) (Table 3). Furthermore, the peptide-primed Th cells were also cross-reactive with HBsAg/p39 (65). This study demonstrated that T- and B-cell sites located on distal areas of the same preS protein could be combined on a single synthetic molecule and serve as an effective immunogen relevant to native protein-specific T and B cells.

Vaccination with nucleocapsid as well as envelope (S or preS2) antigens has been reported to protect against HBV infection (84, 85). Because antibodies to HBcAg are not virus neutralizing, the mechanism of protection by HBcAg is unknown. However, an interrelationship between the immune responses to HBsAg and HBcAg has recently been reported. HBcAg-specific T cells

Table 3 Composite Synthetic Immunogens Comprised of T-cell and B-cell Recognition Sites

T site[a]	B site (preS2)	Antipeptide		Antinative	Ref.
		T site	B site		
PreS2 120–132–133–145[b]		0	+ +	+ +	15, 63
PreS1 12–21–133–151		0	+ +	+ +	65
HBc 120–140–133–143		+ + +	+ +	+ +	75
PreS2 151–174–133–143 (NH$_2$)		+ + +	+ +	±	15
PreS2 151–174–133–143 (COOH)		0	+ + + +	+ + +	15

[a]Composite peptide immunogens were produced in a single synthesis and were tested in strains that could recognize the T-cell component by virtue of their MHC haplotype.
[b]The B-cell site preS2 133–145 is relatively nonimmunogenic when injected alone (63).

are able to provide Th-cell activity for anti-S-, anti-preS2-, and anti-preS1–specific antibody production if HBcAg and the envelope proteins are present within the same particle (i.e., the virion) (86). This phenomenon may contribute to the mechanism of protection by HBcAg vaccination. In view of this, we constructed a synthetic immunogen composed of HBcAg-specific T-cell recognition sites (i.e., residues 120–140) and the preS2 envelope B-cell sites represented by residues 133–143 (75). Strains that can recognize HBc 120–140 at the Th-cell level (i.e., H-$2^{s,b,d}$) respond well to immunization with the composite immunogen, which results in anti-preS2 antibody production and HBcAg-primed Th cells (Table 3). These results demonstrate the feasibility of constructing complex synthetic immunogens that represent multiple proteins of a pathogen and are capable of engaging both T and B cells relevant to protection. Another study has utilized the multiple antigen peptide (MAP) approach to combine B- and T-cell determinants derived from the S region and the preS2 region of HBsAg (62). This system allows for the construction of multivalent synthetic immunogens.

In each of the previous examples of composite T- and B-cell synthetic immunogens, the immunogenicity correlated with the MHC haplotype of the responding strain due to MHC-restricted T-cell recognition of the T-cell site used. Because T-cell recognition of the preS2 regions is focused on residues 151–174 in strains of seven different MHC haplotypes (14), we reasoned that this sequence would be an efficient synthetic T-cell carrier peptide for multiple strains. Therefore, the preS2 sequence 133–174 appeared to represent an ideal synthetic immunogen because it contained dominant B-cell (133–143) and T-cell (151–174) recognition sites. Although 133–174 was indeed immunogenic in all strains, the antibodies produced were primarily directed towards a T-cell site (i.e., 156–174) and, therefore, were only minimally cross-reactive with HBsAg/GP33 (15). This "defect" was corrected by reversing the orientation of the T- and B-cell sites such that the 133–143 B-cell site was positioned carboxyl-terminally to the 151–174 T-cell site. Immunization with 151–174–(133–143) resulted in efficient anti–133–143 antibody production, which cross-reacted with HBsAg/GP33 (Table 3).

Further analysis revealed that the orientation of the T- and B-cell sites also affected T-cell recognition. Figure 3 represents a summary of our experience with these two synthetic preS2 immunogens. Immunization of B10.S mice with native HBsAg/GP33 elicits antibody production primarily specific for 133–139 (B_1) and to a lesser extent 137–143 (B_2). Two overlapping T-cell recognition sites in the B10.S strain have also been identified as 156–170 (T_1) and 161–174 (T_2) (14). B10.S mice immunized with the synthetic preS2 immunogen 133–174 produce high titer antibody to a unique site, 156–174, and significantly less antibody to B_1 and B_2. Furthermore, the antibody produced is not highly cross-reactive and the native HBsAg/GP33. At the T-cell level, 133–174–primed

Pre-S(2) Region of HBsAg

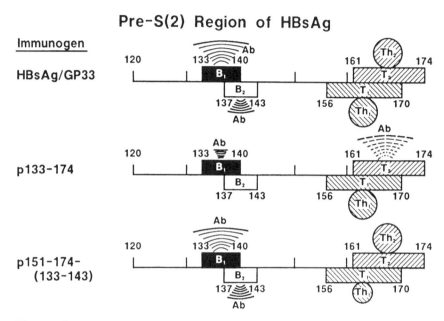

Figure 3 Schematic representation of the T- and B-cell responses to native and synthetic preS2 immunogens. B_1 and B_2 represent dominant antibody-binding sites, and T_1 and T_2 represent dominant T-cell recognition sites in the B10.S strain. The presence of an enriched Th symbol denotes T-cell recognition of the indicated T-cell site. Antibody production is indicated by lines radiating from the B-cell site. (From Ref. 15.)

T cells recognize the T_1 epitope exclusively. Because we wished to duplicate with a synthetic immunogen the immune response to the native preS2 region as closely as possible, these results were unsatisfactory. Immunization with 151–174–(133–143) resulted in a more "nativelike" antibody response directed primarily at sites B_1 and B_2 and highly cross-reactive on native HBsAg/GP33. In contrast to T cells from mice immunized with 133–174, 151–174–(133–143)–primed T cells recognized T_2 preferentially to T_1 (Fig. 3). Both synthetic immunogens were immunogenic in seven of seven murine strains representing seven MHC haplotypes, as opposed to an earlier version of a synthetic preS2 immunogen, 120–145, which is significantly immunogenic in only three of six MHC haplotypes. The enhanced number of responder strains observed with the newer composite peptides reflects the inclusion of the preS2 COOH-terminus, which contains T-cell recognition sites relevant for a number of MHC haplotypes.

Although a "universal" T-cell recognition site probably does not exist, the 148–174 sequence of the preS2 region represents a relatively short sequence (27 residues) recognized by T cells in the context of seven of seven MHC haplotypes tested. Rather than representing one T-cell site recognized in the context of all MHC haplotypes, this sequence contains numerous sites recognized uniquely in the context of each MHC haplotype (14). Presumably proteins from other pathogens contain similar sequences, which may be included in synthetic vaccines to serve as functional T-cell recognition sites relevant for a variety of MHC haplotypes. Therefore, the 151–174–(133–143) composite peptide represents an efficient synthetic preS2 immunogen in the majority of murine MHC haplotypes tested. The 151–174–(133–143) composite synthetic immunogen is currently being tested in chimpanzee protection trials. Our experience with 151–174–(133–143) may also have implications to the design of synthetic vaccines in general. It seems that any combination of synthetic T- and B-cell sites on the same molecule will not guarantee an efficient immunogen that will behave predictably in a diverse recipient population. The orientation of the T- and B-cell determinants and the context of the T-cell site within the larger composite peptide can influence both antibody fine specificity and T-cell fine specificity. The underlying cellular interactions appear complex, and the rational design of effective synthetic vaccines may require a greater understanding of these cellular mechanisms. However, these results also suggest that pathogen-specific immune responses can be effectively mimicked by synthetic immunogens at the level of T- and B-cell recognition.

VII. CHIMERIC PEPTIDE–RECOMBINANT PARTICLE IMMUNOGENS

Another approach to the utilization of synthetic determinants for vaccine design is to couple peptide sequences representing relevant T- or B-cell recognition sites to recombinant proteins derived from the same virus. This can be accomplished by chemical coupling or by recombinant DNA techniques. Two groups have chemically linked preS2 or preS1 peptides to HBsAg/P24 (87) or HBsAg/GP33 (88) particles, respectively (Table 4). In both cases efficient anti–preS antibodies were produced. Moreover, nonresponsiveness to either the peptide or the HBsAg particle could be circumvented due to the additional Th-cell epitopes provided (52).

The enhanced immunogenicity of HBcAg as compared to HBsAg (72), the ability of HBcAg to act as a T-cell-independent antigen (51), and the relevance of HBcAg to protective immunity (84, 85) suggest that HBcAg may represent an ideal carrier moiety for HBV antigens (86). Therefore, a number of investigators have produced recombinant HBcAg chimeric particles containing envelope haptenic sequences inserted at the amino-terminus, at the carboxyl-terminus, or inserted internally into surface loop structures (i.e., surrounding residue 80) of the HBcAg polypeptide (P21) (Table 4). Although some success has been

Table 4 Chimeric Peptide-Recombinant Particle Immunogens

Carrier	Hapten	Method	Ref.
HBsAg/P24	preS2 133–151	chemical	87
HBsAg/GP33	preS1 12–47	chemical	88
HBcAg	S285–330	(COOH)recombinant	89
HBcAg	S285–339	(COOH)recombinant	89
HBcAg	preS1 1–20	(COOH)recombinant	89
HBcAg	preS1 1–36	(COOH)recombinant	89
HBcAg	preS2 120–145	(COOH)recombinant	89
HBcAg	preS1 20–69	(COOH)recombinant	90
HBcAg	preS1 69–106	(COOH)recombinant	90
HBcAg	preS2 120–174	(COOH)recombinant	90
HBcAg	preS2 133–143	(COOH)recombinant	91
HBcAg	preS1 27–53	(INTERNAL)recombinant	92, 116
HBcAg	preS1 12–47	(NH$_2$)recombinant	116

achieved using carboxyl-terminally inserted HBcAg particles (89–91), it appears that localizing the hapten at the amino-terminus or within an internal insertion results in significantly enhanced immunogenicity (i.e., titers $> 1:10^6$) for the carried hapten (92, 116). This is also consistent with the results obtained using HBcAg as a carrier moitey for non–HBV-related haptens (93).

VIII. SUMMARY

There are a number of advantages and disadvantages inherent in the development of synthetic vaccines in general (Table 5). The chemical synthesis of peptide vaccines implies relative purity and safety. Chemical synthesis guarantees an unlimited source of protein for mass vaccination. Synthetic vaccines would be chemically stable and may be dehydrated for storage or delivery to remote areas. Presumably, synthetic vaccines on a large scale would be cost-effective, assuming the costs of development were not exorbitant. There are also a number of more subtle immunological benefits to the use of synthetic vaccines. Although the synthetic vaccine strategy relies on the occurrence of linear B-cell epitopes on protein antigens and/or the ability of peptide-unique antibodies to bind the intact protein and neutralize infectivity, these characteristics have been demonstrated within the HBV system. Synthetic vaccine design can capitalize on the fact that T-cell recognition sites are, for the most part, represented by small peptide fragments. It is clear from many studies that synthetic peptides can adequately

Table 5 Advantages and Disadvantages of Synthetic Vaccine Design

Advantages	Disadvantages
Chemical purity/Safety	Requires amino acid sequence
Unlimited source of material	Requires identification of T- and B-cell
Costs	sites
Stability/Storage/Delivery	Conformational B-cell epitopes
Sequential B-cell epitopes on many	Genetic restriction of T-cell recognition
pathogens	Immunogenicity
T cells recognize peptide fragments	Complexity of protective immune re-
Induction of CTL response	sponse
Defined immunogen	
Exclusion of adverse epitopes	
Adaptability (i.e., mutations)	
Multivalent (intra-interpathogen)	
Immunomodulation (i.e., target antibody)	

Source: Ref. 94.

substitute for the native protein in a number of functionally important situations. Therefore, both T- and B-cell recognitions sites relevant to the native protein can be mimicked by chemical synthesis of small peptides.

A chemically synthesized immunogen represents a defined entity, which can be thoroughly characterized with respect to its antigenicity and immunogenicity. For example, antigenic regions of a protein that activate suppressor mechanisms or are otherwise harmful can be excluded from a synthetic immunogen. A particular Th-cell site, which may elicit an allergic or autoimmune response in some vaccine recipients, could be deleted from the immunogen. Furthermore, a defined synthetic immunogen can be easily altered to accommodate viral mutations. A combination of T- and B-cell sites derived from multiple proteins within HBV can be constructed with synthetic peptides (Table 3). Another application of intrapathogen multivalency would be to combine B-cell epitopes from multiple serotypes of a virus to obtain a broadly cross-reactive vaccine. The adaptability of synthetic and synthetic-recombinant chimeras may be relevant to the possible inclusion of preS epitopes into future-generation HBV vaccines. A number of findings suggest that preS epitopes may be beneficial, including the enhanced immunogenicity of the preS regions (21, 53, 54), the ability to circumvent S and preS2 region nonresponse (21, 22, 54), and the protective nature of preS antibodies (60, 61, 67, 68). However, several preliminary vaccine trials utilizing preS-containing HBsAg recombinant particles have yielded rather mixed results (95–98). One criticism of the proposal to include preS determinants has been that the immunogenicity studies in nonprimate animal species may not pertain to humans (99). In this regard, the preS antigens appear to be immunogenic during HBV infection, and in fact anti-preS antibodies often occur prior to any other HBV-specific antibody (53). The early appearance of preS antibodies may explain their relatively transient nature in infection, since both antigen and antibody occur early during the acute phase and may be cleared rapidly by immune complex formation. Another objection to the inclusion of the preS sequences in future HBV vaccines relates to the presence of the pHSA receptor within the preS2 region. It has been suggested that upon vaccination, pHSA may bind to HBsAg and elicit an antialbumin autoimmune response or downregulate the anti-HBs response (99). This seems unlikely since monomeric (2, 100–102) or naturally occurring polymeric human albumin has not been reported to bind to HBsAg (103). However, a recent study suggested that natural human serum albumin can indeed bind to the preS2 region of HBsAg (104). Because the pHSA receptor site within the preS2 region (105) overlaps with the dominant antibody-binding site (56), it is possible that albumin binding may mask this important antibody site. An efficient interaction between serum albumin and the pHSA receptor within the preS2 region may explain the transient nature of anti-preS2–specific antibody production during infection and possibly the variable anti-preS2 responses among vaccine recipients. This hypothesis is attractive because any apparent compromise in preS2-specific antibody production has been unique to the human response (i.e., all nonhuman animal studies have demonstrated efficient preS2-specific humoral responses), and the pHSA receptor binds only human and chimpanzee albumins. If the presence of the pHSA receptor is proven to interfere with anti-preS2 antibody production, the offending sequences could be deleted from the preS2 region by application of the recombinant or synthetic peptide technologies described previously.

Perhaps the greatest advantage of a synthetic peptide approach will be its potential to modulate the immune response. For example, regions of a protein that are not normally immunogenic and, therefore, have not been subjected to selective pressure by the host's immune system may be targeted for antibody production by the use of synthetic immunogens. Similarly, regions that are not T-cell recognition sites in the native protein by virtue of conditions of antigen processing may activate T-cell responses when presented as small peptide fragments. This would allow priming of a beneficial Th-cell clone, which may be normally "silent." We have recently demonstrated that a synthetic HBeAg-specific Th-cell site injected into HBeAg transgenic mice can circumvent T-cell tolerance to HBeAg and result in seroconversion from HBeAg to anti-HBe status (106). This suggests the possibility of a therapeutic use for peptide antigens in HBV chronic carriers. Another application of synthetic peptide strategy to modulate the immune response may be to selectively combine T- and B-cell recognition sites for use as immunogens. As demonstrated in the HBV system (65), Th-cell fine specificity can affect the fine specificity of the antibody produced. In other words, not all Th-cell clones are equal in their ability to provide help to a given B-cell clone. Altering the Th-cell component of native proteins may qualitatively or quantitatively alter the antibody response. Synthetic immunogens may also provide a means of selectively activating a specific immune cell or T-cell subset. In a circumstance in which a T-cell response to a particular determinant was desired but an antibody response was not (i.e., autoantibody or immunoglobulin Fc receptor–mediated virus-cell interaction), a vaccine consisting of a synthetic T-cell site, which did not induce antibody cross-reactive with the pathogen, would be ideal. Furthermore, the recent findings that peptide fragments can sensitize target cells for lysis by CTL and, indeed, induce CTL in vivo, whereas intact proteins cannot, suggest the possibility that peptide antigens may be used to prime CTL in vivo if an effective delivery system can be devised (107–110). The ability to immunize CTL in vivo with synthetic peptides without the use of infectious virus or vector systems may represent a therapeutic strategy for HBV chronic carriers.

There are also a number of obstacles to the development of synthetic vaccines. An obvious requirement is identification of the T- and B-cell recognition sites of interest. However, one could argue that a detailed characterization of the immunogen, such as is required to identify antibody and T-cell recognition sites, should be performed as a matter of course during the development of any vaccine. Another, at least perceived, limitation is the fact that most antibody recognition sites are of the conformational type that cannot be easily duplicated by the present synthetic peptide technology. This limitation may be resolved in time by advances in peptide chemistry. Until such advances, the question remains whether sequential epitopes, whether immunogenic within the native protein or not, can induce sufficient levels of neutralizing antibody to provide adequate protection from infection. Evidence from a number of systems in addition to HBV suggest that antibody produced to predominantly sequential B-cell epitopes is sufficient to protect against infection.

In terms of T-cell immunity, the limitation of the peptide strategy is clearly not a chemical-structural one in that T-cell antigen recognition and activation can be generally induced by synthetic peptide antigen. The fact that this recognition process involves the dual recognition of MHC gene products as well as the peptide fragment, and that the fine specificity of the T-cell antigenic site is determined by the MHC phenotype of the individual, may present a problem for synthetic peptide vaccine design. Not all individuals will respond to the same T-cell recognition site. For example, in the Th-cell response to the nucleoprotein of HBV, H-2 congenic mice differing only in the MHC focus on different antigenic determinants. Furthermore, T cells of outbred mice "see" one or the other of these defined determinants or novel T-cell sites (unpublished observation). Therefore, a composite synthetic vaccine containing numerous T-cell sites may be required to ensure T-cell responsiveness in an entire outbred population. If one considers that the human MHC is more complex (i.e., has more loci) than the murine, and that there are estimated to be 50–100 different allelic forms of class II molecules in outbred murine populations (111), it will be no small task to identify and include sufficient T-cell sites into a synthetic vaccine. However, this very complexity of the human MHC may actually increase the potential for any given peptide to interact with MHC gene products as discussed previously. The finding that synthetic T-cell sites need not be present on the same molecule as B-cell epitopes (intermolecular Th) as long as they are within the same particulate structure (intrastructural Th) (86) may lessen the burden of delivering multiple T-cell sites per B-cell epitope inasmuch as numerous synthetic T-cell sites may be combined in an artificial particulate structure with a single B-cell epitope displayed on the surface of the particle. A B-cell clone specific for the B-cell epitope on the surface of such a particle could receive Th-cell function from all the Th-cell specificities contained within the particles.

A number of investigators have reported that synthetic peptides are poor immunogens. However, this is a very subjective characterization depending on adjuvant systems, species or strain immunized, form of the antigen (i.e., monomeric, polymeric), inclusion or exclusion of relevant T-cell epitopes, etc. It is possible that this limitation is more a measure of our lack of understanding of what comprises a strong immunogen, rather than an inherent characteristic of peptide immunogens. Another possible limitation of a synthetic peptide vaccine may lie in the characteristic that is most appealing, its intrinsic simplicity. As host-pathogen interactions have become better understood, it is clear that the host immune response can be anything but simple. Multiple antigens on both structural and nonstructural proteins may serve as inducers of Th-cell and/or Ts-cell function, targets for CTL, and sites for neutralizing antibody. Viral clearance may require a myriad network of cellular interactions with differeing specificities. This is not an argument against synthetic vaccines, merely a caution against the assumption that provision of one to several antibody sites on a T-cell carrier will necessarily represent an effective vaccine. More than with any other approach to vaccine development, the application of synthetic antigens to vaccine production requires a thorough knowledge of the mechanisms of protective immunity precisely because a synthetic vaccine must be "engineered" to suit the purpose.

Cumulatively, the studies described in this review suggest that development of a synthetic HBV vaccine is a feasible task. However, the existence of an effective recombinant subunit HBV vaccine raises the question of the necessity of a synthetic-based vaccine. This may ultimately be determined by economic factors. Nevertheless, the knowledge gained from the analysis of synthetic peptide reagents in the HBV system has provided and will continue to provide insights relevant to the development of future generations of HBV vaccines and may serve as a model for the development of synthetic vaccines for diseases in which a recombinant subunit vaccine is not appropriate.

ACKNOWLEDGMENTS

The author wishes to acknowledge the collaborators who have contributed to many of the studies described herein: Janice Hughes, Joyce Jones, Alan McLachlan, Ben Thornton, Ann Moriarty, Richard Lerner, Flörian Schödel, and Darrell Peterson. The author also thanks Rene Lang for editorial assistance. Original work from the author's laboratory summarized in this review was supported by NIH grants AI18391, AI20720, and AI00585 and a grant from the Johnson and Johnson Co.

REFERENCES

1. K. H. Heermann, U. Goldman, W. Schawartz, T. Seyffarth, H. Baumgarten, W. H. Gerlich, Large surface proteins of hepatitis B virus containing the pre-S sequence, *J. Virol. 52:* 396 (1984).

2. A. Machida, S. Kishimoto, H. Ohnuma, K. Baba, Y. Ito, H. Miyamoto, G. Funatsu, K. Oda, S. Usuda, S. Togami, T. Nakamura, Y. Miyakawa, M. Mayumi, A polypeptide containing 55 amino acid residues coded by the pre-S region of hepatitis B virus deoxyribonucleic acid bears the receptor for polymeried human as well as chimpanzee albumin, *Gastroenterology 86:* 910 (1984).

3. K. Takahasi, A. Machida, G. Funatsu, N. Nomura, S. Usuda, S. Aoyagi, K. Tachibana, H. Kiyamoto, M. Imai, T. Nakamura, Y. Miyakawa, M. Mayumi, Immunochemical structure of hepatitis B e antigen in serum, *J. Immunol. 130:* 2903 (1983).

4. D. N. Standring, J-H. Ou, F. R. Masiarz, W. J. Rutter, A signal peptide encoded within the precore region of hepatitis B virus directs the secretion of a heterogenous population of e antigens in *Xenopus* oocytes, *Proc. Natl. Acad. Sci. USA 85:* 8405 (1988).

5. E. R. Unanue, Antigen-presenting function of the macrophage, *Annu. Rev. Immunol. 2:* 395 (1984).

6. E. R. Unanue, P. M. Allen, The basis for the immunoregulatory role of macrophages and other accessory cells, *Science 236:* 551 (1987).

7. D. Hansburg, C. Hannum, J. K. Inman, E. Appella, E. Margoliash, R. H. Schwartz, Parallel cross-reactivity patterns of 2 sets of antigenetically distinct cytochrome C peptides: possible evidence for a presentational model of Ir gene function. *J. Immunol. 127:* 1844 (1981).

8. E. Heber-Katz, D. Hansburg, R. H. Schwartz, The Ia molecule of the antigen-presenting cell plays a critical role in immune response gene regulation of T cell activation, *J. Mol. Cell. Immunol. 1:* 3 (1985).

9. A. M. Solinger, M. E. Ultee, E. Margoliash, R. H. Schwartz, T-lymphocyte

response to cytochrome c. I. Demonstration of a T-cell heteroclitic proliferative response and identification of a topographic antigenic determinant on pigeon cytochrome c whose immune recognition requires two complementing major histocompatibility complex-linked immune response genes, *J. Exp. Med. 150:* 830 (1979).

10. U. Krzych, A. V. Fowler, A. Miller, E. E. Sercarz, Repertoires of T cells directed against a large protein antigen, beta-galactosidase. 1. Helper cells have a more restricted specificity repertoire than proliferative cells, *J. Immunol. 128:* 1529 (1982).

11. I. Berkower, L. A. Matis, G. K. Buckenmeyer, F. R. N. Gurd, D. L. Longo, J. A. Berzofsky, Identification of distinct predominant epitopes recognized in myoglobin specific T cells under the control of different Ir genes and characterization of representative T cell clones, *J. Immunol. 132:* 1370 (1984).

12. D. R. Milich, A. McLachlan, A. Moriarty, G. B. Thornton, Immune response to hepatitis B virus core antigen (HBcAg): localization of T cell recognition sites within HBcAg/HBeAg, *J. Immunol. 139:* 1223, (1987).

13. G. Gammon, N. Shastri, J. Cogswell, S. Wilbur, S. Sadegh-Nasseri, U. Krzych, A. Miller, E. Sercarz, The choice of T-cell epitopes utilized on a protein antigen depends on multiple factors distant from, as well as at the determinant site, *Immunol. Rev. 98:* 53 (1987).

14. D. R. Milich, J. L. Hughes, A. McLachlan, K. E. Langley, G. B. Thornton, J. E. Jones, Importance of subtype in the immune response to the pre-S2 region of the hepatitis B surface antigen: I. T cell fine specificity, *J. Immunol. 144:* 3535 (1990).

15. D. R. Milich, J. E. Jones, A. McLachlan, G. Bitter, A. Moriarty, J. L. Hughes, Importance of subtype in the immune response to the pre-S2 region of the hepatitis B surface antigen: II. Synthetic pre-S2 immunogen, *J. Immunol. 144:* 3544 (1990).

16. S. J. Brett, K. B. Cease, J. A. Berzofsky, Influences of antigen processing on the expression of the T cell repertoire: evidence for MHC-specific hindering structures on the products of processing, *J. Exp. Med. 168:* 357 (1988).

17. M. Sela, Immunological studies with synthetic polypeptides, *Adv. Immunol. 5:* 29 (1966).

18. D. C. Benjamin, J. A. Berzofsky, I. J. East, F. R. N. Gurd, C. Hannum, S. J. Leach, E. Margoliash, J. G. Michael, A. Miller, E. M. Prager, M. Reichlin, E. E. Sercarz, S. J. Smith-Gill, P. E. Todd, A. C. Wilson. The antigenic structure of proteins: a reappraisal, *Ann. Rev. Immunol. 2:* 67 (1984).

19. V. Nussenzweig, R. S. Nussenzweig, Development of a sporozoite malaria vaccine, *Am. J. Trop. Med. Hyg. 35:* 678 (1986).

20. A. R. Neurath, S. B. H. Kent, N. Strick, Location and chemical synthesis of pre-S gene coded immunodominant epitope of hepatitis B virus, *Science 224:* 392 (1984).

21. D. R. Milich, G. B. Thornton, A. R. Neurath, S. B. Kent, M.-L., Michael, P. Tiollais, F. V. Chisari, Enhanced immunogenicity of the pre-S region of hepatitis B antigen, *Science 228:* 1195 (1985).

22. D. R. Milich, A. McLachlan, F. V. Chisari, S. B. H. Kent, G. B. Thornton, Immune response to the pre-S1 region of the hepatitis B surface antigen (HBsAg):

A pre-S1-specific T cell response can bypass nonresponsiveness to the pre-S2 and S regions of the HBsAg, *J. Immunol. 137:* 315 (1986).

23. J. Rosen, Y.-L. Hom, A. Whalley, R. Smith, R. B. Naso, Detection of antibodies to HIV using synthetic peptides derived from the gp41 envelope protein, *Vaccines 87* (R. M. Chanock, R. A. Lerner, F. Brown, H. Ginsberg, eds.), Cold Spring Harbor Laboratory, Cold Spring Harbor, NY, p. 188 (1987).

24. D. D. Ho, M. G. Sarngadharan, M. S. Hirsh, R. T. Schooley, T. R. Rota, R. C. Kennedy, T. C. Chanh, V. L. Sato, Human immunodeficiency virus neutralizing antibodies recognize several conserved domains on the envelope glycoproetins, *J. Virol. 61:* 2024 (1987).

25. J. R. Rusche, K. Javaherian, C. McDanal, J. Petro, D. L. Lynn, R. Grimaila, A. Langlois, R. C. Gallo, L. O. Arthur, P. J. Fischinger, D. P., Bolognesi, S. D. Putney, T. J. Matthews, Antibodies that inhibit fusion of human immunodeficiency virus-related cells bind a 24-amino acid sequence of the viral envelope, gp120, *Proc. Natl. Acad. Sci. USA 85:* 3198 (1988).

26. G. N. Vyas, K. R. Roa, A. B. Ibrahim, Hepatitis associated Australian antigen (HBsAg): A conformational antigen dependent on disulfide bonds, *Science 178:* 1300 (1972).

27. G. A. Cabral, F. Marciano-Cabral, G. A. Frank, Y. Sanchez, F. B. Hollinger, J. L. Melnick, G. R. Dressman, Cellular and humoral immunity in guinea pigs to two major polypeptides derived from hepatitis B surface antigen, *J. Gen. Virol. 38:* 339 (1978).

28. J. W.-K. Shih, J. L. Gerin, Immunochemistry of HBsAg: Preparation and characterization of antibodies to the constituent polypeptides, *J. Immunol. 115:* 634 (1975).

29. R. Arnon, E. Maron, M. Sela, C. B. Anfinsen, Antibodies reactive with a native lysozyme elicited by a completely synthetic antigen, *Proc. Natl. Acad. Sci. USA 68:* 1450 (1971).

30. J. G. Sutcliffe, T. M. Shinnick, N. Green, F.-T., Liu, H. L. Niman, R. A. Lerner, Tapping the immunological repertoire to produce antibodies of predetermined specificity, *Nature 187:* 80 (1980).

31. G. Walter, K.-H. Scheidtmann, A. Carbone, A. P. Laudano, R. F. Doolittle, Antibodies specific for the carboxy- and amino-terminal regions of simian virus 40 large tumor antigen, *Proc. Natl. Acad. Sci. USA 77:* 5197 (1980).

32. M. Z. Atassi, Antigenic structure of myoglobin, *Immunochemistry 12:* 423 (1975).

33. R. Arnon, M. Bustin, E. Calef, S. Chaitchik, J. Haimovich, N. Norvik, M. Sela, Immunological cross-reactivity of antibodies to a synthetic undecapeptide analogous to the amino terminal segment of carcinoembryonic antigen, with the intact protein and with human sera, *Proc. Natl. Acad. Sci. USA 73:* 2123 (1976).

34. J. L. Gerin, H. Alexander, J. W.-K. Shih, R. H. Purcell, G. Dapolito, R. Engle, N. Green, J. G. Sutcliffe, T. M. Shinnick, R. A. Lerner, Chemically synthesized peptides of hepatitis B surface antigen duplicate the d/y specificities and induce subtype-specific antibodies in chimpanzees, *Proc. Natl. Acad. Sci. 80:* 2365 (1983).

35. F. R. Harmon, J. L. Melnick, Synthetic vaccines for viral hepatitis, *Synthetic Vaccines* (R. Arnon, ed.), CRC Press, Inc., Boca Raton, FL, p. 31 (1987).

36. J. W.-K Shih, R. J. Gerety, S. T.-Y Liu, H. Yajima, N. Fuji, M. Nomizu, Y.
     Hayashi, S. Katakura, Immunogenicity of unconjugated synthetic polypeptides of
     hepatitis-B surface antigen, *Modern Approaches to Vaccines* (R. Lerner, F.
     Brown, ed.), Cold Spring Laboratories, Cold Spring Harbor, NY, p. 127 (1983).

37. R. A. Lerner, N. Green, H. Alexander, F.-T, Liu, J. G. Sutcliffe, T. M. Shinnick,
     Chemically synthesized peptides predicted from the nucleotide sequence of the
     hepatitis B virus genome elicit antibodies reactive with the native envelope protein
     of Dane particles, *Proc. Natl. Acad. Sci. USA 78:* 3403 (1981).

38. A. R. Neurath, S. B. H. Kent, N. Strick, Antibody response to two synthetic
     peptides corresponding to residues 45–68 and 69–79 of the major protein of
     hepatitis B surface antigen, *Virus Res. 1:* 321 (1984).

39. G. R. Dreesmann, Y. Sanchez, I. Ionescu-Matiu, J. T. Sparrow, H. R. Six, D. L.
     Peterson, F. B. Hollinger, J. L. Melnick, Antibody to hepatitis B surface antigen
     after a single inoculation of uncoupled synthetic HBsAg peptides, *Nature 295:* 158
     (1982).

40. I. Ionescu-Matiu, R. C. Kennedy, J. T. Sparrow, A. R. Culwell, Y. Sanchez, J.
     L. Melnick, G. R. Dressman, Epitopes associated with a synthetic hepatitis B
     surface antigen peptide, *J. Immunol. 130:* 1947 (1983).

41. C. R. Howard, S. E. Brown, D. N. Hogben, A. J. Zuckerman, I. M. Murray-
     Lyon, M. W. Steward, Analysis of antibody responses to hepatitis B surface
     antigen, *Viral Hepatitis and Liver Disease* (G. N. Vyas, J. L. Dienstag, J. H.
     Hoofnagle, eds.), Grune & Stratton, Inc., Orlando, FL, p. 561 (1984).

42. G. N. Vyas, Molecular immunology of the hepatitis B virus surface antigen,
     Hepatitis B Vaccine (P. Maupas, P. Guesry, eds.), Elsevier, Holland, p. 227
     (1981).

43. A. R. Neurath, S. B. H. Kent, N. Strick, Specificity of antibodies elicited by a
     synthetic peptide having a sequence in common with a fragment of a virus protein,
     the hepatitis B surface antigen, *Proc. Natl. Acad. Sci. USA 79:* 7871 (1982).

44. T. P. Hopp, K. Woods, Prediction of protein antigenic determinants from amino
     acid sequences, *Proc. Natl. Acad. Sci. USA 78:* 3824 (1981).

45. P. K. Bathnagar, E. Papas, H. E. Blum, D. R. Milich, D. Nitecki, M. J. Karels,
     G. N. Vyas, Immune response to synthetic peptide analogues of hepatitis B surface
     antigen specific for the a determinant, *Proc. Natl. Acad. Sci USA 89:* 4400 (1982).

46. S. E. Brown, C. R. Howard, A. J. Zuckerman, M. W. Steward, Affinity of
     antibody response in man to hepatitis B vaccines determined with synthetic
     peptides, *Lancet II:* 184 (1984).

47. E. Celis, D. Ou, L. Otvos, Recognition of hepatitis B virus surface antigen by
     human T-lymphocytes, *J. Immunol. 140:* 1808 (1988).

48. T. Moriyama, S. Guilhot, K. Klopchin, B. Moss, C. A. Pinkert, R. D. Palmiter,
     R. L. Brinster, O. Kanagawa, F. V. Chisari, Immunobiology and pathogenesis of
     hepatocellular injury in hepatitis B virus transgenic mice, *Science 248:* 361 (1990).

49. D. R. Milich, D. L. Peterson, G. G. Leroux-Roels, R. A. Lerner, F. V. Chisari,
     Genetic regulation of the immune response to hepatitis B surface antigen (HBsAg):
     VI. T cell fine specificity, *J. Immunol. 134:* 4203 (1985).

50. D. L. Peterson, D. A. Paul, J. Lam, I. I. E. Tribby, D. T. Achard, Antigenic
     structure of the hepatitis B surface antigen: Identification of the "d" subtype

determinant by chemical modification and use of monoclonal antibodies, *J. Immunol. 132:* 920 (1984).

51. D. R. Milich, A. McLachlan, The nucleocapsid of hepatitis B virus is both a T cell-independent and T cell-dependent antigen, *Science 234:* 1398 (1987).

52. D. R. Milich, G. B. Thornton, A. R. Neurath, S. B. Kent, M. L. Michel, P. Tiollais, F. V. Chisari, Enhanced immunogenicity of the pre-S region of hepatitis B surface antigen, *Science 228:* 1195 (1985).

53. A. R. Neurath, S. B. H. Kent, N. Strick, P. Taylor, C. E. Stevens, Hepatitis B virus contains pre-S gene-encoded domains, *Nature 315:* 154 (1985).

54. D. R. Milich, M. K. McNamara, A. McLachlan, G. Thornton, F. V. Chisari, Distinct H-2 linked regulation of T-cell responses to the pre-S and S regions of the same hepatitis B surface antigen polypeptide allows circumvention of nonresponsiveness to the S region, *Proc. Natl. Acad. Sci. 82:* 8168 (1985).

55. H. Okamoto, M. Imai, S. Usuda, E. Tanaka, K. Tachibana, S. Mishiro, A. Machida, T. Nakamura, Y. Miyakawa, M. Mayumi, Hemagglutination assay of polypeptide coded by the pre-S region of hepatitis B virus DNA with monoclonal antibody: Correlation of pre-S polypeptide with the receptor for polymerized human serum albumin antigens, *J. Immunol. 134:* 1212 (1985).

56. D. R. Milich, A. McLachlan, F. V. Chisari, G. B. Thornton, Two distinct but overlapping antibody binding sites in the pre-S2 region of HBsAg localized within 11 continuous residues, *J. Immunol. 137:* 2703 (1986).

57. M. W. Steward, B. M. Sisley, C. Stanley, S. E. Brown, C. R. Howard, Immunity to hepatitis B: analysis of antibody and cellular responses in recipients of a plasma derived vaccine using synthetic peptides mimicking S and pre-S regions, *Clin. Exp. Immunol. 71:* 19 (1988).

58. A. R. Neurath, P. Adamowicz, S. B. H. Kent, M. M. Riottot, N. Strick, K. Parker, W. Offensperger, M. A. Petit, S. Wahl, A. Budkowska, M. Girard, J. Pillot, Characterization of monoclonal antibodies specific for the pre-S2 region of the hepatitis B virus envelope protein, *Mol. Immunol. 23:* 991 (1986).

59. L. T. Mimms, M. Floreani, J. Tyner, E. Whitters, R. Rosenlof, L. Wray, A. Goetze, V. Sarin, K. Eble, Discrimination of hepatitis B virus (HBV) subtypes using monoclonal antibodies to the pre-S1 and pre-S2 domains of the viral envelope, *Virology 176:* 620 (1990).

60. G. B. Thornton, D. Milich, F. Chisari, K. Mitamura, S. Kent, R. Neurath, R. Purcell, J. Gerin, Immune response in primates to the pre-S2 region of hepatitis-B surface antigen: Identification of a protective determinant, *Vaccines 87* (R. M. Chanock, R. A. Lerner, F. Brown, H. Ginsberg, eds.), Cold Spring Harbor Laboratory, Cold Spring Harbor, NY, p. 77 (1987).

61. Y. Itoh, E. Takai, H. Ohnuma, K. Kitajima, F. Tsuda, A. Machida, A. Mishiro, T. Nakamura, Y. Miyakawa, M. Mayumi, A synthetic peptide vaccine involving the product of the pre-S2 region of hepatitis B virus: Protective efficacy in chimpanzees, *Proc. Natl. Acad. Sci. 83:* 9174 (1986).

62. J. P. Tam, Y.-A. Lu, Vaccine engineering: Enhancement of immunogenicity of synthetic peptide vaccines related to hepatitis in chemically defined models consisting of T- and B-cell epitopes, *Proc. Natl. Acad. Sci. USA 86:* 9084 (1989).

63. D. R. Milich, A. McLachlan, F. V. Chisari, G. B. Thornton, Nonoverlapping T

and B cell determinants on a hepatitis B surface antigen pre-S2 region synthetic peptide, *J. Exp. Med. 164:* 532 (1986).

64. V. Barnaba, A. Franco, A. Alberti, C. Balsano, R. Benevenuto, F. Balsano, Recognition of hepatitis B virus envelope proteins by liver-infiltrating T lympho-ctyes in chronic HBV infection, *J. Immunol. 143:* 2650 (1989).

65. D. R. Milich, A. McLachlan, A. Moriarty, G. B. Thornton, A single 10-residue pre-S1 peptide can prime T cell for antibody production to multiple epitopes within the pre-S1, pre-S2 and S regions of HBsAg, *J. Immunol. 138:* 4457 (1987).

66. A. R. Neurath, S. B. H. Kent, N. Strick, K. Parker, Identification and chemical synthesis of a host cell receptor binding site on hepatitis B virus, *Cell 46:* 429 (1986).

67. A. R. Neurath, N. Strick, B. Seto, M. Girard, Antibodies to synthetic peptides from the pre-S1 region of the hepatitis B virus (HBV) envelope (env) protein are virus-neutralizing and protective, *Vaccine 7:* 234 (1989).

68. G. B. Thornton, A. M. Moriarty, D. R. Milich, J. W. Eichberg, R. H. Purcell, J. L. Gerin, Protection of chimpanzees from hepatitis-B virus infection after im-munization with synthetic peptides: identification of protective epitopes in the pre-S region, *Vaccines 89* (F. Brown, T. Channock, H. Ginsberg, R. Lerner, eds.), Cold Spring Harbor Laboratory, Cold Spring Harbor, NY, p. 467 (1989).

69. K, Kuroki, M. Floreani, L. T. Mimms, D. Ganem, Epitope mapping of the pre-S1 domain of hepatitis B virus large surface protein, *Virology 176:* 604 (1990).

70. Y. Jin, J. W.-K, Shih, I. Berkower, Human T-cell response to the surface antigen of hepatitis B virus (HBsAg), *J. Exp. Med. 168:* 293 (1988).

71. D. R. Milich, Genetic and molecular basis for T- and B-cell recognition of hepatitis B viral antigens, *Immunol. Rev. 99:* 71 (1987).

72. D. R. Milich, A. McLachlan, S. Stahl, P. Wingfield, G. B. Thornton, J. L. Hughes, J. Jones, Comparative immunogenicity of hepatitis B virus core and E antigens, *J. Immunol. 141:* 3617 (1988).

73. M. Inoue, S. Kakumu, K. Yoshioka, Y. Tsutsumi, T. Wakita, M. Arao, Hepatitis B core antigen-specific IFN-y production of peripheral blood monouclear cells in patients with chronic hepatitis B virus infection, *J. Immunol. 142:* 4006 (1989).

74. C. Ferrari, A. Penna, A. Bertoletti, A. Valli, A. D. Antoni, T. Giuberti, A. Cavalli, M.-A. Petit, F. Fiaccadori, Cellular immune response to hepatitis B virus-encoded antigens in acute and chronic hepatitis B virus infection, *J. Im-munol. 145:* 3442 (1990).

75. D. R. Milich, J. L. Hughes, A. McLachlan, J. L. Hughes, G. B. Thornton, A. Moriarty, Synthetic hepatitis B immunogen comprised of nucleocapsid T-cell sites and an envelope B-cell epitope, *Proc. Natl. Acad. Sci. USA 85:* 1610 (1988).

76. D. R. Milich, T- and B-cell recognition of hepatitis B viral antigens, *Immunol. Today 9:* 380 (1988).

77. T. Wakita, S. Kakumu, Y. Tsutsumi, K. Yoshioka, A. Machida, M. Mayumi, Gamma-interferon production in response to hepatitis B core protein and its synthetic peptides in patients with chronic hepatitis B virus infection, *Digestion 47:* 149 (1990).

78. G. Colucci, Y. Beazer, C. Cantaluppi, C. Tackney, Identification of major

hepatitis B core antigen (HBcAg) determinant by using synthetic peptides and monoclonal antibodies, *J. Immunol. 141:* 4376 (1988).

79. J. Salfeld, E. Praff, M. Noah, H. Schaller, Antigenic C-terminus and functional domains in core antigen and e antigen from hepatitis B virus, *J. Virol. 63:* 798 (1989).

80. F. Schödel, T. Weimer, H. Will, HBV: Molecular biology and immunology, *Biotest Bull 4:* 68 (1990).

81. J. L. Gerin, R. H. Purcell, R. A. Lerner, Use of synthetic peptides to identify protective epitopes of the hepatitis-B surface antigen, *Vaccines 85:* (R. A. Lerner, R. A. Lerner, F. Brown, H. Ginsberg, eds.), Cold Spring Harbor Laboratory, Cold Spring Harbor, NY, p. 235 (1985).

82. E. Emini, V. Larson, J. Eichberg, P. Conrad, V. M. Garsky, D. R. Lee, R. W. Ellis, W. J. Miller, C. A. Anderson, R. J. Gerety, Protective effect of a synthetic peptide comprising the complete pre-S2 region of the hepatitis B virus surface protein, *J. Med. Virol. 28:* 7 (1989).

83. J. A. Berzofsky, A. Bensussan, K. B. Cease, J. F. Bourge, R. Cheynier, Z. Lurhuma, J. J. Salaun, R. C. Gallo, G. M. Shearer, D. Zagury, Antigenic peptides recognized by T lymphocytes from AIDS viral envelope-immune humans, *Nature 334:* 706 (1988).

84. E. Tabor, R. J. Gerety, Possible role of immune responses to HBcAg in protection against hepatitis B infection, *Lancet 1:* 172 (1984).

85. K. Murray, S. A. Bruce, A. Hinnen, P. Wingfield, P. Van Erd, A. deReus, H. Schellekens, Hepatitis B virus antigen made in microbial cells immunize against viral infection, *EMBO J. 3:* 645 (1984).

86. D. R. Milich, A. Mclachlan, G. B. Thornton, J. L. Hughes, Antibody production to the nucleocapsid and envelope of the hepatitis B virus primed by a single synthetic T cell site, *Nature 329:* 547 (1987).

87. F. Tsuda, Y. Akahane, S. Usuda, T. Nakamura, Y. Miyakawa, M. Mayumi, A synthetic peptide coded for by the pre-S2 region of hepatitis B virus for adding immunogenicity to small spherical particles made of the product of the S-gene, *Molec. Immun. 24:* 523 (1987).

88. A. R. Neurath, N. Strick, M. Girard, Hepatitis B virus surface antigen (HBsAg) as carrier for synthetic peptides having an attached hydrophobic tail, *Molec. Immun. 26:* 53 (1989).

89. S. J. Stah, K. Murray, Immunogenicity of peptide fusions to hepatitis B virus core antigen, *Proc. Natl. Acad. Sci. USA 86:* 6283 (1989).

90. G. P. Borisova, I. Berzins, P. M. Pushko, P. Pumpen, E. J. Gren, V. V. Tsibinogin, V. Loseva, V. Ose, R. Ulrich, H. Siakkou, H. A. Rosenthal, Recombinant core particles of hepatitis B virus exposing foreign antigenic determinants on their surface, *FEBS Lett. 259:* 121 (1989).

91. F. Schödel, D. R. Milich, H. Will, Hepatitis B virus nucleocapsid/pre-S2 fusion proteins expressed in attenuated *Salmonella* for oral vaccination, *J. Immunol. 145:* 4317 (1990).

92. F. Schödel, H. Will, D. R. Milich, Hybrid hepatitis B virus core/pre-S particles expressed in live attenuated *Salmonellae* for oral immunization, *Vaccines 91* (R.

M. Chanock, H. S. Ginsberg, F. Brown, R. A. Lerner, eds.), Cold Spring Harbor Laboratory, Cold Spring Harbor, NY, p. 319 (1991).

93. M. J. Francis, G. Z. Hastings, A. L. Brown, K. G. Grace, D. J. Rowlands, F. Brown, B. E. Clarke, Immunological properties of hepatitis B core antigen fusion proteins, *Proc. Natl. Acad. Sci. USA 87:* 2545 (1990).

94. D. R. Milich, Synthetic peptides: prospects for vaccine development, *Sem. Immunol. 2:* 307 (1990).

95. Y. Fujisawa, S. Kuroda, P. M. C. A. Van Eerd, H. Schellekens, A. Kakinuma, Protective efficacy of a novel hepatitis B vaccine consisting of M (pre-S2 + S) protein particles (a third generation vaccine), *Vaccine 8:* 193 (1990).

96. M. De Wilde, T. Rutgers, T. Cabezon, P. Hauser, O. Van Opstal, N. Harford, F. Van Wijnendaele, P. Desmons, M. Comberbach, P. Roelants, P. Voet, A. Delem, J. Pêtre, PreS containing HBsAg particles from *Saccharomyces cerevisiae, Viral Hepatitis and Liver Disease* (F. B. Hollinger, S. M. Lemon, H. S. Margolis, eds.); Williams & Wilkins, Baltimore, MD. pp. 732 (1991).

97. H. A. Thoma, G. Kapfer, E. Koller, A. E. Hemmerling, Does the pre-S2 have the same effects in improving the HBV immune response compared to pre-S1? *Viral Hepatitis and Liver Disease* (F. B. Hollinger, S. M. Lemon, H. S. Margolis, eds.), Williams & Wilkins, Baltimore, MD. pp. 736 (1991).

98. S. Iino, H. Suzuki, Y. Akahane, M. Mayumi, Phase II study of recombinant HB vaccine containing the S and pre-S2 antigens, *Viral Hepatitis and Liver Disease* (F. B. Hollinger, S. M. Lemon, H. S. Margolis, eds.), Abstract Vol. p. 119 (1990).

99. U. Hellstrom, S. Sylvan, M. Kuhns, V. Sarin, Absence of pre-S2 antibodies in natural hepatitis B virus infection, *Lancet 2:* 889 (1986).

100. S. N. Thung, M. A. Gerber, Albumin receptors on hepatitis B virus and antibodies to albumin, *Liver 1:* 75: (1981).

101. D. R. Milich, T. Gottfried, G. N. Vyas, Characterization of the interaction between polymerized human albumin and hepatitis B surface antigen, *Gastroenterology 81:* 218 (1981).

102. P. Pontisso, A. Alberti, F. Bortolotti, G. Realdi, Virus-associated receptors for polymerized human serum albumin in acute and in chronic hepatitis B virus infection, *Gastroenterology 84:* 220 (1983).

103. M. W. Yu, J. S. Finlayson, J. W-K. Shih, Interaction between various polymerized human albumins and hepatitis B surface antigen, *J. Virol. 55:* 736 (1985).

104. B. Krone, A. Lenz, K.-H Heermann, M. Seifer, L. Xuangyong, W. H. Gerlich, Interaction between hepatitis B surface proteins and monomeric human serum albumin, *Hepatology 11:* 1050 (1990).

105. Y. Fujisawa, Y. Itoh, T. Miyazaki, M. Kobayashi, T. Asano, Synthesis in yeast and characterization of HBsAg modified P31 particles, *Molecular Biology of Hepatitis B Viruses,* Cold Spring Harbor Laboratory, Cold Spring Harbor, NY, abstract (1986).

106. D. R. Milich, A. McLachlan, A. K. Raney, R. Houghten, G. B. Thornton, T. Maruyama, J. L. Hughes, J. E. Jones, Autoantibody production in HBeAg transgenic mice elicited with a self T cell peptide and inhibited with non-self peptides, *Proc. Natl. Acad. Sci. USA 88:* 4348 (1991).

107. F. R. Carbone, M. J. Bevan, Induction of ovalbumin-specific cytotoxic T cells by in vivo peptide immunization, *J. Exp. Med. 169:* 603 (1989).

108. G. Y. Ishioka, S. Colon, C. Miles, H. M. Grey, R. W. Chesnut, Induction of class I MHC-restricted, peptide-specific cytolytic T lymphocytes by peptide priming in vivo, *J. Immunol., 143:* 1094 (1989).

109. K. Deres, H. Schild, K-H. Wiesmuller, G. Jung, H-G. Rammensee, In vivo priming of virus specific cytotoxic T lymphocytes with synthetic lipopeptide vaccine, *Nature 342:* 561 (1989).

110. P. Aichele, H. Hengartner, R. M. Zinkernagel, M. Schulz, Antiviral cytotoxic T cell response induced by in vivo priming with a free synthetic peptide, *J. Exp. Med. 171:* 1815 (1990).

111. J. Klein, F. Figueroa, Polymorphiom of the mouse H-2 loci, *Immunol. Rev. 60:* 23 (1981).

112. C. Ferrari, A. Bertoletti, A. Penna, A. Cavalli, A. Valli, G. Missale, M. Pilli, P. Fowler, T. Giuberti, F. V. Chisari, F. Fiaccadori, Identification of immodominant T cell epitopes of the hepatitis B virus nucleocapsid antigen, *J. Clin. Invest. 88:* 214 (1991).

113. M. Imai, M. Nomura, T. Gotanda, T. Sano, K. Tachibana, H. Miyamoto, K. Takahashi, S. Toyama, Y. Miyakawa, M. Mayumi, Demonstration of two determinants on hepatitis B e antigen by monoclonal antibodies, *J. Immun. 128:* 69 (1982).

114. M. Sallberg, U. Ruden, B. Wahren, M. Noah, L. O. Magnius, Human and murine B-cells recognize the HBeAg/Beta (or HBe2) epitope as a linear determinant, *Mol. Immun. 28:* 719 (1991).

115. A. Penna, F. Chisari, A. Bertoletti, G. Missale, P. Fowler, T. Giuberti, F. Fiaccadori, C. Ferrari. Cytotoxic T lymphocytes recognize an HLA-A2-restricted epitope within the hepatitis B virus nucleocapsid antigen, *J. Exp. Med. 174:* 1565 (1991).

116. F. Schödel, A. Moriarty, D. Peterson, J. Zheng, J. Hughes, H. Will, D. Leturcq, J. McGee, D. Milich. The position of heterologous epitopes inserted in hepatitis B virus core particles determines their immunogenicity, *J. Virol 66:* 106 (1992).

20

Potential Future Recombinant Vaccines

Tineke Rutgers, Pierre Hauser, and Michel De Wilde

SmithKline Beecham Biologicals, Rixensart, Belgium

I. INTRODUCTION

Currently licensed recombinant hepatitis B vaccines consist of HBsAg particles and have been shown to be both safe and efficacious. The particles are purified from *Saccharomyces cerevisiae* transformed with a plasmid carrying the gene for the major (S) surface protein of hepatitis B virus (HBV) (1, 2) or from cell culture supernatants of Chinese hamster ovary (CHO) cells transfected with DNA encoding the PreS+S regions of the HBV genome (3). The yeast system produces lipoprotein particles containing the S protein, while the CHO system produces particles containing the S and middle (M) protein in a ratio of about 2:1. The purified HBs(S) or HBs(S,M) lipoprotein particles are formulated as vaccines by adsorption on to aluminum hydroxide (RECOMBIVAX HB, Merck Sharp & Dohme; ENGERIX B, SmithKline Beecham Biologicals; GENHEVAC B, Pasteur Mérieux Serum et Vaccins). The vaccine is administered by intramuscular injection, and a primary immunization course consists of three inoculations. The introduction of these recombinant hepatitis B vaccines constituted a major breakthrough as the current availability of unlimited quantities of safe and effective vaccines has opened the way to global control and possible eradication of hepatitis B.

Incentives for further development of recombinant hepatitis B vaccines may be found in the improvement of cost-effectiveness of production, simplification of the immunization schedule or administration, further improvement in efficacy, and in prevention of the emergence of escape mutants or protection against variant viruses (see also Chapter 18).

In addressing these issues, recombinant technology may well make a further contribution. Developing high-level production sytems for more immunogenic vaccines can be expected to influence cost-effectiveness and immunization schedules. Broadening the immune response by inclusion of additional protective and T-helper epitopes may induce protection in those persons who respond poorly or not at all to the current vaccines. A broader immune response may also provide protection against variant viruses and prevent the emergence of escape mutants. Furthermore, built-in adjuvanticity may be provided by introducing immunostimulatory sequences into the immunogen. Finally, the development of an oral vaccine may offer advantages for mass vaccination programs.

II. ALTERNATIVE PRODUCTION SYSTEMS

A. Yeast-Based Production Systems

Large-scale production of HBs(S) particles in *S. cerevisiae* has been achieved with constitutive promoter-driven gene expression and using multicopy plasmids to obtain high levels of expression (1, 2) (see also Chapter 4). At high cell density, plasmid maintenance, distribution, and stability may pose problems in such expression systems during fermentation (4, 5). Several alternative approaches based on integration of expression cassettes into chromosomal DNA, inducible promoters, and other yeasts have been developed. Expression systems developed in the methylotrophic yeasts *Pichia pastoris* (6) and *Hansenula polymorpha* (7) and based on methanol-regulated promoters and integrated expression cassettes have shown to be able to produce HBs(S) particles at levels two to five times higher than the first-generation *S. cerevisiae* systems (1, 2) under large-scale fermentation conditions. Depending on the immunogenic properties of the HBs(S) particles purified from these systems, *P. pastoris* and/or *H. polymorpha* may provide an economically advantageous alternative production system.

B. Higher Eukaryotic Production Systems

Expression of the gene for the S protein and secretion of HBs(S) particles has been demonstrated in a variety of higher eukaryotic expression systems. In contrast to the yeast expression systems where the S protein is produced only in its nonglycosylated form, a proportion of the S protein secreted from higher eukaryotic cells is glycosylated in a manner similar to the plasma-derived protein as judged by molecular size and endoglycosidase sensitivity. The exact nature and linkage of the sugar residues in the N-linked glycan is likely to depend on the cell type used for production. Glycosylation of the S protein, however, does not seem to influence the immunogenicity of the particles, as comparative clinical trials of plasma- and yeast-derived vaccines have demonstrated similar immunogenicity and efficacy. Thus glycosylation does not appear to be an inherent advantage of higher eukaryotic expression systems.

Stable expression of the S gene and secretion of HBs(S) particles was achieved in CHO cells early in the development of recombinant hepatitis B vaccines by transfection with a plasmid carrying the S gene under control of the SV40 early promoter (8). The CHO-derived HBs(S) showed excellent immunogenic potency in mice and chimpanzees. In addition, chimpanzees vaccinated with the cell culture–derived HBs(S) were protected from infection with HBV of either subtype (9). Another expression system based on mouse fibroblasts stably transformed with a bovine papillomavirus–derived vector system has been developed into a large-scale mammalian cell–derived HBs(S) production process. In a clinical trial (10) comparing this mammalian cell–derived recombinant vaccine (Betagen, Connaught Lab.) with a plasma-derived vaccine (HEPTAVAX B, Merck Sharp & Dohme), no significant differences in seroconversion rates were observed between the two vaccines. The geometric mean titer of the antibody response was, however, significantly lower for the recombinant vaccine, and the response was related to age and sex. Higher responses in females and in younger age groups have been observed in trials with other hepatitis B vaccines.

Insertion of the coding sequence for the S protein in vaccinia virus and generation of infectious recombinant virus was achieved in 1983. Cells infected with the recombinant virus synthesized and secreted HBs(S) particles (11). Recently, researchers in the People's Republic of China used a recombinant vaccinia virus system for the production of HBs(S) particles (12). The S gene was placed under control of the vaccinia 7.5–kD promoter and inserted into the vaccinia thymidine kinase gene of the Chinese vaccine strain Tian-Tan. Primary chicken embryo cells (CEC) were used as host cell. Particles purified from the CEC culture supernatants have undergone limited phase I and II clinical trials. Seroconversion rates were similar to those obtained with an equal dose of commercial yeast-derived vaccine, but the kinetics and titers of the antibody responses have not yet been reported.

As the potency and efficacy of mammalian cell–derived HBs(S) appears to be similar to that of the yeast-derived product, the choice of production system for recombinant HBs(S) depends mainly on economic and safety considerations. Mammalian cell systems usually employ expression vectors that carry sequences derived from oncogenic viruses such as SV40 or bovine papilloma viruses, while the host cell is a virus-transformed continuous cell line and/or may carry indigenous viruses. The yeast system with its higher production levels and greater safety (no oncogenic elements are utilized) has become, therefore, the system of choice for the first generation of recombinant HBs(S) vaccines (13, 14). A risk-to-benefit assessment of future mammalian cell–derived hepatitis B vaccines should be performed in view of the potential alternative production systems.

Several other expression systems are still in the experimental stage. Recombinant baculoviruses have been isolated that express the S gene upon infection of insect cells (15, 16). The S protein synthesized in insect cells was glycosylated with a high-mannose N-linked chain, while a complex-type oligosaccharide is present on plasma-derived HBsAg or mammalian cell culture–derived HBs(S) particles. The S protein was partially assembled into lipoprotein particles, which were, however, not efficiently secreted (16). It is possible that the baculovirus expression vector system may be developed further into an efficient production system as methods for large-scale insect cell propagation are under development.

III. ADDITIONAL EPITOPES

A. PreS epitopes

One approach for the development of a new generation of vaccines is to include additional protective B-cell and/or T-helper epitopes. The current yeast-derived vaccines were conceived when only the S protein in the envelope of HBV had been identified. Recent advances in the molecular biology of HBV have resulted in the identification of two minor components of the viral envelope: the middle (M) and large (L) surface proteins (17). These proteins share the S protein sequence at their carboxy terminus and contain additional domains at the amino terminus. The M protein contains an additional domain of 55 amino acids (preS2 domain), the L protein contains in addition to the preS2 domain, a further amino-terminal sequence of 119 (or 108 depending on subtype) amino acids (preS1 domain). The preS domains are immunogenic and elicit antibody responses in humans during natural HBV infection. The anti-preS antibodies often appear prior to any other HBV-specific antibody. The contribution of the preS domains to a protective immune response in humans is not resolved, but there is evidence to indicate that they may be suitable vaccine components (Fig. 1) (see also Chapters 3 and 19).

1. B-Cell Epitopes

Protective B-cell epitopes within the preS domains were demonstrated by both neutralization (18, 19) and immunization (19–22) experiments in chimpanzees. Incubation of HBV with rabbit antiserum raised against synthetic peptides preS2 (120–145) or preS1 (21–47) prior to injection into susceptible chimpanzees resulted in prevention of infection, indicating that the antipeptide sera contain virus-neutralizing antibodies. Active immunization of chimpanzees with synthetic peptides preS2 (120–174), preS2 (120–145), preS2 (133–151), preS1 (12–47), or preS1 (94–117) resulted in protection against HBV challenge. Furthermore, an attachment site for the binding of HBV to human hepatocytes (23) and other cells susceptible to infection (24) has been identified within the preS1 (21–47) sequence. Antibodies that interfere with HBV binding to its host cell would be

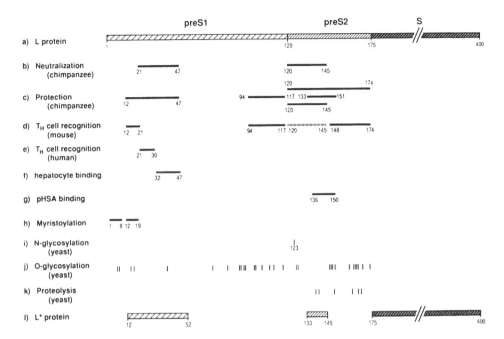

Figure 1 Amino acid sequences implicated in activities contained in the preS region. Numbers indicate amino acid residues based on 119 amino acid residues in the preSl domain. (a) Large envelope protein of HBV (adw) composed of preS1, preS2, and S domains. (b) Synthetic peptides capable of inducing virus-neutralizing antibodies (18, 19). (c) Synthetic peptides inducing protective immunity (19–22). (d) T-helper cell recognition sites determined in mouse model (41–45). (e) T-helper cell recognition site determined in human vaccine recipients (C. Ferrari, personal communication). (f) Hepatocyte-binding site (23,111). (g) pHSA-binding site (28,29). (h) Sequence required for myristoylation of residues 2 or 13 (33,80). (i) N-Glycosylation observed in yeast expression systems (57). (j) Potential O-glycosylation sites utilized in yeast expression systems (55–57). (k) Proteolytic cleavage sites observed in yeast expression systems (55,80). (l) Sequences contained in L* protein (80). (Adapted from Ref. 80.)

expected to be neutralizing. An alternative or synergic host cell recognition mechanism has been proposed based on the observation that a region within the preS2 domain has an affinity for glutaraldehyde polymerized human serum albumin (pHSA) (25). Since pHSA also has an affinity to liver cells, it has been postulated that pHSA mediates HBV–host cell interactions. Although binding of native human serum albumin to the preS2 domain was also demonstrated (26), the functional significance of these in vitro observations remains unresolved. Binding of HSA in vivo may prevent recognition by neutralizing antibodies, and HSA binding to vaccines containing the pHSA-binding site may mask those epitopes that induce a protective antibody response. Moreover, concerns have been raised with respect to the binding of a self-component (serum albumin) to vaccines containing the pHSA-binding site with the possibility of induction of autoimmunity or tolerance phenomena (27). The pHSA-binding site has not been exactly identified, but current evidence indicates that the region spanning residues 136–147/140–150 is involved (28, 29). Another observation of as yet undetermined biological significance is an in vitro immunological cross-reactivity between the preS1 (21–47) sequence and human IgA (30). At present, the relevance of this observation to the generation of autoantibodies by preS1-containing vaccines is unknown.

In addition to the continuous preS epitopes detected with the aid of synthetic peptides, evidence for the existence of discontinuous preS1 epitopes based on differences in reactivity of sera from HBV patients towards denatured or native antigens has been described (31, 32). If such discontinuous epitopes contribute to protection, vaccines should contain the relevant domains in their native conformation. One element that may influence conformation is the amino-terminal myristic acid acylation of the L protein (33). The hydrophobic fatty acid moiety would interact with the lipid component of the particles, imposing secondary-tertiary folding on the L polypeptide chain.

2. T-Cell Epitopes

The human antibody response to HBsAg is T-cell dependent, and low or nonresponsiveness of vaccine recipients has been associated, at least in part, with HLA phenotype (34–37).

Extensive studies in a mouse model (38) have demonstrated that the immune responses to the S, preS2, and preS1 domains are independently regulated by MHC class II molecules. Furthermore, the T-cell response to one domain provides T-cell helper function for multiple B-cell epitopes present on S, preS2, and preS1. Although immunization of mice with preS-containing HBsAg did not result in an enhancement of the anti-S response in S-responder mice, immunization of S-nonresponder mice resulted in induction of both anti-preS and anti-S antibodies (39–41). At present, the crucial question as to whether this mechanism of circumvention of nonresponsiveness is also valid in humans has not yet been resolved.

In the mouse model, T-cell recognition sites were defined within the C-terminal half of the preS2 region (preS2 (148–174)). T-cell recognition was dependent on the H-2 haplotype of the mouse strain and was HBV subtype specific (42). A T-cell recognition site has been localized in synthetic peptide preS2 (120–145), more specifically to residues 120–132. However, T cells from mice that were primed in vivo with peptide 120–145 did not respond to native recombinant HBs(S,M) in in vitro proliferation assays (43). In contrast, Neurath et al. (44) reported that S-nonresponder mice preimmunized with peptide 120–

145 showed enhanced antibody responses to subsequent immunization with preS2-containing plamsa-derived HBsAg as compared to control mice. In the preS1 region T-cell recognition sites were mapped to the (12–21) and (94–117) sequences (41,45).

In humans, the preS1 domain appears to be an efficient T-cell immunogen. A high proportion of CD4-positive T-cell clones isolated from high responders to plasma-derived vaccine (HEVAC B, Pasteur Mérieux Serum et Vaccines) were preS1 specific, although the vaccine contained only traces of preS1 (46). In two vaccinees, the dominant T-cell recognition site has been identified to the N-terminal residues (21–30) of the preS1 sequence (C. Ferrari, personal communication). Jin et al. (47) isolated a preS1 (21–28)–specific T-cell clone from a plasma-derived vaccine recipient. The CD8-positive T-cell line responded to peptide (21–28) in association with MHC class I antigens, indicating that vaccination with HBsAg may induce both MHC class II and MHC class I-restricted-T cells. Barnaba et al. (48) isolated both CD8-positive and CD4-positive cytotoxic T-cell clones recognizing preS2 (120–134) peptide from lymphocytes infiltrating the liver during chronic hepatitis. HBsAg-specific B-cells pulsed with very low concentrations of HBsAg were efficiently and selectively lysed by the CTL clones (49). To what extent such CTL activity can be induced upon vaccination with preS containing vaccines is presently unknown.

3. PreS2-Containing Recombinant Vaccines

As *S. cerevisiae* had proven its utility as host for the production of HBs(S) particles, several groups expressed the coding sequences for the M and L protein by a similar expression system (50–60). The M protein produced was recovered from yeast extracts as typical lipoprotein particles of about 22 nm diameter (HBs(M)). Antigenicity studies showed that the preS2 sequences were accessible to several different preS2-specific monoclonal antibodies, but the S-specific antigenicity, as measured by commercially available polyclonal antibody assay (AUSRIA II, Abbott), was low compared to HBs(S) particles, indicating that the preS2 sequences are exposed on the exterior of the HBs(M) particles and partially mask the S epitopes (53,57). The majority of the M protein was glycosylated. Like the M protein in plasma-derived HBsAg, the yeast-derived protein carried an N-linked glycan at the glycosylation site located in the preS2 region. In one case outer-chain mannose addition was reported, which was prevented by expressing the M protein in a *S. cerevisiae mnn9* mutant strain (59). However, unlike the plasma-derived M protein, the M protein produced in *S. cerevisiae* also carried a variety of short O-linked mannose chains (55–57). These O-linked chains may modify the antigenic and immunogenic properties of the particles. Furthermore, the preS2 moiety exposed on the exterior of the particle appeared particularly sensitive to proteolytic degradation (51,53–55,57). Production of HBs(M) in a peptidase-deficient strain *(pep 4-3)* of *S. cerevisiae* partially reduced the degradation problem (55,57). Itoh and Fujisawa eliminated from the M gene a sequence coding for six amino acids (163–168), which included the most sensitive degradation site. The HBs(M) particles produced showed enhanced resistance to yeast proteases (60).

Immunogenicity studies showed that HBs(M) particles produced in *S. cerevisiae* are capable of inducing both anti-S and anti-preS2 antibodies in guinea pigs (61) and mice (54,61,62). ED_{50} values (54,61) and antibody titers (61,62) of the anti-S response in mice were similar to those obtained with plasma-derived HBsAg or yeast-derived HBs(S). Secondary immunization of guinea pigs (61) or mice (62) resulted in a considerable increase in both anti-S and anti-preS2 antibody titers. Immunization of SJL/J S-nonresponder mice with HBs(M) induced significant amounts of anti-S antibodies, at levels considerably higher than those obtained in response to yeast-derived HBs(S) (61). The circumvention of nonresponsiveness to S in S-nonresponder mice by vaccination with HBs(M) confirmed the results of Milich et al. (40). In African green monkeys induction of both anti-S and anti-preS2 antibodies was observed after administration of each of three doses of HBs(M) vaccine (54). The kinetics of the anti-S antibody response was similar to that observed for HBs(S) vaccine. However, the anti-preS2 antibody response was not boosted after administration of the third dose and was transient and relatively weak. Similar low boosting effects and weak responses were reported by De Wilde et al. (62). In chimpanzees receiving three doses of HBs(M) at 4-week intervals, the immunogenicity of either 10- or 40-μg doses was similar to 10-μg doses of yeast-derived HBs(S) in terms of the anti-S antibody response (63). As in monkeys, the anti-preS2 antibody response was not boosted on administration of the third dose. In those animals immunized with 40-μg vaccine dosage, the anti-preS2 antibodies appeared 2 weeks after the first dose, earlier than the anti-S antibodies, reached a maximum 2 weeks after the second dose, and were well maintained at that level during the next 35 weeks. However, animals receiving the 10-μg dose regime showed a rapid decline of anti-preS2 antibody levels. It appears that high doses of HBs(M) may be required to obtain a persistent anti-preS2 antibody response.

In a healthy young adult human population, comparison of equal doses of HBs(M) and HBs(S) resulted in a significant lower anti-S seroconversion rate and GMT in the HBs(M) vaccinees (62). Most (88%) of the HBs(M) vaccinees seroconverted for anti-preS2, but titers were low and the anti-preS2 response did not appear earlier than the anti-S response. On the contrary, after one dose none of the vaccinees had a measurable anti-preS2 response, while 37% were positive for antibodies to S. Importantly, nonresponders to the S domain did occur in the group receiving the HBs(M) vaccine. The nonresponders to S did not respond to preS2 either. In general, a positive correlation was observed between the anti-S and anti-preS2 responses, suggesting that the presence of preS2 sequences in the HBs(M) vaccine dose not lead to circumvention of nonresponsiveness to the S domain in the human population. Gerety and West (64) reported a dose-response study of HBs(M) particles. A dose range of 12–48 μg HBs(M) was compared to 10 μg HBs(S). Slightly higher anti-S seroconversion rates and GMTs were obtained in the groups that received HBs(M) vaccines, although a classical dose response was not observed. In this study, 100% of the volunteers receiving the HBs(M) vaccine seroconverted to anti-S positivity. The majority of recipients of HBs(M) vaccine had an anti-preS2 response, which, however, did not appear earlier than the anti-S response.

Limited clinical trials in nonresponder groups have given different results. In five nonresponders to either plasma-derived HBsAg or yeast-derived HBs(S) vaccine, two further doses of HBs(M) vaccine did not induce significant titers of anti-S antibodies (62). In contrast, in a preliminary report Iino et al. (65) mentioned 95% seroconversion (anti-S alone, 10%; anti-preS2 alone, 25%; or both, 60%) in a nonresponder group (20 volunteers) to plasma-derived HBsAg after immunization with two doses of HBs(M). Titers of these antibody responses were not reported.

The relatively poor results obtained with HBs(M) particles produced in *S. cerevisiae* might be related to this particular production system, e.g., over-glycosylation of the M protein or producing particles containing only the M protein. Particles containing both the S and M proteins (HBs(S,M)) are secreted from CHO cells transfected with a plasmid carrying the preS and S sequences (3). The purified particles contain 20% glycosylated M protein, 20% glycosylated S protein, and 60% nonglycosylated S protein. A vaccine containing inactivated HBs(S,M) particles has been licensed in France. Clinical trials (66) with the vaccine (GENHEVAC B, Pasteur Mérieux Serum et Vaccins) have demonstrated its safety. No antibodies to serum albumin or liver proteins could be detected in those recipients tested. Transaminase levels remained normal in all vaccinees, indicating that vaccines containing preS2 sequences that include the pHSA binding site do not induce liver damage or autoimmunity. Anti-S seroconversion rates and GMT levels were lower than those obtained with an equal dose of plasma-derived vaccine. Higher doses of HBs(S,M) (10 or 20 μg) were capable of inducing anti-S antibody GMTs similar to the standard dose (5 μg) of plasma-derived vaccine from the same manufacturer. Nonresponsiveness to the S antigen was observed at about the same frequency in all groups receiving either the HBs(S,M) or plasma-derived vaccine. While most vaccinees seroconverted with respect to preS2 the anti-preS2 response appeared earlier than the anti-S response in only a small number receiving the highest dosage. A strong positive correlation was observed between the anti-S and anti-preS2 antibody titers, suggesting that the responses to the two domains are interdependent in humans.

Cumulatively, the results obtained thus far in humans with preS2-containing recombinant vaccines appear disappointing in view of the results obtained in the mouse model. PreS2-containing recombinant vaccines are safe and immunogenic but seem to provide few advantages over the existing HBs(S) vaccines. From the preliminary data cited above it appears as if recombinant vaccines containing additional preS2 sequences induce anti-S titers that are lower than those seen with equivalent amounts of plasma-derived or yeast-derived HBs(S) vaccines. Moreover, the mechanism of circumvention of nonresponsiveness to the S domain by the addition of T-helper epitopes contained in the preS2 domain does not seem to be operative in humans. Nonresponse to the S domain still occurs at about the same frequency. The HBs(M) and HBs(S,M) vaccines induce an anti-preS2 response, which does not appear significantly earlier than the anti-S response and whose persistence has not yet been determined. Theoretically, the broader immune response induced by HBs(M) or HBs(S,M) could provide protection against viruses mutated in the antigenic S domain implicated in neutralization. No experimental evidence to support this notion has been generated thus far.

4.   PreS1-Containing Recombinant Vaccines

The L protein expressed in *S. cerevisiae* could not be recovered in the typical lipoprotein particle form. Instead, heterogeneous lipoprotein structures were obtained (52,53,57,58), and masking of the S epitopes in these structures was almost complete. A proportion of the L molecules was overglycosylated compared to the natural HBV L protein. An N-linked high-mannose glycan was present at the N-glycosylation site in the preS2 domain, and the molecule was extensively O-glycosylated. From the above, it became apparent that coexpression and coassembly of S, M, and L proteins would be necessary to obtain an immunogen exposing all the relevant B-cell epitopes in their most natural conformation and relative density.

This was achieved in *S. cerevisiae* by integrating expression cassettes for each of the HBV surface proteins into the genome in a defined relative ratio (67). A similar coexpression of the S and L genes from different genome-integrated expression cassettes was applied to produce composite (S,L) particles in *H. polymorpha* (7).

In mammalian expression systems, production of L protein at levels higher than a few percent of total HBV surface protein (S+M+L) production led to inhibition of secretion of the composite (S,M,L) particles (68–71). Two reports describe secretion and purification from transfected mouse cells of HBs(S,M,L) particles that have 5–15% L protein content (72,73). Such particles may be useful to analyze the contribution of the preS1 domain to immunogenicity in humans.

In general, the results obtained in yeast and mammalian expression systems indicate that producing antigen with a high content of preS1 epitopes would require redesigning the antigen with respect to its immunological characteristics and with the limitations of the particular expression system in mind.

In mammalian cells such an approach was reported by Hemmerling et al. (74). Mouse cells cotransfected with plasmids carrying expression cassettes for a preS1 (9–36 or 9–67)-S fusion protein and a preS2 (120–175 or 134–162)-S fusion protein secreted particles displaying preS1-, preS2-, and S-specific antigenicity. The principle of cotransfection with different expression cassettes encoding desired epitopes has been applied to the development of a candidate vaccine containing immunologically important preS1, preS2, and S epitopes, including both the *adw* and *ayw* subtypes (75). The candidate vaccine (HEPA-GENE-3) has entered clinical trials, and preliminary results have been communicated (76–79). Compared to yeast-derived HBs(S) vaccines, substantially higher anti-S responses were reported to be induced by this candidate vaccine, both in a healthy adult group and in elderly volunteers. Moreover, 100% of the vaccinees were claimed to respond to HEPA-GENE-3 even in the elderly, a group that in general responds less well to currently licensed vaccines. Details on the vaccine's composition and immunogenicity have not been revealed.

For production in *S. cerevisiae* a modified L protein (L* protein) was designed (Fig. 1) that would retain the immunologically important B and T-helper epitopes, be myristoylated, not contain the pHSA binding site, and would be less susceptible to yeast-related overglycosylation and proteolytic degradation (80). Yeast cells were engineered to produce an L* protein (containing amino acid residues 12–52 of the preS1 domain, residues 133–145 of the preS2 domain, and the complete S domain (residues 175–400)) together with the S protein in the same cell. The L* protein produced was myristoylated, and a minority of the molecules were glycosylated with a high-mannose type N-linked glycan. The L* protein demonstrated remarkable stability during expression and recovery. Composite (S,L*) particles were formed that contain the two proteins in a S:L* ratio of 3:1 (62,80) (Fig. 2), have the typical spherical HBsAg structure, and display preS1, preS2, and S antigenicity. Importantly, the particles were well recognized by both a monoclonal antibody recognizing a virus-neutralizing conformational S epitope and a monoclonal antibody with specificity for the hepatocyte-binding site. The particles were unable to bind pHSA (62). These HBs(S,L*) particles were found to be immunogenic in mice and monkeys, inducing similar or higher titers of anti-S antibodies than yeast-derived HBs(S) antigen (62). Strong antibody responses to the preS1 sequences were obtained in both animal species, while the anti-preS2 responses was relatively low. The HBs(S,L*) particles are undergoing clinical evaluation of their safety and immunogenicity.

B. Core Epitopes

Hepatitis B core antigen (HBcAg) is a potent immunogen eliciting high levels of antibodies in experimental animals and humans. Antibodies to HBcAg are not protective and may even be detrimental, delaying viral clearance and promoting persistent infection (81). However, immunization of chimpanzees with HBcAg/

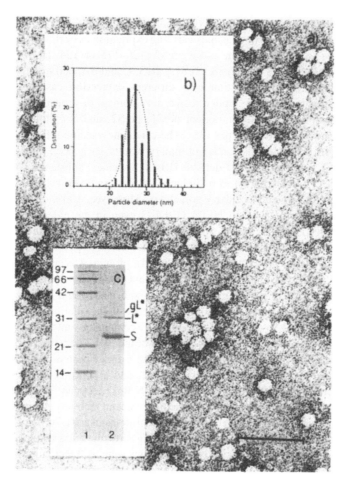

Figure 2 (a) Electron micrograph of purified HBs(S,L*) particles. Magnification ×
180,000. Bar = 100 nm. (b) Size distribution of purified HBs(S,L*) particles. One
hundred particles were analyzed by planimetry. (c) Coomassie brilliant blue staining of
proteins from purified HBs(S,L*) particles separated by SDS-polyacrylamide gel electrophoresis. Lane 1: molecular mass markers. Lane 2: HBs(S,L*) particles. gL*: glycosylated form of L* protein. Electron microscopy and size analysis was performed by Dr. C.
Remacle, Catholic University of Louvain, Belgium.

HBeAg resulted in partial or complete protection against HBV challenge (82–
84). The mechanisms involved have not been elucidated but are assumed to be
mediated by cellular immunity mechanisms. Induction of HBcAg-specific T-
helper cells which provide functional help to HBsAg-specific B cells may offer
an explanation for the protective effect of HBcAg/HBeAg immunization. Such a

mechanism has been proposed to be operative in a mouse model (38,85). Mice primed with HBcAg and challenged with HBV produced anti-S, anti-preS2, and anti-preS1 antibodies, while primed mice challenged with a mixture of HBcAg and HBsAg produced no anti-HBsAg. The proposed mechanism of intermolecular/intrastructural T-cell help involves internalization of the virion by HBsAg-specific B cells, processing and presentation of viral peptides (including core peptides) in the context of MHC class II molecules, and stimulation of HBsAg-specific B cells by HBcAg-specific T-helper cells. Since HBcAg-priming of a mouse strain nonresponsive to the S domain of the viral envelope resulted in anti-S antibody production, the HBcAg-specific T-helper cell stimulation represents another mechanism for circumventing HBsAg nonresponsiveness. Thus, if such mechanism is functional in humans, improvement of HBV vaccine efficacy may result from engineering HBcAg/HBeAg T-helper epitopes into recombinant HBsAg particles. However, examination of the specificity of the T-cell recognition showed dependence on the H-2 haplotype of the mouse strain. Each mouse strain recognized multiple but distinct sites within the HBcAg/HBeAg sequence (86). In a human outbred population a multitude of distinct T-cell sites may be necessary to cover the HLA genotypes. Identification of HBcAg T-cell recognition sites in 18 acute hepatitis B patients of different HLA haplotypes demonstrated three different sequences which were recognized by a majority of patients (C. Ferrari, personal communication), and it is possible that a limited number of T-cell epitopes could cover human HLA-dependent T-cell recognition in a majority of people. A further analysis of the human T-cell response to HBcAg is required to evaluate the potential risks and benefits of HBcAg sequences as a vaccine component. Experiments in the mouse model have recently demonstrated that in utero exposure to HBeAg or neonatal exposure to HBcAg induces tolerance to HBcAg/HBeAg at the T-cell level (87). A correlation between these observations in the mouse model and the human situation where infants born to HBeAg-positive mothers almost invariably become persistently infected was suggested. Since a major target group for hepatitis B vaccination comprises neonates of HBeAg-positive mothers, further studies on the immunogenicity and tolerogenicity of HBcAg/HBeAg and the relationship to the induction of protective levels of anti-HBsAg antibodies are required before inclusion of HBcAg/HBeAg sequences in a vaccine for neonates can be envisaged.

IV. NOVEL VACCINES BASED ON VIRAL ANTIGENS OTHER THAN THE S PROTEIN

Vaccines may be designed based on viral antigens other than the S protein. The immunogenic properties of the preS region of the envelope proteins and HBcAg/HBeAg have been mentioned above. The immune response to the other viral proteins, the polymerase and X gene products, have been less well studied. Antibodies to the polymerase and X gene products were detected in sera from acute and chronic HBV patients (88–91). So far, a T-cell immune response has not been described. The significance of an immune response to these proteins with respect to protection and vaccine development is currently unknown.

The only viral antigen other than the S protein shown to elicit a protective antibody response is the preS region of the viral envelope proteins. Vaccines based on the relevant B- and T-cell epitopes of the preS region only may be considered and indeed are subject of synthetic vaccine design (see Chapter 19). Additionally, the relevant B-cell epitopes may be engineered into various carrier moieties for efficient antigen presentation.

HBcAg is a very potent immunogen eliciting both T-cell-dependent and T-cell-independent antibody responses (92). These properties have led to the utilization of HBcAg as carrier moiety for other epitopes: for example, a peptide of the foot and mouth disease virus capsid fused to HBcAg particles showed enhanced immunogenicity as compared to other carrier systems (93). Fusions made carboxy-terminally, replacing the arginine-rich nucleic acid–binding domain of HBcAg, are still capable of forming particles. Sequences encoding B-cell epitopes of the hepatitis B envelope proteins from the preS2 or preS1 domains have also been fused to the HBcAg-coding sequence (94, 95). The particles displayed HBcAg, HBeAg, and preS antigenicity. Rabbits immunized with the fusion protein particles responded to both the carrier (anti-HBcAg and anti-HBeAg) and the fusion peptide sequences (anti-preS2 or anti-preS1).

The possibility of creating composite particles displaying several different protective B-cell epitopes to broaden the immune response to a particular pathogen or to develop a multivalent vaccine has been envisaged (85). However, the development of the HBcAg carrier concept for human vaccine applications in general, and to HBV vaccines in particular, is hampered by concerns regarding the immunological properties of HBcAg discussed above and by the affinity of the core protein for nucleic acids. Deletion of the nucleic acid-binding domain from the protein does not completely prevent nucleic acid encapsidation into the particles (96).

In general, any candidate vaccine based on antigens other than the S protein has to demonstrate its efficacy in humans before a license is granted. However, efficacy trials in high-risk populations with any vaccine based on novel concepts may be considered unethical in view of the current availability of safe and effective vaccines.

V. LIVE RECOMBINANT VACCINES

Vaccinia virus has been utilized extensively to generate live recombinant vaccine candidates (97,98), with the S gene of HBV being one of the first foreign genes inserted into the vaccinia virus genome (11). Rabbits inoculated intradermally with the live recombinant vaccinia virus seroconverted rapidly and high anti-S antibody titers were induced. Chimpanzees receiving a single intradermal vaccination developed no significant antibody response, but the animals were nevertheless protected from clinical signs of hepatitis after an intravenous challenge with HBV (99). Recombinant vaccinia virus that synthesized the M protein induced both anti-S and anti-preS2 antibody titers in rabbits inoculated intradermally (100). Intradermal inoculation of rabbits with recombinant vaccinia virus that synthesized the L protein induced antibodies to the preS1 and S domains. The production of anti-S antibodies was delayed compared to the kinetics of anti-S antibody production induced by S recombinant vaccinia virus (101). To demonstrate the possibility of engineering multivalent vaccines, a single vaccinia virus recombinant has been generated which expressed the influenza hemagglutinin, herpes simplex virus gD protein, and the S protein of HBV. Rabbits inoculated intradermally with this triple vaccinia virus recombinant seroconverted to all three antigens (102). A yet unresolved issue is whether previous vaccination against smallpox or a recombinant vaccinia virus will preclude the induction of an immune response to a revaccination with another recombinant virus (102–104).

The application of vaccinia recombinant viruses as live vaccines in humans is highly controversial. Low costs, ease of administration, potency at single inoculation and stability without refrigeration are all advantages for mass vaccination programs. However, serious adverse reactions to vaccinia virus, especially in young children, the main target group for hepatitis B vaccination, preclude the live recombinant vaccinia approach. Further understanding of the factors involved in viral virulence may lead to the possibility of engineering vaccine strains that are safe and effective.

Live recombinant adenovirus vaccines provide the convenience of oral administration. Current adenovirus vaccines given orally as enteric-coated tablets cause asymptomatic intestinal infection in humans and induce immunity against adenovirus respiratory disease. Recombinant adenoviruses carrying the S gene of HBV in the adenovirus E3 region replicated efficiently in human cell lines and HBsAg particles were secreted from the infected cells (105,106). Preclinical testing of recombinant adenovirus vaccines has been difficult due to the lack of suitable animal models. However, Lubeck et al. (106) showed that chimpanzees are susceptible to enteric infection by wild-type human adenovirus of serotype 7 and by recombinant type 4 and 7 adenoviruses. Enteric-coated gelatin capsules containing lyophilized recombinant adenovirus carrying the S gene of HBV were administered orally to chimpanzees (106), and relatively low anti-S responses of a transient nature were induced. Upon intravenous HBV challenge, chimpanzees that had received a booster immunization showed partial or complete protection against acute clinical hepatic disease. As in the HBV challenge study of chimpanzees immunized with the recombinant vaccinia virus expressing the S gene of

HBV (99), the animals were not protected from HBV infection. Like recombinant vaccinia virus, the acceptance of recombinant adenovirus as a human vaccine candidate depends on further evaluation of such vaccines with respect to induction of immunity in the presence of preexisting immunity to adenoviruses and on the pathogenic properties of the recombinants. One specific concern is the oncogenic potential of adenoviruses.

Bacteria have also been envisaged as live carriers of antigens from heterologous pathogens. As the protective epitopes of HBV are relatively well defined, these epitopes have been used to test the approach. Genetic insertion of preS2 epitopes into the outer membrane protein LamB of *Escherichia coli* resulted in cell surface exposure of the preS2 epitopes. The intravenous or intraperitoneal administration of the live recombinant bacteria to mice induced antibodies against both preS2 and the LamB protein as well as antibodies against other *E. coli* antigens (107,108).

The potent immunogenicity of *Salmonella* vaccine strains and their ability to induce immune responses after oral administration has attracted interest in their use as oral delivery system for heterologous antigens. PreS2 and S epitopes have been genetically inserted into the *Salmonella* flagellin protein, and hybrid flagella were expressed in an attenuated *Salmonella* strain. Animals immunized orally with the live recombinant bacteria developed serum antibodies to the HBV epitopes (109). Development of *Salmonella* or other bacterial delivery systems to induce an immune response appropriate for a particular pathogen depends on the ability to engineer attenuated strains that are both safe and effective.

VI. CONCLUSION

Currently licensed recombinant hepatitis B vaccines have established a remarkable safety and efficacy record. In the short term, efforts should be concentrated on a wider application of these vaccines, and large immunization campaigns aimed at newborns and young children, especially in intermediate and high HBV prevalence regions, should be considered. In this respect, studies on simultaneous administration of hepatitis B vaccine with BCG and DTP-polio vaccine have shown encouraging results (110).

Since the introduction of the first generation of recombinant vaccines, the development of more immunogenic and efficacious immunogens has been actively pursued. Over the last 5 years, efforts have been mainly concentrated on the analysis of the contribution of the preS domains to protective immunity. Research in this area has led to several experimental vaccines currently undergoing clinical evaluation. Preliminary results on the preS2 domain have been disappointing as the potency of preS2-containing recombinant vaccines was generally lower than that of currently available recombinant HBs(S) vaccines, and occasional cases of nonresponsiveness to vaccination were still found.

Results from trials with vaccines containing the preS1 domain are not yet available. Inclusion of T-helper epitopes from the core protein has been proposed as yet another way to reduce the percentage of nonresponders. T-cell sites recognized by humans are currently being defined, and this knowledge may lead to the development of new vaccine candidates. In the long term there is a possibility that oral vaccines capable of inducing a long-lasting protective systemic immunity may be developed. Diverse approaches towards this goal are in early experimental stages but are still a long way from clinical testing as fundamental safety issues have yet to be resolved.

ACKNOWLEDGMENTS

The authors thank Nigel Harford and Jean Pêtre for many helpful discussions and critical reading of the manuscript. We are especially grateful to Catherine Van Roy and Hélène Monnig for expert preparation of the manuscript. Research at SmithKline Beecham Biologicals was supported in part by the Walloon Region (STN 1109).

REFERENCES

1. P. Valenzuela, A. Medina, W. J. Rutter, G. Ammerer, and B. D. Hall, Synthesis and assembly of hepatitis B virus surface antigen particles in yeast, *Nature, 298*:347–350 (1982).

2. N. Harford, T. Cabezon, M. Crabeel, E. Simoen, A. Rutgers, and M. De Wilde, Expression of hepatitis B surface antigen in yeast, *Develop. Biol. Standard., 54*:125–130 (1983).

3. M. L. Michel, P. Pontisso, E. Sobczak, Y. Malpiece, R. E. Streeck, and P. Tiollais, Synthesis in animal cells of hepatitis B surface antigen particles carrying a receptor for polymerized human serum albumine, *Proc. Natl. Acad. Sci. USA, 81*:7708–7712 (1984).

4. S. B. Primrose, P. Derbyshire, I. M. Jones, M. Nugent, and W. Tacon, Hereditary instability of recombinant DNA molecules, *Soc. Gen. Microbiol., 10*:63–67 (1983).

5. F. Srienc, J. L. Campbell, and J. E. Bailey, Analysis of unstable recombinant *Saccharomyces cerevisiae* population growth in selective medium, *Biotechnol. Bioeng., 28*:996–1006 (1986).

6. J. M. Cregg, J. F. Tschopp, C. Stillman, R. Siegel, M. Akong, W. S. Craig, R. G. Buckholz, K. R. Madden, P. A. Kellaris, G. R. Davis, B. L. Smiley, J. Cruze, R. Torregrossa, G. Velicelebi, and G. P. Thill, High-level expression and efficient assembly of hepatitis B surface antigen in the methylotrophic yeast, *Pichia pastoris, Biotechnology, 5*:479–485 (1987).

7. Z. A. Janowicz, K. Melber, A. Merckelbach, E. Jacobs, N. Harford, M. Comberbach, and C. P. Hollenberg, Simultaneous expression of the S and L surface

antigens of hepatitis B, and formation of mixed particles in the methylotrophic yeast, *Hansenula polymorpha, Yeast, 7:* 431–443 (1991).

8. E. J. Patzer, C. C. Simonsen, G. R. Nakamura, R. D. Hershberg, T. J. Gregory, and A. D. Levinson, Characterization of recombinant-derived hepatitis B surface antigen secreted by a continuous cell line, *Viral Hepatitis and Liver Disease,* (G. N. Vyas, J. L. Dienstag, and J. H. Hoofnagle, eds.), Grune and Stratton, Inc., Orlando, FL, pp. 477–485 (1984).

9. E. J. Patzer, G. R. Nakamura, R. D. Hershberg, T. J. Gregory, C. Crowley, A. D. Levinson, and J. W. Eichberg, Cell culture derived recombinant HBsAg is highly immunogenic and protects chimpanzees from infection with hepatitis B virus, *Biotechnology, 4:*630–636 (1986).

10. M. L. Halliday, J. G. Rankin, N. J. Bristow, R. A. Coates, P. N. J. Corey, and A. C. Strickler, A randomized double-blind clinical trial of a mammalian cell-derived recombinant DNA hepatitis B vaccine compared with a plasma-derived vaccine, *Arch. Intern. Med., 150:*1195–1200 (1990).

11. G. L. Smith, M. Mackett, and B. Moss, Infectious vaccinia virus recombinants that express hepatitis B virus surface antigen, *Nature, 302:*490–495 (1983).

12. Y. Wang, Z.-P. Li, Y.-R. Han, K. Zhao, Z.-H. Hu, and H.-M. Li, A subunit vaccine for hepatitis B produced by a recombinant vaccinia virus, *Vaccines 90* (F. Brown, R. M. Chanock, H. S. Ginsberg, and R. A. Lerner, eds.), Cold Spring Harbor Laboratory Press, Cold Spring Harbor, NY, pp. 187–191 (1990).

13. J. Stephenne, Recombinant versus plasma-derived hepatitis B vaccines: Issues of safety, immunogenicity and cost-effectiveness, *Vaccine, 6:*299–303 (1988).

14. M. R. Hilleman, History, precedent, and progress in the development of mammalian cell culture systems for preparing vaccines: Safety considerations revisited, *J. Med. Virol., 31:*5–12 (1990).

15. C. Y. Kang, D. H. L. Bishop, J.-S. Seo, Y. Matsuura, and M. Choe, Secretion of particles of hepatitis B surface antigen from insect cells using a baculovirus vector, *J. Gen. Virol., 68:*2607–2613 (1987).

16. R. E. Lanford, V. Luckow, R. C. Kennedy, G. R. Dreesman, L. Notvall, and M. D. Summers, Expression and characterization of hepatitis B virus surface antigen polypeptides in insect cells with a baculovirus expression system, *J. Virol., 63:*1549–1557 (1989).

17. K. H. Heermann, U. Goldmann, W. Schwartz, T. Seyffarth, H. Baumgarten, and W. H. Gerlich, Large surface proteins of hepatitis B virus containing the pre-S sequence, *J. Virol., 52:*396–402 (1984).

18. A. R. Neurath, S. B. H. Kent, K. Parker, A. M. Prince, N. Strick, B. Brotman, and P. Sproul, Antibodies to a synthetic peptide from the preS 120–145 region of the hepatitis B virus envelope are virus neutralizing, *Vaccine, 4:*35–37 (1986).

19. A. R. Neurath, B. Seto, and N. Strick, Antibodies to synthetic peptides from the preS1 region of the hepatitis B virus (HBV) envelope (env) protein are virus-neutralizing and protective, *Vaccine, 7:*234–236 (1989).

20. Y. Itoh, E. Takai, H. Ohnuma, K. Kitajima, F. Tsuda, A. Machida, S. Mishiro, T. Nakamura, Y. Miyakawa, and M. Mayumi, A synthetic peptide vaccine involving the product of the pre-S(2) region of hepatitis B virus DNA: Protective efficacy in chimpanzees, *Proc. Natl. Acad. Sci. USA, 83:*9174–9178 (1986).

21. E. A. Emini, V. Larson, J. Eichberg, P. Conard, V. M. Garsky, D. R. Lee, R. W.

Ellis, W. J. Miller, C. A. Anderson, and R. J. Gerety, Protective effect of a synthetic peptide comprising the complete preS2 region of the hepatitis B virus surface protein, *J. Med. Virol., 28:*7–12 (1989).

22. G. B. Thornton, A. M. Moriarty, D. R. Milich, J. W. Eichberg, R. H. Purcell, and J. L. Gerin, Protection of chimpanzees from hepatitis B virus infection after immunization with synthetic peptides: identification of protective epitopes in the pre-S region, *Vaccines 89* (R. A. Lerner, H. Ginsberg, R. M. Chanock, and F. Brown, eds.), Cold Spring Harbor Laboratory Press, Cold Spring Harbor, NY, pp. 467–471 (1989).

23. A. R. Neurath, S. B. H. Kent, N. Strick, and K. Parker, Identification and chemical synthesis of a host cell receptor binding site on hepatitis B virus, *Cell, 46:*429–436 (1986).

24. A. R. Neurath, N. Strick, P. Sproul, H. E. Ralph, and J. Valinsky, Detection of receptors for hepatitis B virus on cells of extrahepatic origin, *Virology, 176:*448–457 (1990).

25. M. Imai, Y. Yanase, T. Nojiri, Y. Miyakawa, and M. Mayumi, A. receptor for polymerized human and chimpanzee albumins on hepatitis B virus particles co-occurring with HBeAg, *Gastroenterology, 76:*243–247 (1979).

26. B. Krone, A. Lenz, K.-H. Heerman, M. Seifer, L. Xuangyong, and W. H. Gerlich, Interaction between hepatitis B surface proteins and monomeric human serum albumin, *Hepatology, 11:*1050–1056 (1990).

27. U. Hellström and S. Sylvan, Should pre-S coded peptides be used in hepatitis B vaccines? *Lancet, i:*389–390 (1986).

28. B. Krone, W. H. Gerlich, K. H. Heermann, A. Lenz, X. Lu, M. Seifer, and R. Tomssen, Significance of pre-S antigens for hepatitis B vaccines, *Progress in Hepatitis B Immunization* (P. Coursaget and M. J. Tong, eds.), Colloque IN-SERM/John Libbey Eurotext Ltd., Paris/London Vol. 194, pp. 21–33 (1990).

29. M.-A. Petit, S. Dubanchet, F. Capel, P. Voet, C. Dauguet, and P. Hauser, HepG2 cell binding activities of different hepatitis B virus (HBV) isolates: Inhibitory effect of anti-HBs and anti-preS1 (21–47), *Virology, 180:*483–491 (1991).

30. A. R. Neurath and N. Strick, Antigenic Mimicry of an immunoglobulin A epitope by a hepatitis B virus cell attachment site, *Virology, 178:*631–634 (1990).

31. K.-H. Heermann, F. Kruse, M. Seifer, and W. H. Gerlich, Immunogenicity of the gene S and Pre-S domains in hepatitis B virions and HBsAg filaments, *Intervirology, 28:*14–25 (1987).

32. A. Alberti, W. H. Gerlich, K.-H. Heermann, and P. Pontisso, Nature and display of hepatitis B virus envelope proteins and the humoral immune response, *Springer Semin. Immunopathol., 12:*5–23 (1990).

33. D. H. Persing, H. E. Varmus, and D. Ganem, The preS1 protein of hepatitis B virus is acylated at its amino terminus with myristic acid, *J. Virol., 61:*1672–1677 (1987).

34. M. Walker, W. Szmuness, C. Stevens, and P. Rubinstein, Genetics of anti-HBs responsiveness. I. HLA-DR7 and non-responsiveness to hepatitis vaccination, *Transfusion, 21:*601 (1981).

35. D. E. Craven, Z. L. Awdeh, L. M. Kunches, E. J. Yunis, J. L. Dienstag, B. G. Werner, B. F. Polk, D. R. Syndman, R. Platt, C. S. Crumpacker, F. Grady and C. A. Alper, Non-responsiveness to hepatitis B vaccine in health careworkers. Re-

sults of revaccination and genetic typings, *Ann. Intern. Med.*, *105*:356–360 (1987).

36. J. Y. Weissman, M. M. Tsuchiyose, M. J. Tong, R. Co, K. Chin, R. B. Ettenger, Lack of response to recombinant hepatitis B vaccine in nonresponders to the plasma vaccine, *JAMA*, *260*:1734–1738 (1988).

37. C. A. Alper, M. S. Kruskall, D. Marcus-Bagley, D. E. Craven, A. J. Katz, S. J. Brink, J. L. Dienstag, Z. Awdeh, and E. J. Yunis, Genetic prediction of nonresponse to hepatitis B vaccine, *N. Engl. J. Med.*, *321*:708–712 (1989).

38. D. R. Milich, T- and B-cell recognition of hepatitis B viral antigens, *Immunol. Today*, *9*:380–386 (1988).

39. D. R. Milich, G. B. Thornton, A. R. Neurath, S. B. Kent, M.-L. Michel, P. Tiollais, and F. V. Chisari, Enhanced immunogenicity of the pre-S region of hepatitis B surface antigen, *Science*, *228*:1195–1199 (1985).

40. D. R. Milich, M. K. McNamara, A. McLachlan, G. B. Thornton, and F. V. Chisari, Distinct H-2-linked regulation of T-cell responses to the pre-S and S regions of the same hepatitis B surface antigen polypeptide allows circumvention of nonresponsiveness to the S region, *Proc. Natl. Acad. Sci. USA*, *82*:8168–8172 (1985).

41. D. R. Milich, A. McLachlan, F. V. Chisari, S. B. H. Kent, and G. B. Thornton, Immune response to the pre-S(1) region of the hepatitis B surface antigen (HBsAg): A pre-S(1) specific T cell response can bypass nonresponsiveness to the pre-S(2) and S regions of HBsAg, *J. Immunol.*, *137*:315–322 (1986).

42. D. R. Milich, J. L. Hughes, A. McLachlan, K. E. Langley, G. B. Thornton, and J. E. Jones, Importance of subtype in the immune response to the pre-S(2) region of the hepatitis B surface antigen, *J. Immunol.*, *144*:3535–3543 (1990).

43. D. R. Milich, A. McLachlan, F. V. Chisari, and G. B. Thornton, Nonoverlapping T and B cell determinants on a hepatitis B surface antigen (HBsAg) pre-S(2) region synthetic peptide, *J. Exp. Med.*, *164*:532–547 (1986).

44. A. R. Neurath, S. B. H. Kent, N. Strick, D. Stark, and P. Sproul, Genetic restriction of immune responsiveness to synthetic peptides corresponding to sequences in the pre-S region of the hepatitis B virus (HBV) envelope gene, *J. Med. Virol.*, *17*:119–125 (1985).

45. D. R. Milich, A. McLachlan, A. Moriarty, and G. B. Thornton, A single 10-residue pre-S(1) peptide can prime T cell help for antibody production to multiple epitopes within the pre-S(1), pre-S(2), and S regions of HBsAg, *J. Immunol.*, *138*:4457–4465 (1987).

46. C. Ferrari, A. Penna, A. Bertoletti, A. Cavalli, A. Valli, C. Schianchi, and F. Fiaccadori, The preS1 antigen of hepatitis B virus is highly immunogenic at the T cell level in man, *J. Clin. Invest.*, *84*:1314–1319 (1989).

47. Y. Jin, W.-K. Shih, and I. Berkower, Human T cell response to the surface antigen of hepatitis B virus (HBsAg), *J. Exp. Med.*, *168*:293–306 (1988).

48. V. Barnaba, A. Franco, A. Alberti, C. Balsano, R. Benvenuto, and F. Balsano, Recognition of hepatitis B virus envelope proteins by liver-infiltrating T lymphocytes in chronic HBV infection, *J. Immunol.*, *143*:2650–2655 (1989).

49. V. Barnaba, A. Franco, A. Alberti, R. Benvenuto, and F. Balsano, Selective killing of hepatitis B envelope antigen-specific B cells by class I-restricted, exogenous antigen-specific T lymphocytes, *Nature*, *345*:258–260 (1990).

50. P. Valenzuela, D. Coit, and C. H. Kuo, Synthesis and assembly in yeast of hepatitis B surface antigen particles containing the polyalbumin receptor, *Biotechnology, 3*:317–320 (1985).

51. Y. Itoh, T. Hayakawa, and Y. Fujisawa, Expression of hepatitis B virus surface antigen P31 gene in yeast, *Biochem. Biophys, Res. Comm., 138*:268–274 (1986).

52. P. Dehoux, V. Ribes, E. Sobczak, and R. E. Streeck, Expression of the hepatitis B virus large envelope protein in *Saccharomyces cerevisiae, Gene, 48*:155–163 (1986).

53. T. Imamura, M. Araki, A. Miyanohara, J. Nakao, H. Yonemura, N. Ohtomo, and K. Matsubara, Expression of hepatitis B virus middle and large surface antigen genes in *Saccharomyces cerevisiae, J. Virol., 61*:3543–3549 (1987).

54. R. W. Ellis, P. J. Kniskern, A. Hagopian, L. D. Schultz, D. L. Montgomery, R. Z. Maigetter, D. E. Wampler, E. A. Emini, D. Wolanski, W. J. McAleer, W. M. Hurni, and W. J. Miller, Preparation and testing of a recombinant-derived hepatitis B vaccine consisting of Pre-S2 + S polypeptides, *Viral Hepatitis and Liver Disease* (A. J. Zuckerman, ed.), A. R. Liss, New York, pp. 1079–1086 (1988).

55. K. E. Langley, K. M. Egan, J. M. Barendt, C. G. Parker, and G. A. Bitter, Characterization of purified hepatitis B surface antigen containing pre-S(2) epitopes expressed in *Saccharomyces cerevisiae, Gene, 67*:229–245 (1988).

56. M. Kobayashi, T. Asano, M. Utsunomiya, Y. Itoh, Y. Fujisawa, O. Nishimura, K. Kato, and A. Kakinuma, Recombinant hepatitis B virus surface antigen carrying the pre-S2 region derived from yeast: purification and characterization, *J. Biotechnology, 8*:1–22 (1988).

57. T. Rutgers, T. Cabezon, N. Harford, D. Vanderbrugge, M. Descurieux, O. Van Opstal, F. Van Wijnendaele, P. Hauser, P. Voet, and M. De Wilde, Expression of different forms of hepatitis B virus envelope proteins in yeast, *Viral Hepatitis and Liver Disease* (A. J. Zuckerman, ed.), A. R. Liss, New York, pp. 304–308 (1988).

58. P. J. Kniskern, A. Hagopian, P. Burke, N. Dunn, E. A. Emini, W. J. Miller, S. Yamazaki, and R. W. Ellis, A candidate vaccine for hepatitis B containing the complete viral surface protein, *Hepatology, 8*:82–87 (1988).

59. P. J. Kniskern, A. Hagopian, W. J. Miller, S. Yamazaki, and R. W. Ellis, Eur. Patent. Appl. 89201381.4, EPO Pub. No. 0344864 (1989).

60. Y. Itoh and Y. Fujisawa, Synthesis in yeast of hepatitis B virus surface antigen modified P31 particles by gene modification, *Biochem. Biophys. Res. Commun., 141*:942–948 (1986).

61. M. Hazama, M. Takaoki, K. Ohfune, S. Hinuma, and Y. Fujisawa, Immunogenicity of a new type of yeast-derived hepatitis B vaccine consisting of M (pre-S2 + S) protein particles, *Vaccine, 7*:567–573 (1989).

62. M. De Wilde, T. Rutgers, T. Cabezon, P. Hauser, O. Van Opstal, N. Harford, F. Van Wijnendaele, P. Desmons, M. Comberbach, P. Roelants, A. Safary, G. Wiedermann, F. Ambrosch, P. Voet, A. Delem, and J. Petre, PreS containing HBsAg particles from *Saccharomyces cerevisiae:* Production, antigenicity and immunogenicity, *Proceedings of the 1990 International Symposium on Viral Hepatitis and Liver Disease* (F. B. Hollinger, S. M. Lemon, and H. S. Margolis, eds.), William & Wilkins, Baltimore, MD, pp. 732–736 (1991).

63. Y. Fujisawa, S. Kuroda, P. M. C. A. Van Eerd, H. Schellekens, and A. Kaki-

numa, Protective efficacy of a novel hepatitis B vaccine consisting of M (pre-S2 + S) protein particles (a third generation vaccine), *Vaccine*, 8:192–198 (1990).

64. R. J. Gerety and D. J. West, Current and future hepatitis B vaccines, *Progress in Hepatitis B Immunization* (P. Coursaget and M. J. Tong, eds.) Colloque INSERM/ John Libbey Eurotext Ltd., Paris/London Vol. 194, pp. 215–225 (1990).

65. S. Iino, H. Suzuki, Y. Akahane, and M. Mayumi, Phase II study of recombinant HB vaccine containing the S and preS2 antigens, *The 1990 International Symposium on viral Hepatitis and Liver Disease*, Houston, TX, p. 119 (abstract 292) (1990).

66. F. Tron, F. Degos, Chr. Bréchot, A.-M. Couroucé, A. Goudeau, F.-N. Marie, Ph. Adamowicz, P. Saliou, A. Laplanche, J.-P. Benhamou, and M. Girard, Randomized dose range study of a recombinant hepatitis B vaccine produced in mammalian cells and containing the S and preS2 sequences. *J. Infect. Dis.*, 160:199–204 (1989).

67. E. Jacobs, T. Rutgers, P. Voet, M. Dewerchin, T. Cabezon, and M. De Wilde, Simultaneous synthesis and assembly of various hepatitis B surface proteins in *Saccharomyces cerevisiae, Gene*, 80;279–292 (1989).

68. D. H. Persing, H. E. Varmus, and D. Ganem, Inhibition of secretion of hepatitis B surface antigen by a related presurface polypeptide, *Science*, 234:1388–1391 (1986).

69. A. McLachlan, D. R. Milich, A. K. Raney, M. G. Riggs, J. L. Hughes, J. Sorge, and F. V. Chisari, Expression of hepatitis B virus surface and core antigens: Influence of pre-S and precore sequences, *J. Virol.*, 61:683–692 (1987).

70. J. H. Ou and W. J. Rutter, Regulation of secretion of the hepatitis B virus major surface antigen by the pre-S1 protein, *J. Virol.*, 61:782–786 (1987).

71. K. L. Molnar-Kimber, V. Jarocki-Witek, S. K. Dheer, S. K. Vernon, A. J. Conley, A. R. Davis, and P. P. Hung, Distinctive properties of the hepatitis B virus envelope proteins, *J. Virol.*, 62:407–416 (1988).

72. B. W. Youn and H. Samanta, Purification and characterization of pre-S-containing hepatitis B surface antigens produced in recombinant mammalian cell culture, *Vaccine*, 7:60–68 (1989).

73. H. Samanta and B. W. Youn, Expression of hepatitis B virus surface antigen containing the pre-S region in mammalian cell culture system, *Vaccine*, 7:69–76 (1989).

74. A. E. Hemmerling, J. Fuchs, G. Steichele, and H. A. Thoma, Comparison of the entire pre-S peptide sequence to selected epitope sequences in a new hepatitis B vaccine development, *Progress in Hepatitis B Immunization* (P. Coursaget and M. J. Tong, eds.) Colloque INSERM/John Libbey Eurotext Ltd., Paris/London Vol. 194, p. 93 (1990).

75. H. A. Thoma, A. E. Hemmerling, and H. Hötzinger, Evaluation of immune response in a third generation hepatitis B vaccine containing pre-S proteins in comparative trials, *Progress in Hepatitis B Immunization* (P. Coursaget and M. J. Tong, eds.), Colloque INSERM/John Libbey Eurotext Ltd., Paris/London vol. 194, pp. 35–42 (1990).

76. H. A. Thoma, G. Käpfer, E. Koller, and A. E. Hemmerling, Does the pre-S2 have the same effects in improving the HBV immune response compared to pre-S1? *The*

1990 International Symposium on Viral Hepatitis and Liver Disease, Houston, TX, p. 118 (abstract 286) (1990).

77. H. A. Thoma, Clinical evidence that only pre-S1 can bypass hepatitis-B non-responsiveness, *The 1990 International Symposium on Viral Hepatitis and Liver Disease*, Houston, TX, p. 118 (abstract 287) (1990).

78. D. Poma, H. Hötzinger, A. Wischnik, and H. Thoma, The superior immunogenicity of a pre-S1 containing HBV vaccine compared to a S-vaccine in comparative clinical trials, *The 1990 International Symposium on Viral Hepatitis and Liver Disease*, Houston, TX, p. 118 (abstract 288) (1990).

79. H. A. Thoma, D. Poma, and A. E. Hemmerling, Improvement of the hepatitis-B immune response through pre-S incorporation with specific respect to elderly, *The 1990 International Symposium on Viral Hepatitis and Liver Disease*, Houston, TX, p. 119 (abstract 289) (1990).

80. T. Cabezon, T. Rutgers, R. Biemans, D. Vanderbrugge, P. Voet, and M. De Wilde, A new hepatitis B vaccine containing pre-S1 and pre-S2 epitopes from *Saccharomyces cerevisiae*, *Vaccines 90* (F. Brown, R. M. Channock, H. S. Ginsberg, and R. A. Lerner, eds.), Cold Spring Harbor Laboratory Press, Cold Spring Harbor, NY, pp. 199–203 (1990).

81. M. Pignatelli, J. Waters, A. Lever, S. Iwarson, R. Gerety, and H. C. Thomas, Cytotoxic T-cell responses to the nucleocapsid proteins of HBV in chronic hepatitis—evidence that antibody modulation may cause protracted infection, *J. Hepatol.*, *4*:15–21 (1987).

82. K. Murray, S. A. Bruce, A. Hinnen, P. Wingfield, P. A. C. M. van Eerd, A. de Reus, and H. Schellekens, Hepatitis B virus antigens made in microbial cells immunise against viral infection. *EMBO J.*, *3*:645–650 (1984).

83. S. Iwarson, E. Tabor, H. C. Thomas, P. Snoy, and R. J. Gerety, Protection against hepatitis B virus infection by immunization with hepatitis B core antigen, *Gastroenterology*, *88*:763–767 (1985).

84. K. Murray, S. A. Bruce, P. Wingfield, P. A. C. M. van Eerd, A. de Reus, and H. Schellekens, H. Protective immunization against hepatitis B with an internal antigen of the virus, *J. Med. Virol.*, *23*:101–107 (1987).

85. D. R. Milich, A. McLachlan, G. B. Thornton, and J. L. Hughes, Antibody production to the nucleocapsid and envelope of the hepatitis B virus primed by a single synthetic T cell site, *Nature*, *329*:547–549 (1987).

86. D. R. Milich, A. McLachlan, A. Moriarty, and G. B. Thornton, Immune response to hepatitis B virus core antigen (HBcAg): Localization of T cell recognition sites within HBcAg/HBeAg, *J. Immunol.*, *139*:1223–1231 (1987).

87. D. R. Milich, J. E. Jones, J. L. Hughes, J. Price, A. K. Raney, and A. McLachlan, Is a function of the secreted hepatitis B e antigen to induce immunologic tolerance in utero? *Proc. Natl. Acad. Sci. USA*, *87*:6599–6603 (1990).

88. M. Stemler, J. Hess, R. Braun, H. Will, and C. H. Schroeder, Serological evidence for expression of the polymerase gene of human hepatitis B virus in vivo, *J. Gen. Virol.*, *69*:698–693 (1988).

89. L. J. Chang, J. Dienstag, D. Ganem, and H. Varmus, Detection of antibodies against hepatitis B virus polymerase antigen in hepatitis B virus-infected patients, *Hepatology*, *10*:332–335 (1989).

90. J. Hess, M. Stemler, H. Will, C. H. Schröder, J. Kühn, and R. Braun, Frequent detection of antibodies to hepatitis B virus X-protein in acute, chronic and resolved infections, *Med. Microbiol. Immunol.*, *177*:195–205 (1988).

91. M. Stemler, T. Weimer, Z. X. Tu, D. F. Wan, M. Levrero, C. Jung, G. R. Pape, and H. Will, Mapping of B-cell epitopes of the human hepatitis B virus X protein, *J. Virol.*, *64*:2802–2809 (1990).

92. D. R. Milich, and A. McLachlan, The nucleocapsid of hepatitis B virus is both a T-cell-independent and a T-cell-dependent antigen, *Science*, *234*:1398–1401 (1986).

93. B. E. Clarke, S. E. Newton, A. R. Caroll, M. J. Francis, G. Appleyard, A. D. Syred, P. E. Highfield, D. J. Rowlands, and F. Brown, Improved immunogenicity of a peptide epitope after fusion to hepatitis B core protein, *Nature, 330*:381–384 (1987).

94. S. J. Stahl and K. Murray, Immunogenicity of peptide fusions to hepatitis B virus core antigen, *Proc. Natl. Acad. Sci. USA, 86*:6283–6287 (1989).

95. F. Schödel, T. Weimer, and H. Will, Recombinant HBV core particles carrying immunodominant B-cell epitopes of the HBV pre-S2 region, *Vaccines 90* (F. Brown, R. M. Chanock, H. S. Ginsberg, and R. A. Lerner, eds.), Cold Spring Harbor Laboratory Press, Cold Spring Harbor, NY, pp. 193–198 (1990).

96. F. Birnbaum and M. Nassal, Hepatitis B virus nucleocapsid assembly: Primary structure requirements in the core protein, *J. Virol.*, *64*:3319–3330 (1990).

97. M. Mackett, Vaccinia virus as a vector for delivering foreign antigens, *Sem. Virol.*, *1*:39–47 (1990).

98. D. E. Hruby, Vaccinia virus vectors: New strategies for producing recombinant vaccines, *Clin. Microbiol. Rev.*, *3*:153–170 (1990).

99. B. Moss, G. L. Smith, J. L. Gerin, and R. H. Purcell, Live recombinant vaccinia virus protects chimpanzees against hepatitis B, *Nature, 311*:67–69 (1984).

100. K. C. Cheng, and B. Moss, Selective synthesis and secretion of particles composed of the hepatitis B virus middle surface protein directed by a recombinant vaccinia virus: Induction of antibodies to pre-S and S epitopes, *J. Virol., 61*:1286–1290 (1987).

101. K. C. Cheng, G. L. Smith, and B. Moss, Hepatitis B virus large surface protein is not secreted but is immunogenic when selectively expressed by recombinant vaccinia virus, *J. Virol., 60*:337–344 (1986).

102. M. E. Perkus, A. Piccini, B. R. Lipinskas, E. Paoletti, Recombinant vaccinia virus: Immunization against multiple pathogens, *Science, 229*:981–984 (1985).

103. J. F. Rooney, C. Wohlenberg, K. J. Cremer, B. Moss, and A. L. Notkins, Immunization with a vaccinia virus recombinant expressing herpes simplex virus type 1 glycoprotein D: Long-term protection and effect of revaccination, *J. Virol., 62*:1530–1534 (1988).

104. E. L. Cooney, L. Corey, S. L. Hu, A. Collier, D. Arditti, M. Hoffman, G. Smith, K. Steimer, and P. Greenberg, Enhanced immunogenicity in humans of an HIV subunit vaccine regimen employing priming with a vaccinia gp160 recombinant virus (Vac/Env) by boosting with recombinant HIV envelope glycoprotein (rgp160), International conference on advances in AIDS vaccine development, Third annual meeting of the national cooperative vaccine development groups for AIDS, Clearwater Beach, Florida, poster 21 (1990).

105. J. E. Morin, M. D. Lubeck, J. E. Barton, A. J. Conley, A. R. Davis, and P. P. Hung, Recombinant adenovirus induces antibody response to hepatitis B virus surface antigen in hamsters, *Proc. Natl. Acad. Sci. USA, 84:*4626–4630 (1987).

106. M. D. Lubeck, A. R. Davis, M. Chengalvala, R. J. Natuk, J. E. Morin, K. Molnar-Kimber, B. B. Mason, B. M. Bhat, S. Mizutani, P. P. Hung, and R. H. Purcell, Immunogenicity and efficacy testing in chimpanzees of an oral hepatitis B vaccine based on live recombinant adenovirus, *Proc. Natl. Acad. Sci. USA, 86:* 6763–6767 (1989).

107. A. Charbit, E. Sobczak, M.-L. Michel, A. Molla, P. Tiollais, and M. Hofnung, Presentation of two epitopes of the preS2 region of hepatitis B virus on live recombinant bacteria, *J. Immunol., 139:*1658–1664 (1987).

108. C. Leclerc, A. Charbit, A. Molla, and M. Hofnung, Antibody response to a foreign epitope expressed at the surface of recombinant bacteria: Importance of the route of immunization, *Vaccine, 7:*242–248 (1989).

109. J. Y. Wu, S. Newton, A. Judd, B. Stocker, and W. S. Robinson, Expression of immunogenic epitopes of hepatitis B surface antigen with hybrid flagellin proteins by a vaccine strain of *Salmonella, Proc. Natl. Acad. Sci. USA, 86:*4726–4730 (1989).

110. P. Coursaget, B. Yvonnet, E. Relyveld, A. Brizard, C. Bourdil, L. Bringer, E. Jeannée, S. Guindo, I. Diop-Mar, and J. P. Chiron, Simultaneous injection of hepatitis B vaccine with BCG, diphtheria and tetanus toxoids, pertussis and polio vaccines, *Progress in Hepatitis B Immunization* (P. Coursaget and M. J. Tong, eds.), Colloque INSERM/John Libbey Eurotext Ltd., Paris/London Vol. 194, pp. 319–324 (1990).

111. A. R. Neurath, S. B. H. Kent, N. Strick, and K. Parker, Delineation of contiguous determinants essential for biological functions of the pre-S sequence of the hepatitis B virus envelope protein: Its antigenicity, immunogenicity and cell-receptor recognition, *Ann. Inst. Pasteur, 139:*13–38 (1988).

Index

About the Editor

RONALD W. ELLIS is Executive Director of Virus & Cell Biology at Merck Research Laboratories, West Point, Pennsylvania. He is the author or coauthor of over 100 articles and 20 review chapters in the fields of vaccines, infectious diseases, molecular and cellular biology, virology, and experimental oncology, and the editor of the book *Vaccines: New Approaches to Immunological Problems*. Dr. Ellis received the B.A. degree (1974) in biology from the University of Chicago, Illinois, the Ph.D. degree (1979) from Cornell University, Ithaca, New York, and the M.B.A. degree (1981) from the University of Maryland, College Park.

Printed and bound by CPI Group (UK) Ltd, Croydon, CR0 4YY

17/10/2024

01775700-0016